Sleep Science

Sleep Science

EDITED BY HAWLEY MONTGOMERY-DOWNS

OXFORD
UNIVERSITY PRESS

OXFORD
UNIVERSITY PRESS

Oxford University Press is a department of the University of Oxford. It furthers
the University's objective of excellence in research, scholarship, and education
by publishing worldwide. Oxford is a registered trade mark of Oxford University
Press in the UK and certain other countries.

Published in the United States of America by Oxford University Press
198 Madison Avenue, New York, NY 10016, United States of America.

Library of Congress Cataloging-in-Publication Data
Names: Montgomery-Downs, Hawley, editor.
Title: Sleep science / edited Hawley Montgomery-Downs.
Description: New York : Oxford University Press, 2020. |
Includes bibliographical references and index.
Identifiers: LCCN 2019054127 (print) | LCCN 2019054128 (ebook) |
ISBN 9780190923259 (paperback) | ISBN 9780190923273 (epub) |
ISBN 9780197523308
Subjects: LCSH: Sleep—Psychological aspects. | Consciousness.
Classification: LCC BF1071 .S5854 2020 (print) | LCC BF1071 (ebook) |
DDC 154.6—dc23
LC record available at https://lccn.loc.gov/2019054127
LC ebook record available at https://lccn.loc.gov/2019054128

9 8 7 6 5 4 3 2 1

Printed by Marquis, Canada

CONTENTS

On the first day of class in the very first undergraduate sleep course I taught, a student asked, "Are we going to nap in this class?" The answer—then and now—was a qualified "no." The purpose of the class wasn't sleeping per se, but every semester I went on to explain that if my students were having trouble staying awake, then they weren't going to learn much from being there. In that case, I encouraged them to put their heads down, or even stretch out on the floor, for some much-needed sleep. I also explained that by doing so, they were agreeing to be observed—that the rest of us will take the opportunity to test their arousal threshold, observe their reduced muscle tone, and watch for eye movements. With regret, I've never had a student fall asleep in class.

Over the 20 years that I've been teaching sleep courses, the "Will we nap?" question has disappeared. I interpret this as a testament to the marked advances in this field of scientific inquiry and to the extent that it no longer needs defending as an important subject in university-level behavioral and biological sciences training. The first-day question has now become "Why do we sleep?" With no spoilers, I can answer this question before you even start reading Chapter 1. The short answer is, because if we don't sleep, we die. I'm sorry to be so morbid, but it's true—much of this book will explain, in graphic, scientific detail, the many ways that not sleeping well or enough can sickness, inure, and even kill.

The slightly more nuanced answer to the "Why we sleep?" question is to consider the parallel: Why are we awake? We are awake because there are things we must do, that we can only do, while fully conscious. These things include eating, using the bathroom, and reproducing (ignore for now that each of these behaviors can also occur during disordered sleep!) The answer to the "Why we sleep?" question is the same: we sleep because there are things we only do when we are in sleep's altered state of consciousness. This book is an introduction to the incredible feats we, and all animals, accomplish while we sleep.

One delightful surprise I've had from editing this book has been getting a front-row seat to the latest sleep research advances. Indeed, I learned something fascinating from the authors of each chapter herein—I hope you enjoy these discoveries as much as I have. So, set your alarm (to make sure you go to bed on time, obviously!) and prepare for the strange, wonderful world of what is known about sleep. We're depending on you to help solve some of the remaining mysteries.

ACKNOWLEDGMENTS

I've had the great fortune to work on this project alongside many remarkable professionals—I am tremendously grateful to each of them. Sarah Harrington and Hayley Singer at Oxford University Press were the driving forces behind getting this book started and finished, respectively. The book would not have been remotely possible without the generous commitments of time and intellect by those who crafted each of its chapters. I am also truly grateful to all the students who have chosen to enroll in my course Psychobiology of Sleep. I am also deeply indebted to those who have taught me to how to teach—in chronological order, they have been my parents Yvonne Norrbom and Ronald Downs; my mentors John Morgan, Evelyn Thoman, Victor Deneberg, David Miller, Ralph Lydic, and David Gozal; and my children Shea, Bryn, and Owen. Finally, the information in this book exists thanks to the contributions of worldwide sleep investigators, trainees, technicians, reviewers, technology developers, funding agencies, politicians, advocates, educators, taxpayers, and research participants.

CONTRIBUTORS

Sabra M. Abbott, MD, PhD
Northwestern University Feinberg
School of Medicine

Shilpa M. Agraharkar, MD
Psychiatrist

Marco Angriman, MD
Central Hospital of Bolzano

Hrayr Attarian, MD
Northwestern University Feinberg
School of Medicine

Fiona C. Baker, PhD
SRI International

Siobhan Banks, PhD
University of South Australia

Argelinda Baroni, MD
NYU Langone Health

Chiara Bartolacci, PhD
Sapienza University of Rome

Bei Bei, PhD, PsyD
Monash University

Oliviero Bruni, MD
Pediatric Sleep Center at Sapienza
Sapienza University of Rome

Stephanie Claudatos, BS
SRI International and Palo Alto
University

Ian M. Colrain, PhD
SRI International and University
of Melbourne

Keren Armoni Domany, MD
Tel Aviv University

Jeanne F. Duffy, MBA, PhD
Brigham and Women's Hospital and
Harvard Medical School

Jason G. Ellis, PhD
Northumbria University

Raffaele Ferri, MD
Oasi Research Institute IRCCS

Luigi De Gennaro, PhD
Sapienza University of Rome

Kevin Gipson, MD
Massachusetts General Hospital

Marc P. Halperin, MD
NYU Langone Health

Sarah M. Honaker, PhD, DBSM
Indiana University School
of Medicine

Rosemary S. C. Horne, PhD, DSc
Monash University

Defne Inhan, BSc
New York University Shanghai

Kathryn M. Johnson, AS, R.EEG/EPT.,
RPSGT, FASET
St. Mary's Sleep Center

John D. Kennedy
University of Adelaide

Kurt Lushington, MPsych, PhD
University of South Australia

Anastasia Mangiaruga, PhD
University of Bologna

Carolina Z. Marcus, MD
University of Rochester
Medical Center

Jennifer L. Marsella, MD
University of Rochester
Medical Center

Alfred J. Martin
University of Adelaide

James J. McKenna, PhD
University of Notre Dame, Emeritus,
and Santa Clara University

Jacob E. Medina, BS
Ridley-Tree Cancer Center

Maria Grazia Melegari, MD
Sapienza University of Rome

Yvonne Pamula, PhD
Adelaide Women's and
Children's Hospital

Rafael Pelayo, MD
Stanford Center for Sleep Sciences
and Medicine

Kevin R. Peters, PhD
Trent University

Alexandria M. Reynolds, PhD
University of Virginia's College at Wise

Jason Rihel, PhD
University College London

Serena Scarpelli, PhD, IRCCS
Fondazione Santa Lucia

Michael K. Scullin, PhD
Baylor University

Katherine M. Sharkey, MD, PhD,
FAASM, FACP
Warren Alpert Medical School of
Brown University

Jess P. Shatkin, MD, MPH
New York University Grossman
School of Medicine

Karen Spruyt, PhD
University Claude Bernard Lyon

Riva Tauman, MD
Sleep Medicine Center, Tel Aviv
Souraski Medical Center and
Tel Aviv University

Kristin P. Tully, PhD
University of North Carolina
at Chapel Hill

Erin J. Wamsley, PhD
Furman University

Amy R. Wolfson, PhD
Loyola University

Crystal L. Yates, PhD
University of South Australia

Margaret Yu, MD
Northwestern University Feinberg
School of Medicine

Massimiliano de Zambotti, PhD
SRI International

Terra Ziporyn, PhD
Start School Later

PART I

Normative Adult Sleep

Sleep and Consciousness

DEFNE INHAN AND JESS P. SHATKIN ■

He that sleeps feels not the tooth-ache.

—WILLIAM SHAKESPEARE

INTRODUCTION

Roughly one-third of our lifetime is—or should be—spent asleep; yet, despite the expansive scientific knowledge gained in many fields (i.e., psychology, neurophysiology) about our wake state, only relatively recently have we begun to catch up with the study of sleep. As Tom Roth, former editor of the journal *Sleep*, put it, "it's analogous to going to Mars with a third of the Earth's surface still unexplored" [1].

Sleep is a strange experience, playing tricks on our consciousness. Sometimes within only a couple minutes of dozing off, we can go through a plethora of vivid and complex experiences. Alternatively, we may lapse into what feels like a total absence of consciousness, a jump in time, waking after a long slumber with no memory of the last 8 hours. Sleep does not bend time, but without a doubt, it alters our consciousness. It is, therefore, no surprise that most people enjoy sleeping—when we sleep, we no longer feel the toothache, headache, or the heartache that we suffer when awake.

Today, with the help of the electroencephalogram (EEG), magnetic resonance imaging, and other tools, we are able to study our brains and bodies as we sleep. We now recognize consistent patterns of neuronal activity that tell us when we are awake, when we are asleep, and when we are dreaming. Long before our EEGs, magnetic resonance imaging, and other scientific tools allowed us to delve into the inner recesses of the brain, however, we had many ideas about why and how we sleep.

In this chapter, we will describe how our understanding of sleep has changed over time, from early myths and theories to brilliant discoveries of modern science. We will take a close look at sleep architecture and what our brains, bodies, and minds experience as we move through the sleep cycle. Finally, we will explore how we lose consciousness and disconnect from our environment during sleep.

EARLY THEORIES OF SLEEP

Many ancient cultures saw sleep as a time for the soul to travel between worlds and communicate with spirits [2]. Other cultures saw in sleep a social function, one in which dreams could be shared and provide a rich source of valuable information. The Bible is replete with stories of prophets whose dreams foretold the future and guided leaders to victory. In Greek mythology, the goddess Nyx (Night) and the god Erebus (Darkness) came together to create the brothers Hypnos (Sleep) and Thanatos (Death). Many cultures saw a similar kinship between sleep and death, which look quite similar to an outside observer, and these ideas helped to shape some of the early theories about sleep. Alcmaeon, a Greek physician, theorized that sleep was a loss of consciousness that occurred when blood drained from vessels on the surface of the body. Aristotle believed that vapors released from food during digestion in the stomach rose to the heart, what he thought to be the body's seat of intelligence, to cause sleep; and Galen, the second-century Greek physician, believed that the 4 body humors were rebalanced by sleep.

For generations, sleep was generally viewed as a passive process, in many ways similar to coma, intoxication, hypnosis, anesthesia, or hibernation [3]. Almost 2,000 years after the Ancient Greeks, Scottish physician Robert MacNish opened his book, *The Philosophy of Sleep*, with the thought, "Sleep is the intermediate state between wakefulness and death; wakefulness is regarded as the active state of all the physical and intellectual functions, and death as that of their total suspension" [4]. To most thinkers, sleep was what happened in the dark and still of the night, in the absence of sensory input.

As the 20th century came into view, many scientists believed that sleep was the result of an unidentified hypnotoxin. During the day, the hypnotoxin theory suggested, the body accumulated toxins and fatigue products, which were eliminated during sleep. The longer we stayed awake, the sleepier we became. Yet to anyone who has stayed up all night (i.e., "pulled an all-nighter"), this theory makes little intuitive sense; how is it possible that we can stay up all night, accumulating more and more sleep debt, becoming sleepier and sleepier, but then regain much of our energy when the day begins?

Enter Nathaniel Kleitman, the first true sleep scholar (see Figure 1.1). If the hypnotoxin theory were true, he reasoned, then sleep deprived subjects would gradually feel more and more tired the longer they stayed awake, and anyone pulling an all-nighter would feel much worse by 10 AM than they would at 3 AM; yet Kleitman observed the exact opposite in his subjects. Kleitman, as it turned

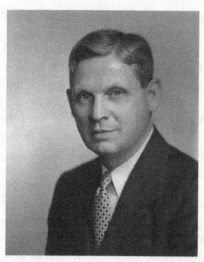

Figure 1.1 Nathaniel Kleitman pioneered modern day sleep research, including the discovery of REM sleep with his student, Eugene Aserinsky.
SOURCE: Photo obtained from the University of Chicago Photographic Archive, apf1-03484, Special Collections Research Center, University of Chicago Library.

out, was partly right and partly wrong. While his observations would later help form our understanding of the body's inherent circadian rhythm (also see Chapter 4 of this volume), the work of Ishimori, Legendre, and Pieron would convince us that a hypnotoxin, now understood to be the neurotransmitter adenosine, also contributes to our need for sleep. In a series of thoughtful experiments, these three scientists obtained cerebrospinal fluid from sleep deprived dogs and then injected this cerebrospinal fluid into well-rested dogs, which resulted in the rested dogs falling asleep [5–7].

Kleitman's assertion that sleep was not solely the result of a tired and overworked brain calling it a day, or night, was a radical departure. With Kleitman at the helm, the era of sleep discovery was just beginning. Kleitman and his team, and those who followed, would challenge not only our understanding of sleep, but also our conception of our awake consciousness.

A prominent physical manifestation of rapid eye movement (REM) sleep is openly visible to anyone who looks at the eyes of a sleeping human. Yet this behavior was hidden in plain sight for thousands of years, until Kleitman's doctoral student, Eugene Aserinsky, stumbled upon it in the lab [8]. Aserinsky was initially studying infant sleep under Kleitman's supervision. After months of tedious observations, he detected a 20-minute period during each infant's sleep when the eye movements ceased, after which the infant usually woke up. Exploiting his observation, he was able to impress mothers standing near the cribs by predicting when their babies would wake up. "The mothers were invariably amazed at the accuracy of my prediction and equally pleased by my impending departure," he once wrote [1, p. 215].

Following his study of infants, Aserinsky decided to study sleeping adults. His first subject was his son, Armond. Aserinsky had tinkered with an old Offner Dynograph (an early prototype of an EEG machine) that he had found in the lab's basement, which he adapted to detect both his son's brainwaves and eye movements. Once calibrated, the inkwriter moved in sync with Armond's eyes. Hours after Armond fell asleep—and much graph paper later—Aserinsky noticed the ink writer moving back and forth in the adjacent room, indicating that Armond's brain was awake. Expecting him to be up and looking around, Aserinsky went to check on Armond only to find his eyes shut: Armond was fast asleep [1].

Initially bewildered, Aserinsky thought the old machine was dysfunctional, oblivious that he was on the verge of discovering a phenomenon so important that some would designate it the "third state of being," following wakefulness and sleep [9]. After replicating the study and the same outcome with different subjects, Aserinsky's doubts vanished. "In one of the earliest sleep sessions, I went into the sleep chamber and directly observed the eyes through the lids at the time that the sporadic eye movement deflections appeared on the polygraph record," Aserinsky recalled later in the *Journal of the History of the Neurosciences*. "The eyes were moving vigorously, but the subject did not respond to my vocalization. There was no doubt whatsoever that the subject was asleep despite the EEG that suggested a waking state" [1].

The discovery of REM sleep, which Aserinsky originally intended to call "Jerky Eye Movement Periods," or JEM, was the revolution that led to sleep science—yet it was merely the first step in unraveling a much more complicated mystery [10]. Within a few years, William Dement, then a medical student in Kleitman's lab, would discover that sleep was cyclical in nature. At the time, researchers studying the brain during waking periods were not willing to squander expensive graph paper and ink by running an EEG while their patients slept. After all, they reasoned, sleep is a passive state, and nothing other than a quiet brain would be evident on EEG. Encouraged by Aserinsky's observation of the pendulous eye movements sometimes observed during sleep, Dement, however, decided to run a continuous all-night sleep study. What emerged from his studies were five distinct patterns of brain activity occurring with regular frequency over the course of the night. These patterns would eventually be named non-REM stages 1 (N1), 2 (N2), 3 (N3), and 4 (N4) and REM. With the discovery of REM sleep and a firm understanding that the brain constructs an orderly pattern of activity throughout the sleep period (instead of being simply "turned off"), the notion of sleep as a passive process was entirely debunked, and the stage was set for delving deeper into the secrets of sleep [11].

Today, we use polysomnography (*polus* for "many," *somnus* for "sleep," and *graphein* for "to write"; abbreviated PSG) to assess the many physiological changes our bodies undergo during sleep. Polysomnography monitors many body functions, including brain activity (EEG), eye movements (electrooculogram, or EOG), skeletal muscle activity (electromyography, or EMG), heart rate (electrocardiogram, or ECG), and blood oxygen carrying capacity (also see Chapter 22 of this volume). Each of these body functions is differentially affected as we proceed from wakefulness through each stage of non-REM, and then to REM sleep. To better understand precisely how our consciousness changes throughout a 24-hour period, let's follow Laura, a typical young adult, through her typical day.

WAKEFULNESS

It's been a long day, and Laura is ready to conclude it with a good night's sleep. As Laura reads a few pages of an exciting new mystery novel on the couch before getting into bed, her brain remains correspondingly busy, producing many high-frequency (12–30 Hz), low-voltage beta waves, emanating diffusely from throughout her brain. With all of this alert beta activity going on, Laura does not feel sleepy. So, she wisely dims the lights and, for now, replaces her mystery novel with a relaxing picture book of classic art. As she begins to feel sleepy, she puts her book aside and gets into bed. Laura will spend approximately 5% of her sleeping period awake at the beginning of the night and during regular, brief awakenings throughout the night, as do all typical adults. Upon closing her eyes, the beta waves slow and diminish and are largely replaced by alpha waves (8–13 Hz), which indicate that she is awake and relaxed, with eyes closed. Alpha waves emanate from the occipital lobe, indicating a lack of visual input. Soon after, her muscles relax, her breathing slows, and she falls asleep (Figure 1.2).

NON-REM STAGE 1 SLEEP

N1 sleep technically begins when alpha waves disappear from the EEG reading. Laura's eye movements are now slow and rolling. Her muscle tone is relaxed. She briefly experiences a falling sensation (from whence comes the term "falling asleep") and some dream-like imagery. These hypnagogic hallucinations are entirely normal and lack the dramatic story and bizarre imagery of the dreams she will soon experience; the thoughts in her head during this brief episode may bear some loose connection to the book she was just reading or to some experiences from her day. Suddenly, the falling sensation intensifies, causing her to kick her legs unintentionally. This "hypnic jerk" startles her awake for a moment before she falls back into N1 sleep. Her connection to the environment around her decreases rapidly, yet her arousal threshold remains low (i.e., she would be easy to awaken). If she were to awaken at this moment, she may deny that she were ever asleep.

Laura's brain, however, does not lie. If we were to look at her EEG during N1 sleep, we would see a clear change in her neuronal activity. Alpha waves have disappeared, although they may come and go periodically throughout the night, and theta waves (3–7 Hz) have become predominant. Theta waves originate in the hippocampus and diffusely throughout the cortex. They also show up during relaxed wakeful states, such as when we daydream or engage in repetitive tasks like jogging or swimming laps, and are thought to play a role in creativity and

EEG Sleep Patterns

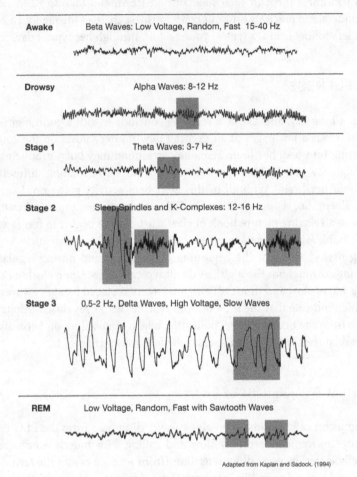

Awake   Beta Waves: Low Voltage, Random, Fast 15-40 Hz

Drowsy   Alpha Waves: 8-12 Hz

Stage 1   Theta Waves: 3-7 Hz

Stage 2   Sleep Spindles and K-Complexes: 12-16 Hz

Stage 3   0.5-2 Hz, Delta Waves, High Voltage, Slow Waves

REM   Low Voltage, Random, Fast with Sawtooth Waves

Adapted from Kaplan and Sadock. (1994)

Figure 1.2 Brain wave patters during wake and each sleep stage.

achieving states of "flow" [12]. Increasing the theta-to-alpha ratio during wakefulness has, in fact, been shown to enhance creativity in music and dance performance [13]. Laura will spend roughly 2% to 5% of her night in N1 sleep.

NON-REM STAGE 2 SLEEP

After a short time in N1 sleep (typically fewer than 10 minutes), Laura progresses to N2 sleep. The slow, pendular eye movements have disappeared, and Laura's muscle tone reduces further. N2 is characterized by the appearance of K-complexes and sleep spindles. K-complexes resemble an isolated tsunami wave in the midst of a calm sea. They originate diffusely from within the cortex and are typically triggered by external (e.g., noises in the sleeping environment, such as a dog's bark) or internal (e.g., digestion) stimuli, appearing as isolated, high-voltage, sharp negative waves, followed by a slower positive component. K-complexes are thought to aid in suppressing cortical arousal, thereby allowing Laura to stay asleep.

By contrast, sleep spindles follow a sinusoidal rhythm of 12 to 14 Hz, waxing and waning for 1 or 2 seconds. They occur about every 10 to 30 seconds in both N2 and N3 sleep (although they are difficult to see in the EEG tracing during N3). Sleep spindles emanate from within the thalamus and are thought to be important for the transfer of information from the hippocampus (which acts as a site of recently learned information) into the memory cortex (which acts as the site of long-term memory; also see Chapter 7 of this volume). The more sleep spindles we experience during sleep, the more we learn and remember. After 20 minutes or so of N2, which comprises roughly 50% of the total sleep period, Laura starts drifting into N3.

NON-REM STAGE 3 SLEEP

Laura's brain and body are now sufficiently relaxed to further let go engagement with the environment and enter N3 sleep. Also known as "slow-wave sleep" and "delta sleep," N3 is characterized by high-voltage, low-frequency (or delta) waves (roughly 2 Hz), which produce the most restful and rejuvenating sleep of the evening. Laura's muscle tone relaxes further, and her eyes remain still. During N3 sleep, more of Laura's neurons will fire in synchrony, like hundreds of millions of soldiers marching perfectly in time with one another, which accounts for the high-voltage waves. Sleep spindles and K-complexes may or may not be seen on the EEG due to the predominance of high-voltage waves, but they occur often. Fast frequency ripples, occurring at 100 to 200 Hz, and lasting about 200 msec, coincide with sleep spindle activity and the transfer of information from the hippocampus to the memory cortex.

Deep sleep, N3, is essential for many physiological processes. Numerous hormones vital to Laura's daily functioning are released during N3 sleep, such as growth hormone-releasing hormone, prolactin, and thyroid-stimulating hormone. If we were to awaken her during N3, Laura would be groggy and confused, in the midst of what is termed "sleep inertia." If the phone were to ring and she were to answer after awakening from N3, it is likely that she would have no memory of the event in the morning. N3 will account for roughly 13% to 23% of Laura's total sleep and is concentrated in the first half of the sleep period. After roughly 30 minutes in her first N3 phase of the evening, the delta waves begin to diminish, and signs of N2 sleep re-emerge for about 10 more minutes before she drifts into REM sleep. (Until recently, slow-wave sleep was divided into stages N3 and N4, where the EEG in N3 was comprised of less than 50% delta waves and the EEG in N4 was comprised of more than 50% delta waves. Because this distinction proved to be of no clinical value, the American Academy of Sleep Medicine eliminated all reference to N4 in 2007 and now considers all deep sleep N3.)

RAPID EYE MOVEMENT SLEEP

It's been around 80 minutes since Laura fell asleep. Her skeletal muscle tone has diminished dramatically and is almost entirely absent. Her eyes now begin to move swiftly back and forth; Laura has entered REM sleep. REM, also called "paradoxical sleep" because the characteristic sawtooth electrical brain waves resemble beta waves of the awake state, is so-called for the saccadic eye movements once recognized so plainly by Eugene Aserinsky. The brain activity is generally of low-voltage and mixed frequency, signifying that many parts of the brain are active at the same time. Although her brain is much more active than during N3 sleep, Laura's arousal threshold is almost as high in REM as it was in N3. If we were to wake Laura during REM sleep, she would almost certainly report vivid and bizarre thoughts with full-fledged stories centered around herself; in other words, Laura would be dreaming (also see Chapter 6 of this volume).

REM sleep can be described in terms of both *tonic* and *phasic* events. Tonic aspects are manifested by an active brain and a general loss of muscle tone, while the phasic aspects represent the irregular bursts of eye movements and skeletal muscle twitches. Given the relaxed state of our skeletal muscles, REM proves to be an excellent time of day for cell repair and immune system operations. REM also appears important for procedural memory (e.g., how we learn to perform various actions, such as riding a bicycle or playing the guitar), and may have an evolutionary purpose that we are only now beginning to understand (also see Chapter 2 of this volume). While REM comprises about 25% of sleep in adults like Laura (mostly concentrated toward the end of the sleep period or the early morning hours), REM accounts for approximately 50% of sleep in infants. It is believed that this intensity of REM (called "active sleep" in young infants; also see Chapter 8 of this volume) is necessary to further stimulate the infant's developing brain in the first year of life, which would have otherwise been too big to deliver through the pelvis of a bipedal female human [14].

DREAMING

Dreams are an essential and unique occurrence of consciousness during sleep and perhaps one of the most mysterious of human experiences. Why would evolution paralyze us, enable our sexual arousal system, and make us watch vivid, often disturbing or frightening, sometimes amusing, and occasionally enlightening images from within our minds each time we sleep? This question has bewildered scientists, philosophers, religious leaders, and each of us throughout the entirety of human history. To be fair, the brain is an extremely efficient organ, and it is hard to imagine that we would dream for roughly 2 hours each night, or approximately 8% of our lives, for absolutely no reason. Current theories suggest that, among other things, N3 and REM work together to enhance our memory function and learning. While N3 weeds out unnecessary neural connections, occurs earlier in the sleep period, and moves memory information from short-term storage in the hippocampus to long-term storage in the memory cortex, REM strengthens those new neural connections that enhance our memory, occurs later in the sleep period, and integrates new memories with our backlog of collected memories from the past [15].

On a strictly neurological level, we now know that the visual, perceptual, and emotional centers of the brain are active during REM dreams, while the frontal cortex is largely quiet. This effect allows us to watch our dreams and feel many emotions without the aid of the frontal cortex to make sense of it all. REM is not the only stage of sleep in which we dream, but it is the stage in which our dreams are the most hallucinogenic. This topic will be explored in greater depth in Chapter 6 of this volume.

THE SLEEP CYCLE

Following a short REM phase of perhaps 10 to 15 minutes, the first being the shortest of the sleep period, Laura shifts and moves around in her bed. Laura will almost certainly awaken briefly between sleep cycles, but unless she stays awake for more than a few minutes, she is unlikely to have a memory of the event. Due to these small awakenings between sleep cycles, no one truly sleeps through the night. The fact is, however, that because these awakenings are typically just a few minutes in length, most of us do not remember them and so believe that we have not awoken during our sleep. Once Laura falls back to sleep, the classic signs of REM sleep are gone. She enters N1 once again and restarts the cycle of sleep that will repeat itself another three to five times throughout the sleep period, each cycle lasting approximately 90 to 120 minutes. Her longest REM periods may eventually reach up to 30 minutes in length. Myriad other neural and physiological events will occur throughout the night (see Chapter 4 of this volume). Most notably, Laura's body temperature, which began to decrease about an hour before her usual bedtime, drops still further throughout the night, ultimately cascading to a nadir of 1.8°F below normal about 4 to 5 hours after going to sleep. The temperature drop, which occurs at a predictable time based upon our circadian rhythm and happens whether or not we are asleep, is thought to be necessary for energy conservation (also see Chapter 4 of this volume; Figure 1.3).

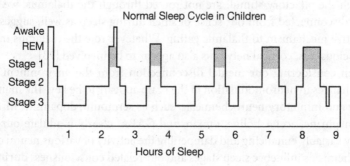

Figure 1.3 A normal sleep cycle for a child.

SLEEP AND CONSCIOUSNESS

Our obvious disconnection from the environment is the key characteristic that separates sleep from waking consciousness [16]. Throughout the sleep period, we demonstrate no meaningful response to external stimuli, unless the stimuli breach our arousal threshold, as would the ringing of an alarm clock. As we move through each successive NREM stage, further into the sleep cycle, our arousal threshold increases, making it more and more difficult to awaken us. Despite the robust brain activity and vivid sensory experiences of REM, a second notable paradox is that our disconnection from the environment largely persists.

Early sleep researchers experimented to see whether external stimuli could be incorporated into their subjects' dreams. Although some invasive stimuli such as a spray of water, pressure on the limbs, or meaningful words had a higher chance of incorporation into the dream reports upon waking [17–19], most stimuli failed to be incorporated, even when the subjects slept with their eyes taped open and objects were illuminated in front of them [20].

Despite the many things we have learned about sleep in recent years, we remain unsure of its purpose. Is it to restore us to homeostasis? Conserve energy via thermoregulation? Consolidate learning and memory? Help infants' brains to grow fully, program species-specific behaviors, or even, perchance, to dream? These questions are only beginning to be answered. We are, however, perhaps further along in our understanding of how we disconnect from consciousness and the external environment during sleep. One widely considered theory suggests that the thalamus limits sensory information from reaching our frontal cortex, rendering us unaware of our surroundings during sleep [16].

The "thalamic gating" theory is attractive, yet sleep proves to be a much more complex phenomenon. Several lines of evidence challenge the thalamic gating model for sensory disconnection during sleep. The most compelling evidence is that neuronal activity in the primary auditory cortex (A1), a part of the auditory cortex that initially receives information from the thalamus, is comparable in both sleep and wakefulness [16, 21, 22]. In addition, the event-related potentials (measured brain responses that result directly from a specific sensory, cognitive, or motor event) are also preserved during sleep, further challenging the notion that the thalamus stops the relay of information to the cortex during sleep. Finally, although the olfactory stimuli are not routed through the thalamus, we remain largely disconnected from our sense of smell during sleep as well, suggesting an alternative mechanism to thalamic gating. Whatever role the thalamus may play in consciousness, cortical networks also appear to be involved [23].

When considering our mental disconnection from the environment during sleep, changes in neuromodulation in the brain appears to be key. The many stimulatory and inhibitory neurochemicals, such as serotonin, dopamine, histamine, norepinephrine, acetylcholine, orexin, and GABA, clearly modulate our awareness. By variably enhancing and dampening the activity of various neural circuits, these chemicals influence sleep stages and our related consciousness during these stages. More specifically, levels of norepinephrine, serotonin, histamine, and orexin are significantly reduced in REM sleep as compared to the awake state, indicating that they may be playing particularly important roles in incorporating sensory stimuli into our conscious experience [16].

Clearly, the brain's relative isolation from the environment and the shifting of our consciousness during sleep are processes that involve highly complicated, cyclical sequence of events. Being a somewhat new field built upon the combination of accidental discoveries and thoughtfully posed questions, sleep science is growing in scope. Yet, just a handful of decades after the discovery of REM sleep, the dark of the night remains full of mysteries. It is clear that sleep is crucial to our survival, but how exactly sleep keeps us alive and well-functioning is unclear, indicating a multifaceted answer that will take many more decades to elucidate.

CONCLUSION

While sleep was historically believed to be a passive phenomenon, the discovery of REM sleep changed everything. Sleep cycles were soon after identified and characterized by regular patterns of neural, endocrine, and behavioral activity. Not surprisingly, the study of sleep has also enhanced our understanding of consciousness.

REFERENCES

1. Brown C. The stubborn scientist who unraveled the mystery of the night. The Smithsonian. https://www.smithsonianmag.com/science-nature/the-stubborn-scientist-who-unraveled-a-mystery-of-the-night-91514538/. Published 2003. Accessed May 17, 2019.
2. Domhoff GW. Senoi dream theory: Myth, scientific method, and the dreamwork movement. Dreamresearch.net. https://dreams.ucsc.edu/Library/senoi2.html. Published 2003. Accessed May 17, 2019.
3. Dement WC. History of sleep physiology and medicine. In: Kryger MH, Roth T, Dement WC, eds. *Principles and Practice of Sleep Medicine*. 4th ed. Philadelphia, PA: Elsevier; 2005:1–12.
4. MacNish R. *The Philosophy of Sleep*. New York, NY: D. Appleton; 1834.
5. Ishimori, K. True cause of sleep: a hypnogenic substance as evidenced in the brain of sleep-deprived animals. *Tokyo Igakkai Zasshi*. 1909;23:429–459.
6. Legendre R, Pieron H. Le problème des facteurs du sommeil: resultats d'injections vasculaires et intracerebrales de liquids insomniques. *CR Soc Biol*. 1910;68:1077–1079.
7. Kleitman N. *Sleep and Wakefulness*. Chicago, IL: University of Chicago Press; 1939.
8. Aserinsk E, Kleitman N. Regularly occurring periods of eye motility, and concomitant phenomena, during sleep. *Science*. 1953;118:273–274.

9. Chow HM, Horovitz SG, Carr WS, et al. Rhythmic alternating patterns of brain activity distinguish rapid eye movement sleep from other states of consciousness. *PNAS*. 2013;110:10300–10305.

10. Aserinsky E. Memories of famous neuropsychologists. *J Hist Neurosci*. 1996;5:213–227.

11. Pelayo R, Dement W. History of sleep physiology and medicine. In: Kryger MH, Roth T, Dement WC, eds. *Principles and Practice of Sleep Medicine*. 6th ed. Philadelphia, PA: Elsevier; 2017:3–14.

12. Csikszentmihalyi M. *Flow: The Psychology of Optimal Experience*. New York, NY: Harper & Row; 1990.

13. Gruzelier J. A theory of alpha/theta neurofeedback, creative performance enhancement, long distance functional connectivity and psychological integration. *Cogn Process*. 2008;10:101–109.

14. Mirmiran M. The importance of fetal/neonatal REM sleep. *Eur J Obstet Gynecol Reprod Biol*. 1986;21:283–291.

15. Rasch B, Born J. About sleep's role in memory. *Physiol Rev*. 2013;93:681–766.

16. Nir Y, Massimini M, Boly M, Tononi G. Sleep and consciousness. In: Cavanna A, Nani A, Blumenfeld H, Laureys S, eds. *Neuroimaging of Consciousness*. Berlin: Springer; 2013:133–182.

17. Dement, W. The occurrence of low voltage, fast electroencephalogram patterns during behavioral sleep in the cat. *Electroen Clin Neuro*. 1958;10:291–296.

18. Berger RJ. Experimental modification of dream content by meaningful verbal stimuli. *Br J Psychiat*. 1963;109:722–740.

19. Koulack D. Effects of somatosensory stimulation on dream content. *Arch Gen Psychiat*. 1969;20:718–725.

20. Rechtschaffen A., Foulkes D. Effect of visual stimuli on dream content. *Percept Mot Skills*. 1965;20:1149–1160.

21. Pena JL, Perez-Perera L, Bouvier M, Velluti RA. Sleep and wakefulness modulation of the neuronal firing in the auditory cortex of the guinea pig. *Brain Res*. 1999;816:463–470.

22. Issa EB, Wang X. Sensory responses during sleep in primate primary and secondary auditory cortex. *J Neurosci*. 2008;28:14467–14480.

23. Schredl M, Atanasova D, Hormann K, Maurer JT, Hummel T, Stuck BA. Information processing during sleep: the effect of olfactory stimuli on dream content and dream emotions. *J Sleep Res*. 2009;18:285–290.

2

Sleep Across the Animal Kingdom

JASON RIHEL ∎

INTRODUCTION: SLEEP VARIABILITY — IMPLICATIONS FOR SCIENCE

Sleep is highly variable across the animal kingdom. If you have ever had a pet, visited a farm, or gone to the zoo, you've probably already realized this. For example, while a typical adult human sleeps around 8 hours a night, domesticated cats can rack up more than 13 hours of sleep a day. You're probably also aware that the timing of sleep varies dramatically from one animal species to the next. Some species, like humans, sleep predominately at night, while others, like owls, slumber during the day and prowl about in the dark. Most other features of sleep are also malleable across species. Sleep location can vary from the tops of trees to the edge of cliffs to deep, underground burrows. Animals contort into a variety of sleeping postures, from lying down on the back to curled up tight in a ball, or even standing up. The structure of sleep is also varied, with some animals, like humans, tending to sleep in long continuous periods and others, like mice, preferring many short naps. The proportion of dream-rich rapid eye movement (REM) sleep that different animals get each day or night is also highly variable. Evolution has clearly tinkered with sleep to allow for the exploitation of diverse environmental niches.

A complete understanding of sleep variation is of fundamental scientific importance. To account for how the properties of sleep have developed over evolutionary time, we must be able to properly identify and measure sleep even in the simplest of animals. Only then are we able to pinpoint which aspects of sleep are evolutionarily most ancient—and therefore likely to be related to sleep's core biological functions—and which elements are more recent inventions, serving the needs of more complex brains and bodies. At the same time, any theories of sleep's form and function must be able to account for the great diversity of sleep timing and amount across the animal kingdom. After all, if an animal can forego supposedly critical features of sleep, to what extent can those features really be vital for life? These two opposing views of sleep across the animal kingdom—universality of sleep on one end, diversity and malleability on the other—sit in tension but also complement each other to provide a clearer scientific understanding of sleep's structure and function.

SLEEP IS CONSERVED ACROSS THE ANIMAL KINGDOM—A NEW UNDERSTANDING OF SLEEP

If you open a sleep-related textbook prior to the early 2000s, you will likely read that sleep is restricted to mammals and birds and that reptiles (controversially) exhibit some primitive aspects of sleep. Yet, naturalists and philosophers had been describing sleep in a large range of animals going back thousands of years. In 350 BCE, Aristotle, in his treatise *On Sleep and Sleeplessness*, declared that "almost all other animals are clearly observed to partake in sleep, whether they are aquatic, aerial, or terrestrial, since fishes of all kinds, and mollusks, as well as all others which have eyes, have been seen sleeping." (Aristotle, *On Sleep and Sleeplessness*, translated by J. I. Beare). The previous consensus that all animals sleep changed when researchers began to measure brain activity in humans and other animals with electroencephalographic (EEG) and other sophisticated recordings and discovered the neuronal orchestra that accompanies the various stages of sleep, from the slow waves characteristic of non-REM sleep to the active brain and muscle paralysis of dreaming REM sleep (also see Chapter 1 of this volume). These discoveries provided clear electrophysiological correlates for an animal's behavioral state and provided a powerful new way to distinguish an animal or human that is sleeping from one that is quietly awake but immobile. It also allowed for the identification and quantification of the two distinct stages: NREM and REM sleep. Armed with EEG recording capability, researchers looked for signs of sleep in the brains of other species. They mostly failed to find it. These experiments led to the concept that sleep did not arise in evolutionary history until after the emergence of reptiles, with the additional elaboration of REM sleep occurring only in birds and mammals.

However, there are several problems with simply using the EEG as a readout for sleep in other species. One issue is that the major signals of the sleep and wake EEG arise from the neocortex, a relatively recent evolutionary invention that is not present even in other vertebrates like fish and frogs, let alone species like worms, insects, and mollusks. This means that the electrical signals that can be generated by the brain look very different from one species to another. Thus, an animal may very well enter a state of sleep, but the electrical signatures of that state will not look the same as they do in birds and mammals. Another problem with using only electrophysiological criteria to define sleep is that, even in mammals and birds, EEG features that normally correlate with sleep can occasionally be found in animals that are awake, and vice versa. The EEG is not always a perfect readout of behavioral state [1]. A final problem is technical: electrical recordings of the brain are experimentally difficult, requiring fairly invasive laboratory techniques that

- Period of *inactivity*
- Species specific sleep *posture* and *location*
- *Elevated arousal threshold* to stimuli
- *Reversible* with strong stimuli
- Restricted to *specific times* (Circadian)
- *Increased after deprivation* (Homeostatic)

Figure 2.1 Behavioral criteria of sleep.

are often only suitable for recording from larger brains. Stress from the experimental setup may prevent an animal in laboratory conditions from entering behavioral states like sleep that they would normally exhibit in their natural habitat. This means that an experimenter might easily miss sleep states, especially if they record for only a few hours and in constant lighting conditions.

To get around this problem, Campbell and Tobler, elaborating on ideas from Nathaniel Kleitman and Henri Peiron in the early 1900s, suggested a series of behavioral criteria that could be applied to define sleep in other species (Figure 2.1) [2]. Using these criteria, researchers have greatly expanded the list of animals that sleep to include species from nearly every animal phyla with a nervous system, from jellyfish to worms to flies to fish (Figure 2.2). Some researchers have even used these criteria to suggest that cortical neurons in a dish are capable of exhibiting sleep-like states [3]! Identifying a behavioral sleep state in such a diverse range of animals has revealed that many of the fundamental mechanisms that regulate sleep in humans are also at play in other animals. In other words, sleep follows many of

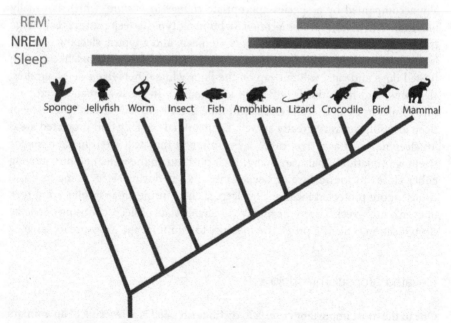

Figure 2.2 Behavioral criteria allow inclusion of species from nearly every animal phyla with a nervous system.

the same rules, is governed by several similar brain mechanisms, and is regulated by a multitude of similar biochemical and molecular interactions in almost every animal that has been carefully examined.

At its core, sleep is a sustained period of behavioral quiescence. This inactive period can be short, on the order of seconds for some types of microsleeps and minutes for a brief nap, or long, as in a sustained night of sleep. However, a period of inactivity by itself is insufficient to distinguish sleep from quiet, immobile wakefulness. The additional criteria used to define sleep are (i) an animal usually adopts a species-specific change in posture for sleeping; (ii) sleep regularly occurs in a species-appropriate location that is often distinct from waking behaviors; (iii) sleep is associated with an increased arousal threshold and unresponsiveness to stimuli, although strong enough stimuli can awaken the animal; (iv) sleep is usually under control of the 24-hour circadian clock; and (v) depriving an animal of sleep leads to an increase in the subsequent intensity or amount of sleep. Not every criterion is of equal importance for defining a state of behavioral sleep. Of these, the most important criteria are the reversible elevation in arousal threshold and the increase in sleep after a period of extended wakefulness or sleep deprivation; as we shall see, even these criteria can apparently be violated under unique circumstances.

Species-Appropriate Sleep Posture and Location

Sleep can be distinguished from quiet wakefulness in part because sleep is usually accompanied by a species-appropriate *change in posture*, which is usually undertaken in a *sleep-specific location*. In humans, typical sleep postures can range from lying down on their back, side, or stomach, and a typical sleeping location is a bed. Animals have a huge range of sleep postures. Many animals, like domesticated dogs and cats, will curl up on the floor while others like horses, giraffes, elephants, and many birds will sleep standing up. In most animals, sleep posture results from an overall relaxation of the muscles called "atonia." The type of sleep location can vary greatly as well. Land animals usually find protected areas for sleeping, such as a tree, cave, or burrow, and they will often make nests for sleeping. Aquatic animals can change their position on the water column, moving either closer to the surface or deeper into the sea during sleep. Some fish also choose more protected locations to sleep, such as inside an anemone, coral reef, or even a shipwreck. Given the highly vulnerable state of sleep, choosing a specific sleep location is likely a protective measure to minimize the exposure to danger.

Elevated Arousal Threshold

One of the most important criteria to distinguish sleep is a lowering of an animal's ability to respond to the environment, across a range of stimuli. A sleeping animal has a higher *arousal threshold*; that is, it takes a more intense or sustained stimulus to arouse a sleeping animal than one that is quietly awake. An increased arousal threshold can be measured as a slower response time (i.e., a longer response latency), which many of us have experienced when we sluggishly respond to our alarm clocks in the morning. A change in arousal threshold may also be observed by slowly increasing the intensity of a stimulus, such as the loudness of a sound or the pressure of a touch, until an animal rouses. A sleeping animal will typically fail to respond (or do so at a lower rate) to a stimulus intensity that easily elicits a response in an awake animal.

Importantly, this change in arousal threshold during sleep applies across multiple senses simultaneously. Multimodal changes in arousal threshold are more likely to demonstrate that the brain has switched into a sleep state, as opposed to just single sensory systems losing sensitivity because of natural daily fluctuations. To take one slightly trivial example, animals that close their eyes when awake may be less sensitive to a visual stimulus, but hearing will be unaffected. During sleep, all the sensory systems show a change in responsiveness.

Reversibility

To be considered sleep, inactive states must be rapidly *reversible*, with very strong stimuli able to wake the animal, despite the increase in arousal threshold. If an immobile animal cannot respond to any kind of stimulus, they might be paralyzed, in a coma, or in the specialized states of hibernation or torpor, during which mammals have dramatically lowered metabolic rates and temperature. This reversibility is critical for the survival of an animal, allowing for a rapid switch to the waking state in response to danger, such as a predator. The arousal threshold during sleep may be globally elevated across sensory systems, but particularly salient stimuli—those associated with danger—may still awaken an animal quickly.

Circadian Rhythms of Sleep

If periods of behavioral quiescence associated with an increase in arousal threshold in nonmammalian species are truly episodes of sleep, fulfilling some of the same functions of sleep in mammalian brains, then the timing and duration of these periods of inactivity should also be governed by some of the same rules that govern sleep in humans and other mammals. Two of the very important rules that regulate sleep time and amount are the *circadian rhythm* and the *sleep homeostat*, the components that make up the 2-process model of sleep [4] (see also Chapter 4 of this volume).

The circadian, or about 24-hour, clock, is a critical regulator of sleep timing, typically restricting sleep to certain times of the day relative to the rising and the setting of the sun. This timing of sleep need not be at night, as it typically is in humans, and animals have a variety of sleep times that are evolved to suit their lifestyles and environmental niches. Animals that are awake during the day and asleep at night are said to be *diurnal*, while animals that restrict sleep to the day are *nocturnal*. The timing of sleep and wakefulness can be even more restricted to select times of day, such as the periods of twilight at either dawn or dusk. Animals that restrict their active period to twilight are called *crepuscular*. Animals that restrict their active waking periods to the predawn are *matutinal*, and those limiting activity to just after sunset are *vespertine*.

While circadian behavior normally acts like clockwork to restrict behaviors like sleep to the same window of time each day, this timing is not necessarily stable for a given animal across life stages, different seasons, or in short-term responses to external, environmental stressors. For example, newborn infants of many species do not show any circadian regulation of sleep for the first weeks after birth. In human infants, circadian regulation of sleep is not imposed until approximately 6 weeks of age [5] (also see Chapter 8 of this volume). Other animals, such as those that have evolved to live in caves that do not receive any light from the sun, such as the cavefish, also show no circadian rhythms to sleep/wake behavior [6]. Many species of animal are even capable of completely switching the timing of their sleep–wake rhythms in response to changing light conditions (e.g., when switching from the wild to the lab) or across seasons [7].

Homeostatic Regulation of Sleep

Although circadian regulation of sleep timing is an important factor to consider when assessing inactivity as a sleep-like state, because this regulation can be abolished or dramatically altered during certain life-stages, a 24-hour rhythm is not an absolutely essential sleep component. Much more important is for these periods of inactivity to be under homeostatic regulation, which is the increased drive to go to sleep after a period of extended wakefulness or after sleep deprivation. Animals that are deprived of sleep show a subsequent increase in both the duration and intensity of sleep—as measured by increases in delta power in slow waves in animals with non-REM (NREM) sleep or by increased difficulty awakening an animal. In other words, if an animal's inactive state is akin to sleep, preventing animals from entering this state will subsequently result in more and deeper sleep-like inactive periods (i.e., the animal's arousal threshold will be even higher than normal).

Evidence for sleep homeostasis is considered more important than demonstrating a clear circadian rhythm to describe a behavior as sleep, because, unlike circadian rhythms, which are an internalized adaptation to living on a rotating planet and therefore represent behavioral responses to external cues, sleep homeostasis is driven in response to physiologically altered internal states that have changed in response to extended wakefulness and is therefore most intimately tied to the possible functions of sleep. Moreover, the sleep homeostat can ultimately override the circadian regulation of sleep, driving an animal to sleep at its ecologically inappropriate time, demonstrating that of these 2 processes, homeostatic regulation of sleep is the more fundamental. Interestingly, even lowered

metabolic states like hibernation and torpor are followed by a homeostatic rebound in slow-wave sleep afterwards, highlighting that even profoundly inactive
states are unable to dissipate the homeostatic pressure of sleep [8].

Despite the centrality of sleep homeostasis to sleep, even for this criterion,
one must use caution when applying it to define sleep states. Under unique
conditions, some animals appear capable of avoiding an increase in sleep pressure following sleep deprivation or restriction. For example, during mating
season, sandpiper males are capable of extreme feats of wakefulness, with some
individuals staying awake 95% of the time for 19 days [9]. This is likely under
genetic selection, as males with the most extreme sleep deprivation during this
period produce the most offspring. Similarly, fruit fly males will normally exhibit increased sleep after a period of forced wakefulness, except when kept
awake by receptive females [10]. Flies will also decrease sleep dramatically when
starved and increase foraging behavior to find food. However, after a period of
starvation-induced wakefulness, the flies do not exhibit a strong an increase in
sleep [11]. These examples demonstrate that under special circumstances that
are critical for species survival the regulation of sleep can be decoupled from
the circadian and homeostatic machinery that normally dictates the timing and
duration of sleep.

Let us now examine, by way of important examples, how these sleep criteria
have been used in the past 20 years to vastly expand our appreciation of the near
universality of sleep across the animal kingdom.

SLEEP DIVERSITY ACROSS
PHYLOGENY—NONVERTEBRATES

Jellyfish

The most evolutionarily ancient animals to have an experimentally demonstrated
sleep state are jellyfish, which belong to the Phylum Cnidaria and diverged from
bilateral animals during evolution approximately 600 million years ago. The
"upside-down" jellyfish, *Cassiopeia*, was recently shown to have a sleep state using
the behavioral criteria for sleep [12]. *Cassiopeia* has a characteristic pulsing behavior of their central bell, which generates current for filter feeding and waste
secretion. These pulses occur continuously at a rate of one pulse/second during
the day but much more slowly at night (circadian behavior), with some very long
pauses in activity lasting 10s of seconds. These quiescent states are accompanied
by a change in the jellyfish's arousal threshold, as measured by the increased time
they take to reorient after being suspended in a water column (they prefer to be
attached to rocks or surfaces of aquaria). The inactive periods are also rapidly
reversible, for example, in response to the presence of food. Finally, depriving
Cassiopeia of these night-time inactive states leads to an increased frequency of
rest the following day, demonstrating that these sleep-like states are under homeostatic control.

The discovery of a sleep state in jellyfish was an important conceptual milestone in sleep research because this demonstrated that behavioral sleep is likely a universal phenomenon of animals with a nervous system, even in animals with a simplified neural net (Figure 2.2). Remarkably, jellyfish sleep also appears to be regulated by some of the same mechanisms that regulate sleep in humans, such as the sleep-inducing drugs melatonin and antihistamines [12]. This suggests that the control of sleep is also shared across the animal kingdom over vast evolutionary distances.

Worms

Sleep has been described in the nematode, *C. elegans*, a small roundworm that lives in the soil. *C. elegans* is a very important model system, famed for its optical transparency, its easily manipulated genetics, and its rapid development, making the description of sleep in this system an important scientific discovery because it made available a sophisticated, established research toolkit. As in other species, *C. elegans* has inactive periods that meet most of the criteria for sleep, including changes in arousal threshold and homeostatic regulation following sleep deprivation [13]. However, a few features of *C. elegans* sleep are more unusual. In particular, sleep in this animal is not under the control of a circadian clock. Instead, sleep states are restricted to a developmental window that coincides with the timing of each molt, when the worm sheds its cuticle between each of the four larval stages. This state of complete immobility, known as lethargus, meets the criteria for sleep. Curiously, although the timing of lethargus is developmentally and not circadianally regulated (all four lethargus stages occur within 7–9 hours of development), lethargus is temporally controlled by the worm version of the gene *period*, which is a central component of the molecular machinery that controls the circadian rhythm in both insects and vertebrates [14].

As an adult, *C. elegans* has a short lifespan, typically of only a few weeks, and during adulthood they almost continuously feed or mate. However, in response to stress or changes in food availability, adult worms will also enter immobile periods that include changes in arousal thresholds [15]. Although stress-induced sleep in the worm has not been demonstrated to be homeostatically regulated, this state is regulated by numerous molecular signals regulated to sleep in vertebrates, including several neuropeptides [16]. Stress-induced sleep in the worm may be similar to sleep induced in many other animals, including humans, such as in response to illness.

Insects

Sleep has been demonstrated in a variety of insects, including cockroaches and bees, but by far the most important insect shown to sleep is the fruit fly, *Drosophila melanogaster*. In fact, it was the clear behavioral demonstration of sleep in *Drosophila* in two papers in 2000 that caused the field to re-evaluate sleep in nonmammalian systems [17, 18]. Since those important behavioral observations, the *Drosophila* model has been used to uncover fundamental aspects of sleep regulation, including the identification of genes and neurons that regulate sleep, the role of synaptic plasticity in sleep, and molecular mechanisms of sleep homeostasis.

To observe *Drosophila* sleep, most researchers have borrowed a method that circadian rhythm researchers use to track flies' long-term behavior. (N.B., the molecular 24-hour clockwork was solved using fruit fly genetics, earning Drs. Michael Young, Michael Rosbash, and Jeff Hall the Nobel Prize for Physiology and Medicine in 2017) This method places flies into sealed glass tubes, with food on one end, and their locomotor activity is tracked each time the fly breaks an infrared beam that crosses the middle of the tube. Flies are crepuscular, with peaks of activity in the morning and evening and long periods of inactivity in the middle of the day (which is called the siesta) and especially long periods of inactivity at night. Flies that have not crossed the beam for more than 5 minutes have changes in posture, electrophysiological signatures, an increased arousal threshold, and homeostatic control; thus, this length of inactive time meets the behavioral definition of sleep in *Drosophila* [18]. More modern methods for tracking individual flies using continuous videography promise to further refine this behavioral definition, as flies can now be tracked in every position in the tube, not just when they break the infrared beam [19].

The power of the *Drosophila* model has facilitated many creative experiments that tell us about fundamental aspects of sleep, including the role of sleep in learning and memory, the regulation of synapses, the interaction with infection and sickness, and the importance of sleep in overall viability [20]. For example, despite the widespread assumption that total sleep deprivation leads to death, the fruit fly is, along with the rat, one of the only species for which this has been experimentally demonstrated [18, 21], although recent results have called this conclusion into question [22]. Other experiments in flies have examined the importance of sleep for learning and for healthy aging. Flies have also been used to uncover genes and neuronal circuits that regulate sleep [23]. Remarkably, despite the several hundred million years of evolution separating the common ancestor of flies and humans, many of these genes and circuits are also used to regulate sleep in both species. For example, one of the critical sleep-inducing neurons in the fly brain signals using the insect neuropeptide, allatostatin, which acts through the fly version of the galanin receptor, which also regulates sleep in mammals [24].

SLEEP ACROSS PHYLOGENY—VERTEBRATES

Fish

Fish represent the most primitive vertebrate species known to have sleep states. Despite living in an aquatic environment, the fish species that have been studied most carefully also exhibit states of sleep that satisfy all of the behavioral criteria [25]. Sleep has been most clearly established in the freshwater zebrafish (*Danio rerio*), a small fish with blue and white stripes from the Ganges and Indus river valleys. The zebrafish is popular in home aquariums and has been an important research tool for investigating early development and behavior. Zebrafish develop very rapidly from a single cell into a free-swimming larval stage in just 5 days, when they begin to exhibit sleep behaviors. In zebrafish larvae, which can be tracked by automated video software, sleep is defined as an inactive period that lasts at least 1 minute, as these are associated with an increased arousal threshold to both light and acoustic stimuli [26]. Zebrafish larvae are diurnal, and their bouts of sleep at night are homeostatically regulated. As in humans, sleep is longer and more frequent in younger animals, with progressively less sleep behavior as these animals age. In adult zebrafish, which reach sexual maturity at about three months of age, behavioral sleep can last as few as 6 seconds [27].

As we have seen for other species, the regulation of sleep in zebrafish shares many fundamental features with sleep regulation in humans. One of the most remarkable of these demonstrated so far may be the role of the neuropeptide hypocretin (also known as orexin) in maintaining wakefulness. In humans, the loss of either hypocretin signaling or, more commonly, the loss of the small set of neurons in the hypothalamus that produce hypocretin leads to the sleep disorder narcolepsy, which is characterized by excessive daytime sleepiness and unstable sleep and wake transitions [28]. Zebrafish also produce hypocretin in the hypothalamus, and it is similarly important for maintaining wakefulness in the fish [29, 30]. Other populations of neurons in the zebrafish brain that are critical for regulating sleep in a way similar to that in mammals include sleep-promoting serotonin neurons [31] and the inhibitory neuropeptide galanin-producing neurons [32]. Another advantage of using fish to study sleep is that the effect of drugs can be rapidly tested by adding small molecule compounds to their water. Our recent study of the effects of more than 5500 compounds on larval zebrafish sleep and wake behavior found a broad agreement between drugs that promote or inhibit sleep in fish and in humans [33].

Although the zebrafish is the most experimentally studied fish, there is evidence for sleep in other fish species as well. One particularly interesting species is the eyeless Mexican cavefish, which has been adapted to living not only in the dark but in a low-food availability, low-pH environment [34]. These cavefish species no longer exhibit circadian rhythms of sleep in dark conditions [6]. (N.B., curiously, cavefish can become rhythmic again if given a 24-hour light:dark cycle, demonstrating they can still detect light without eyes.) Cavefish also exhibit dramatically reduced sleep relative to their surface-dwelling relatives [35]. Perhaps this reduced sleep is a specific adaptation to the harsh conditions of living in the cave environment. Another species of fish that deserve additional consideration are sharks. Some species of sharks are considered obligate swimmers because the structure of their gills requires them to continuously swim to generate water flow for the exchange of oxygen (obligate ram ventilators). While this would seem to preclude the possibility of fulfilling the behavioral criteria for sleep, there are documented examples of reef sharks entering inactive states in oxygen rich coastal caves. Despite the name, whether reef sharks in the Sleeping Shark Cave off the coast of Isla Mujeres, Mexico actually fulfill all the behavioral criteria for sleep has not been properly tested.

Amphibians

Amphibians are a diverse class of vertebrates that include frogs, toads, and salamanders. Despite their evolutionary importance as the transition point between aquatic and terrestrial vertebrates, few systematic studies of amphibian sleep using the full suite of behavioral or electrophysiological criteria have been performed [36]. Although inactive periods of behavioral quiescence have been observed in most amphibian species that have been tested, a change in arousal threshold during these states has only been clearly shown in toads and frogs [37], and only one study has examined and found a homeostatic increase in sleep after prolonged wakefulness in the common frog [38]. Although most evidence indicates that amphibians sleep, much more work needs to be performed to characterize sleep in these species, especially in younger animals as they undergo metamorphosis and transition from aquatic to land environments.

Reptiles

Using both electrophysiological and behavioral criteria, most studies have concluded that reptiles, including turtles, crocodilians, and lizards, exhibit sleep [36]. When examined, all these species enter quiescent periods of inactivity, with lowered heart and respiration rates and increases in arousal thresholds in response to stimuli. Studies across these reptiles also have found increases in sleep following periods of sleep deprivation, showing that these states are under homeostatic control. The electrophysiological evidence for sleep in reptiles is more mixed, although most studies have found a reduction in the EEG frequency during these inactive periods that is characteristic of sleep in mammals. The evidence for slow wave sleep is strongest for Crocodylia, with both increased amplitude and reductions in frequency seen in most studies of these species [39]. The scientific consensus is that reptiles sleep.

More controversial is whether reptile sleep can also be divided into two states, an inactive slow-wave sleep (NREM) stage and an electrophysiologically active, muscle atonic paradoxical sleep stage (REM), as seen in mammals and birds. Although a few studies have reported an active EEG and muscle atonia in turtles [40], the best evidence for a REM state has been reported in several species of lizard [36]. Recording from the brains of Australians dragons, Shein-Idelson and colleagues recently demonstrated that at night, during periods of behavioral quiescence and lowered muscle tone, these lizards switch between a slow-wave sleep and a brain-active paradoxical sleep state at a frequency of about 80 seconds [41].

Remarkably, during this paradoxical sleep stage, the dragons even have the characteristic eye movements associated with paradoxical/REM sleep in mammals. The presence of paradoxical/REM sleep in reptiles is an important discovery, showing that REM sleep exists in a cold-blooded species (Figure 2.2). Theories of REM sleep that have postulated that this state evolved to serve some important function associated with warm-bloodedness must therefore be re-examined.

Birds

Bird sleep is behaviorally similar to mammalian sleep, exhibiting all of the sleep criteria, and brain activity measurements show that birds have both slow-wave NREM and paradoxical REM sleep. However, birds have evolved several unusual modifications to both sleep stages, presumably as adaptations for a life of flying and perching in trees. The most remarkable of these adaptations is the ability to engage in unihemispheric slow-wave sleep (USWS); that is, they can sleep one half of their brain at a time! During USWS, while one brain hemisphere is undergoing the slow-wave activity of sleep, the other hemisphere is fully awake and responsive to the environment [42]. During USWS, the eye under control of the awake hemisphere can remain open. Sleeping with one eye open is likely used by birds to maintain awareness of potential predators in the environment. In particular, bird species that sleep on the ground, such as ducks, will position themselves in groups with the outermost birds sleeping with the open eye facing away from the others [43]. In addition, ducks in the middle of the group are more likely to sleep with both hemispheres simultaneously, suggesting that although birds can engage in USWS, they will engage in bi-hemispheric slow wave sleep when given a safe opportunity to do so [44].

Because birds are capable of sleeping with one brain hemisphere at a time when measured on land, it had been widely assumed that USWS is used by birds to engage in long-haul flights that can last many days—hundreds of days in flight have been observed in some species [45]. However, this hypothesis was only recently tested in frigatebirds, which engage in long foraging flights over the ocean lasting up to 2 months, using specialized lightweight EEG recording devices capable of measuring sleep in flight [46]. As predicted, frigatebirds engaged in USWS while in flight. Surprisingly, however, during gliding flight, they also slept with *both* hemispheres at the same time. Overall, while able to sleep in flight, frigatebirds slept less than 10% of the time they slept while on land, suggesting that the vigilance granted by USWS is insufficient for performing all of the necessary attention tasks during flight.

Birds also have modifications to REM sleep. In particular, birds are capable of entering REM sleep without losing muscle tone in the leg muscles required for maintaining a standing posture, on one or both legs, without falling over [42]. This feature appears to be unique to bird REM sleep, as even mammals, like horses and giraffes, that usually enter NREM sleep while standing, must lie down for REM sleep [47, 48]. Although the mechanisms for how birds achieve this is unknown, maintaining posture during REM has likely evolved to keep birds from falling out of trees or other high perches.

Mammals

Sleep has been best studied in mammals, although it is important to note that sleep timing and duration have often been estimated only through behavioral observation of animals in zoos, not in animals' native habitats. Behavioral and EEG studies have revealed NREM and REM sleep stages in almost all mammalian orders, including the egg-laying monotremes of Australia, the echidna and platypus [49, 50]; the exception is whales and dolphins, which have not been reported to have REM sleep [51]. Especially striking is the diversity of sleep duration across mammalian species, with bats sleeping upwards of 20 hours a day and large land mammals like the elephant and giraffe sleeping for just a few hours a night [52, 53]. This cannot be simply explained differences in brain structure or function across the different mammalian orders, because even closely related species can have large differences in total sleep time [54]. For example, among primates, sleep ranges from 8 hours in humans, 10 to 12 hours in lab and wild chimpanzees [55, 56] to upwards of 17 hours in owl monkeys [57]. Likewise, REM sleep amount varies greatly over mammalian species, with domesticated cats achieving more than 3 hours of REM sleep a day, while horses typically obtain less than 1 hour of REM per night [53]. If sleep serves a set of universal, evolutionarily ancient functions, how can sleep achieve these tasks in different animals with such diversity in sleep time and structures?

Several researchers have tried to leverage the diversity of mammalian sleep across species to hone theories of sleep regulation. For example, mammalian metabolic rate is inversely proportional to body size: small animals have a large metabolic rate, and large animals have a small one. It is also true that, in general, mammalian sleep amount is inversely proportional to body size, with the smallest animals sleeping more while the largest animals sleep less, suggesting a link between sleep time and metabolic rate. However, this relationship only holds true for plant-eating herbivores, while carnivores and omnivores show almost no relationship between body size and sleep amount [52]. Expanding on this approach, Drs. Van Savage and Geoffrey West have developed a quantitative model demonstrating that sleep amount across mammals can instead be best described as a function of the metabolic rate of the brain, not the body [58]. Attempts to explain the diversity of REM sleep across mammalian species have been less successful, although the diversity of REM sleep amounts has been used to argue against certain popular theories of the function of REM sleep. For example, REM sleep time does not correlate with intelligence or memory skills; some of the most intelligent animals, whales and dolphins, have no detectable REM [59], raising the possibility that REM sleep is not essential for memory consolidation as has been proposed. As most mammals with REM sleep have more REM during early stages of development than as adults [60], it has been suggested that REM plays

an important role during brain development. More research is needed to establish clear links between the diverse mammalian NREM and REM sleep structure,
timing, and duration with its potential functions.

Most mammals exhibit bi-hemispheric slow-wave sleep, but sea-dwelling
mammals, including dolphins, whales, and seals, have the remarkable ability
to sleep with one side of the brain at a time, as seen in birds. This is very
likely an adaptation to living in an aquatic environment while still needing
to return to the water's surface to breathe. Whale species almost exclusively
exhibit USWS, but mammals like the fur seal, which spend considerable time
on both the land and sea, are capable of switching between USWS while in
the ocean and bi-hemispheric slow-wave sleep when on land [61, 62]. The fur
seal's ability to switch between two types of sleeping patterns is perhaps the
clearest example of the high degree of plasticity of the systems that govern
sleep structure. Given that sleep is a dangerous undertaking for most animals,
since they become less sensitive to their environment, it is still unclear why
the ability to sleep with one brain hemisphere at a time has not evolved in
other land-dwelling species.

CONCLUSION

When researchers have looked carefully, they have shown that sleep is detectable
in almost every animal species. Remarkably, many of the brain chemicals, genes,
and neuronal structures that regulate sleep are also shared across millions of years
of evolution. This suggests that underneath all the diverse modifications that have
been added or subtracted from sleep over the millennia, sleep may serve a set of
fundamental, universal functions. By expanding the menagerie of animals used
to study sleep, researchers are making rapid progress on understanding these core
principles of sleep.

REFERENCES

1. Davis CJ, Clinton JM, Jewett KA, Zielinski MR, Krueger JM. Delta wave
   power: an independent sleep phenotype or epiphenomenon? *J Clin Sleep*. 2011;7(5
   Suppl):S16–S18.
2. Campbell SS, Tobler I. Animal sleep: a review of sleep duration across phylogeny.
   Neurosci Biobehav Rev. 1984;8(3):269–300.
3. Hinard V, Mikhail C, Pradervand S, et al. Key electrophysiological, molecular,
   and metabolic signatures of sleep and wakefulness revealed in primary cortical
   cultures. *J Neurosci*. 2012;32(36):12506–12517.
4. Borbély AA. A two process model of sleep regulation. *Hum Neurobiol*.
   1982;1(3):195–204.
5. McGraw K, Hoffmann R, Harker C, Herman JH. The development of circadian
   rhythms in a human infant. *Sleep*. 199;22(3):303–310.

6. Beale A, Guibal C, Tamai TK, Klotz L, Cowen S, Peyric E, et al. Circadian rhythms in Mexican blind cavefish: *Astyanax mexicanus* in the lab and in the field. *Nat Commun.* 2013;4:2769.

7. Yassumoto TI, Tachinardi P, Oda GA, Valentinuzzi VS. Acute effects of light and darkness on the activity and temperature rhythms of a subterranean rodent, the Anillaco tuco-tuco. *Physiol Behav.* 2019;210:112645.

8. Deboer T, Tobler I. Sleep EEG after daily torpor in the Djungarian hamster: similarity to the effect of sleep deprivation. *Neurosci Lett.* 1994;166(1):35–38.

9. Lesku JA, Rattenborg NC, Valcu M, et al. Adaptive sleep loss in polygynous pectoral sandpipers. *Science.* 2012;337(6102):1654–1658.

10. Beckwith EJ, Geissmann Q, French AS, Gilestro GF. Regulation of sleep homeostasis by sexual arousal. *eLife.* 2017;12(6):e27445.

11. Keene AC, Duboué ER, McDonald DM, et al. Clock and cycle limit starvation-induced sleep loss in Drosophila. *Curr Biol.* 2010;20(13):1209–1215.

12. Nath RD, Bedbrook CN, Abrams MJ, Basinger T, Bois JS, Prober DA, et al. The jellyfish Cassiopea exhibits a sleep-like state. *Curr Biol.* 2017;27(19):2984–2990.e3.

13. Raizen DM, Zimmerman JE, Maycock MH, et al. Lethargus is a Caenorhabditis elegans sleep-like state. *Nature.* 2008;451(7178):569–572.

14. Trojanowski NF, Raizen DM. Call it worm sleep. *Trends Neurosci.* 2016;39(2):54–62.

15. Hill AJ, Mansfield R, Lopez JMNG, Raizen DM, Van Buskirk C. Cellular stress induces a protective sleep-like state in C. elegans. *Curr Biol.* 2014;24(20):2399–2405.

16. Nath RD, Chow ES, Wang H, Schwarz EM, Sternberg PW. *C. elegans* stress-induced sleep emerges from the collective action of multiple neuropeptides. *Curr Biol.* 2016 26;26(18):2446–2455.

17. Hendricks JC, Finn SM, Panckeri KA, et al. Rest in Drosophila is a sleep-like state. *Neuron.* 2000;25(1):129–138.

18. Shaw PJ, Cirelli C, Greenspan RJ, Tononi G. Correlates of sleep and waking in Drosophila melanogaster. *Science.* 2000;287(5459):1834–1837.

19. Gilestro GF. Video tracking and analysis of sleep in Drosophila melanogaster. *Nat Protoc.* 2012;7(5):995–1007.

20. Beckwith EJ, French AS. Sleep in Drosophila and its context. *Front Physiol.* 2019;10:1167.

21. Rechtschaffen A, Bergmann BM, Everson CA, Kushida CA, Gilliland MA. Sleep deprivation in the rat: X. Integration and discussion of the findings. *Sleep.* 1989;12(1):68–87.

22. Geissmann Q, Beckwith EJ, Gilestro GF. Most sleep does not serve a vital function: evidence from Drosophila melanogaster. *Sci Adv.* 2019;5(2):eaau9253.

23. Artiushin G, Sehgal A. The Drosophila circuitry of sleep–wake regulation. *Curr Opin Neurobiol.* 2017;44:243–250.

24. Donlea JM, Pimentel D, Talbot CB, et al. Recurrent circuitry for balancing sleep need and sleep. *Neuron.* 2018;97(2):378–389.e4.

25. Zhdanova IV, Wang SY, Leclair OU, Danilova NP. Melatonin promotes sleep-like state in zebrafish. *Brain Res.* 2001;903(1-2):263–268.

26. Barlow IL, Rihel J. Zebrafish sleep: from geneZZZ to neuronZZZ. *Curr Opin Neurobiol.* 2017;44:65–71.

27. Yokogawa T, Marin W, Faraco J, et al. Characterization of sleep in zebrafish and insomnia in hypocretin receptor mutants. *PLoS Biol.* 2007;5(10):e277.

28. Sakurai T. Orexin deficiency and narcolepsy. *Curr Opin Neurobiol.* 2013; 23(5):760–766.
29. Elbaz I, Yelin-Bekerman L, Nicenboim J, Vatine G, Appelbaum L. Genetic ablation of hypocretin neurons alters behavioral state transitions in zebrafish. *J Neurosci.* 2012;32(37):12961–12972.
30. Prober DA, Rihel J, Onah AA, Sung RJS, Schier AF. Hypocretin/orexin overexpression induces an insomnia-like phenotype in zebrafish. *J Neurosci.* 2006;26:13400–13410.
31. Oikonomou G, Altermatt M, Zhang R-W, et al. The serotonergic raphe promote sleep in zebrafish and mice. *Neuron.* 2019;103(4):686–701.e8.
32. Reichert S, Pavón Arocas O, Rihel J. The neuropeptide galanin is required for homeostatic rebound sleep following increased neuronal activity. *Neuron.* 2019;104(2):370–384.e5.
33. Rihel J, Prober DA, Arvanites A, et al. Zebrafish behavioral profiling links drugs to biological targets and rest/wake regulation. *Science.* 2010;327(5963):348–351.
34. Keene AC, Duboue ER. The origins and evolution of sleep. *J Exp Biol.* 2018;221 (Pt 11):jeb159533.
35. Duboué ER, Keene AC, Borowsky RL. Evolutionary convergence on sleep loss in cavefish populations. *Curr Biol.* 2011;21(8):671–676.
36. Libourel P-A, Herrel A. Sleep in amphibians and reptiles: a review and a preliminary analysis of evolutionary patterns. *Biol Rev.* 2016;91(3):833–866.
37. Hobson JA, Goin OB, Goin CJ. Electrographic correlates of behaviour in tree frogs. *Nature.* 1968;220(5165):386–387.
38. Aristakesian EA, Karmanova IG. [Effects of 6-hour deprivation of protosleep (primary sleep) in the brown frog, Rana temporaria]. *Zh Evol Biokhim Fiziol.* 1998;34(4):510–515.
39. Tisdale RK, Lesku JA, Beckers GJL, Rattenborg NC. Bird-like propagating brain activity in anesthetized Nile crocodiles. *Sleep.* 2018;41(8):zsy105.
40. Ayala-Guerrero F, Calderón A, Pérez MC. Sleep patterns in a chelonian reptile (*Gopherus flavomarginatus*). *Physiol Behav.* 1988;44(3):333–337.
41. Shein-Idelson M, Ondracek JM, Liaw H-P, Reiter S, Laurent G. Slow waves, sharp waves, ripples, and REM in sleeping dragons. *Science.* 2016;352(6285):590–595.
42. Rattenborg NC, van der Meij J, Beckers GJL, Lesku JA. Local aspects of avian non-REM and REM sleep. *Front Neurosci.* 2019;13:567.
43. Rattenborg NC, Lima SL, Amlaner CJ. Facultative control of avian unihemispheric sleep under the risk of predation. *Behav Brain Res.* 1999;105(2):163–172.
44. Rattenborg NC, Lima SL, Amlaner CJ. Half-awake to the risk of predation. *Nature.* 1999;397(6718):397–398.
45. Liechti F, Witvliet W, Weber R, Bächler E. First evidence of a 200-day non-stop flight in a bird. *Nat Commun.* 2013;4:2554.
46. Rattenborg NC, Voirin B, Cruz SM, et al. Evidence that birds sleep in mid-flight. *Nat Commun.* 2016;7:12468.
47. Ruckebusch Y. The relevance of drowsiness in the circadian cycle of farm animals. *Anim Behav.* 1972;20(4):637–643.
48. Tobler I, Schwierin B. Behavioural sleep in the giraffe (*Giraffa camelopardalis*) in a zoological garden. *J Sleep Res.* 1996;5(1):21–32.

49. Siegel JM, Manger PR, Nienhuis R, Fahringer HM, Pettigrew JD. Monotremes and the evolution of rapid eye movement sleep. *Philos Trans R Soc Lond B Biol Sci.* 1998;353(1372):1147–1157.

50. Siegel JM, Manger PR, Nienhuis R, Fahringer HM, Shalita T, Pettigrew JD. Sleep in the platypus. *Neuroscience.* 1999;91(1):391–400.

51. Lyamin OI, Manger PR, Ridgway SH, Mukhametov LM, Siegel JM. Cetacean sleep: an unusual form of mammalian sleep. *Neurosci Biobehav Rev.* 2008;32(8):1451–1484.

52. Siegel JM. Clues to the functions of mammalian sleep. *Nature.* 2005;437 (7063):1264–1271.

53. Zepelin H, Siegel JM, Tobler I. Mammalian sleep. In: Kryger MH, Roth T, Dement WC, eds. *Principles and Practice of Sleep Medicine.* 4th ed. Philadelphia, PA: W. B. Saunders; 2005:91–100.

54. Allada R, Siegel JM. Unearthing the phylogenetic roots of sleep. *Current Biology.* 2008;5:R670–R679. doi:10.1016/j.cub.2008.06.033

55. Bert J, Kripke DF, Rhodes J. Electroencephalogram of the mature chimpanzee: twenty-four hour recordings. *Electroencephalogr Clin Neurophysiol.* 1970; 28(4):368–373.

56. Lodwick JL, Borries C, Pusey AE, Goodall J, McGrew WC. From nest to nest— influence of ecology and reproduction on the active period of adult Gombe chimpanzees. *Am J Primatol.* 2004;64(3):249–260.

57. Suzuki J, Sri Kantha S. Quantitation of sleep and spinal curvature in an unusually longevous owl monkey (*Aotus azarae*). *J Med Primatol.* 2006;35(6):321–330.

58. Savage VM, West GB. A quantitative, theoretical framework for understanding mammalian sleep. *Proc Natl Acad Sci U S A.* 2007;104(3):1051–1056.

59. Siegel JM. The REM sleep-memory consolidation hypothesis. *Science.* 2001;294(5544):1058–1063.

60. Marks GA, Shaffery JP, Oksenberg A, Speciale SG, Roffwarg HP. A functional role for REM sleep in brain maturation. *Behav Brain Res.* 1995;69(1–2):1–11.

61. Lyamin OI, Kosenko PO, Lapierre JL, Mukhametov LM, Siegel JM. Fur seals display a strong drive for bilateral slow-wave sleep while on land. *J Neurosci.* 2008;28(48):12614–12621.

62. Lyamin OI, Mukhametov LM, Siegel JM. Sleep in the northern fur seal. *Curr Opin Neurobiol.* 2017;44:144–151.

3

Systems Physiology During Sleep

MARGARET YU AND HRAYR ATTARIAN ■

INTRODUCTION

Sleep is a crucial aspect of life maintenance. All animals, even the simpler organisms like nematodes, need to enter a state of relative inactivity that promotes homeostatic regulation [1]. In fact, humans spend one-third of their lives asleep. If sleep did not have such an essential function, it would be an evolutionary failure as it leaves the sleeper immensely vulnerable.

Over the course of a sleep period, two distinct states, rapid eye movement (REM) and nonrapid eye movement (NREM) sleep alternate in cycles. During each, the various organ systems undergo distinct physiological changes. This chapter will review each of those systems and their unique changes across the sleep cycle.

NREM sleep is divided into three stages. Stage N1 is the transition from awake to asleep, with initiation of relaxation and gradual slowing of brain wave frequency, as measured by an electroencephalogram (EEG). In stage N2, new types of brain wave patterns emerge. There are sleep spindles (thought to be important for memory consolidation) and K-complexes (induced by external stimulation like a "knock" on the door). During stage N3 sleep, the dominant activity is large amplitude and very slow waves. This stage is thought to play an important role in overall tissue restoration and homeostasis [1–3].

REM is made up of two stages that are less distinct from stages of NREM. These are tonic REM and phasic REM. During the tonic stage, there are no eye movements and all voluntary muscles (other than the diaphragm) are paralyzed. There is atonia, or loss of muscle tone. During the phasic stage, while there is still atonia, there are bursts of muscle twitches and rapid eye movements [1–4].

We will now delineate the physiological changes during both NREM and REM sleep of the different organ systems.

THE NERVOUS SYSTEM

Cerebral Blood Flow

The brain is a highly vascular organ and cerebral blood flow (blood flow to and from the brain) is controlled by a variety of factors including the cerebral metabolic rate and the different needs for glucose and oxygen for energy and cell survival. Cerebral autoregulation, as well as the influence of respiratory blood gases (e.g., percentage of oxygen and carbon dioxide), influence cerebral blood flow [5].

Autoregulation is the ability of the organ to maintain a constant blood flow despite changes in perfusion pressures. Normally, cerebral blood flow is maintained at a mean arterial pressure (MAP) of 60 to 150 mmHg. MAP is defined as the average of the pressure in a person's arteries during one cardiac cycle. It is calculated by doubling the diastolic blood pressure and adding the sum to the systolic blood pressure. This number is then divided by 3. This is considered a better indicator of end organ perfusion than the systolic blood pressure alone [6].

During NREM sleep, there is significant reduction in both blood flow and the cerebral metabolic rate. There is decreased blood flow to the deep structures of the brain (pons, thalamus, and basal ganglia) as well as the spinal cord (Figure 3.1) [5–7].

The thalamic neurons become hyperpolarized during N2, which then generates sleep spindles and K-complex structures. During hyperpolarization, the cell's membrane potential becomes more negative and this inhibits further action potentials, or activations of the cell. This is crucial for being a restorative function of sleep (Figure 3.2) [8].

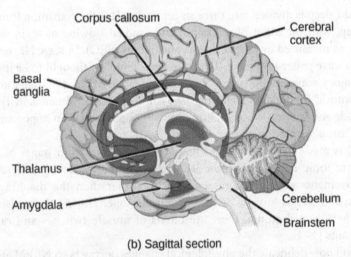

(b) Sagittal section

Figure 3.1 The deep structures of the brain with decreased blood flow during sleep (basal ganglia, thalamus, brainstem).
SOURCE: Openstax, Biology.

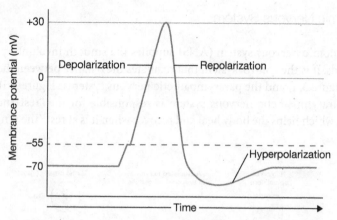

Figure 3.2 Depolarization and hyperpolarization of cells, causing propagation of action potentials.
SOURCE: Openstax, Anatomy and Physiology

During REM, cerebral blood flow and metabolism are comparable to during wakefulness, particularly in the limbic system (which is involved with emotions and memory), as well as the visual association areas, which are involved in dream imagery generation (Figure 3.3).

Autoregulation of intracerebral blood vessels is the brain's ability to maintain relatively constant blood flow, even when there are changing perfusion pressures. This autoregulation is more adversely affected during REM sleep [5].

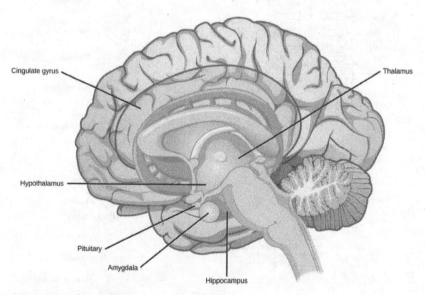

Figure 3.3 The limbic system, involved in dreams.
SOURCE: Openstax, Anatomy and Physiology

Autonomic Nervous System

The autonomic nervous system (ANS) supplies the smooth involuntary muscles and glands. It is the control system that regulates the balance between the sympathetic (Figure 3.4) and the parasympathetic nervous systems (Figure 3.5).

The parasympathetic nervous system is responsible for the "rest-and-digest" pathway, which helps the body heal and recover when it is at rest. The sympathetic

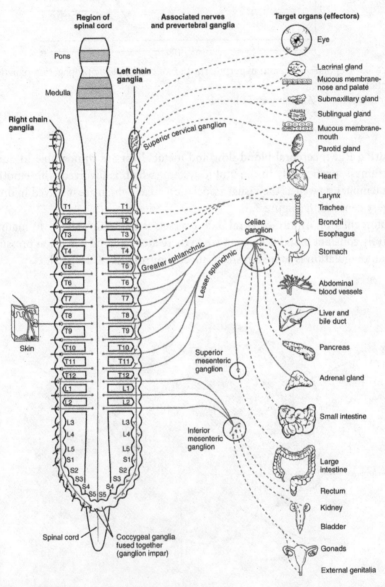

Figure 3.4 The sympathetic autonomic nervous system.
SOURCE: Openstax, Anatomy and Physiology

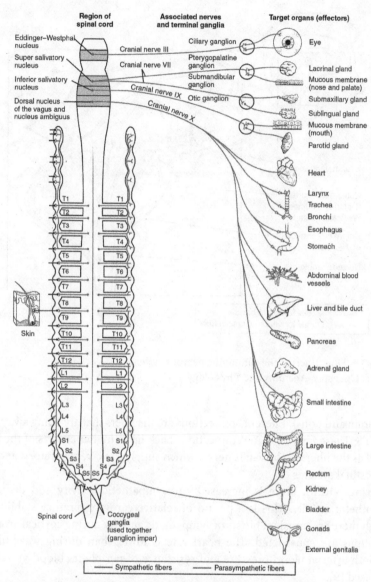

Region of spinal cord	Associated nerves and terminal ganglia	Target organs (effectors)

Eddinger–Westphal nucleus

Cranial nerve III — Ciliary ganglion — Eye

Super salivatory nucleus

Cranial nerve VII — Pterygopalatine ganglion — Lacrinal gland

Inferior salivatory nucleus

Submandibular ganglion — Mucous membrane (nose and palate)

Cranial nerve IX — Otic ganglion — Submaxillary gland

Dorsal nucleus of the vagus and nucleus ambiguus

Cranial nerve X

Sublingual gland

Mucous membrane (mouth)

Parotid gland

Heart

Larynx

Trachea

Bronchi

Esophagus

Stomach

Skin

Abdominal blood vessels

Liver and bile duct

Pancreas

Adrenal gland

Small intestine

Large intestine

Rectum

Kidney

Bladder

Spinal cord — Coccygeal ganglia fused together (ganglion impar)

Gonads

External genitalia

——— Sympathetic fibers   ——— Parasympathetic fibers

Figure 3.5 The parasympathetic autonomic nervous system.
SOURCE: Openstax, Anatomy and Physiology

nervous system is the "fight or flight" pathway, which helps with survival in stressful and dangerous situations. The control center for the ANS is the nucleus tractus solitarius (NTS), which is in the medulla, at the lowest part of the brainstem. The NTS is in direct communication with the central nervous system, as well as the different organ systems that are under ANS control (Figure 3.6) [8].

Afferent connections are the fibers going towards the NTS. Those fibers are from the cardiovascular (CV), respiratory, gustatory, and gastrointestinal systems, as well as descending fibers from the cerebral cortex and upper brainstem

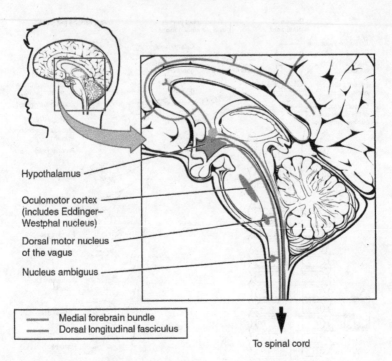

Figure 3.6 Fiber tracts of the autonomic nervous system.
SOURCE: Openstax, Anatomy and Physiology

(midbrain and pons). Efferent connections are the fibers that are going away from the NTS. These fibers include connections back up to higher centers of the brain as well as the fibers of the vagus nerve, which supply the CV, respiratory, and gastrointestinal systems [8].

During NREM, there is increased parasympathetic activity and decreased sympathetic activity. This is a period of relative cardiorespiratory stability, although there are transient bursts of sympathetic activity during cortical arousals. The pupils are constricted. The heart rate is lower than during wakefulness, and both arterial blood pressure and resistance of peripheral blood vessels are decreased [9].

During tonic REM, there are no rapid eye movements. The pupils continue to be constricted, and parasympathetic activity continues to predominant during tonic REM [4, 7].

During phasic REM, there are rapid eye movements. The sympathetic system predominates, and there is autonomic instability, meaning that there can be dramatic fluctuations in blood pressure and heart rate. The pupils are now dilated as there is central inhibition of parasympathetic outflow to the iris [4, 7].

Clinically, this autonomic instability during REM is the reason for an increased risk of death during sleep for patients with cardiopulmonary disorders. In addition, diseases of primary autonomic failure such as multiple system atrophy and familial dysautonomia also worsen during sleep. Patients with obstructive sleep apnea (OSA) have chronically elevated sympathetic activity, which is thought to be a major contributor to the link between OSA and CV and cerebrovascular diseases [9].

THE CARDIOVASCULAR SYSTEM

The CV system includes not just the heart and blood vessels, but also the 5 liters of blood that circulate continuously throughout the body.

During NREM, the heart rate usually decreases by 5% to 8%, and cardiac output is reduced. Systemic blood pressure also decreases but then rises sharply during awakenings. Vagal and baroreceptor control of the CV system is increased, which can make a person more prone to arrhythmias due to the uncoupling of the respiratory and CV systems [1].

During REM, the heart rate becomes highly variable, and, similarly to NREM sleep, cardiac output decreases. Compared to NREM, systemic blood pressure increases in NREM by about 5%. The overall loss of homeostasis during REM makes it a dangerous time for patients with CV disease [1–4]. In fact, REM carries an increased risk of myocardial infarctions, or heart attacks, in the mornings due to the sharp increases in heart rate and blood pressure that occur with awakening [5].

THE ENDOCRINE SYSTEM

The goal of the endocrine system is to secrete hormones that influence the overall functioning of all organs in the body. There are feedback loops built into the endocrine system, and sleep is one of the important factors maintaining proper functioning and integrity of these feedback loops (Figure 3.7) [10].

Some parts of the endocrine system are controlled by the circadian rhythm, while others are related to the different sleep stages. We will address each aspect of sleep's impact on the hormone systems.

Growth Hormone

Secreted by the pituitary, growth hormone (GH) stimulates cell growth and cell regeneration and is also a stress hormone. There is a reliable burst of GH during slow wave sleep (N3) during the first sleep cycle, which occurs shortly after sleep onset. In men, this pulse of GH is often the only secretory pulse over 24 hours. For women, the GH pulses are more frequent, and there may be some that occur during the daytime as well. As we get older, this nocturnal increase in GH decreases, along with the overall decrease in the amount of N3 sleep [4].

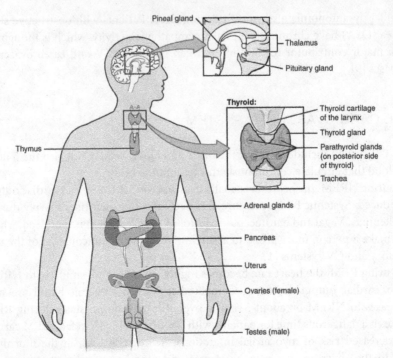

Figure 3.7 Organs involved in the endocrine system.
SOURCE: Openstax, BiologyE.

Adrenocorticotropic Hormone

Adrenocorticotropic hormone (ACTH) is secreted by the pituitary and controls the amount of cortisol secreted from the adrenals. Cortisol is released in response to stress, as well as low blood glucose concentrations. This is under circadian control. The plasma levels of cortisol and ACTH are highest in the early morning, which triggers us to awaken. When we first fall asleep, we experience our lowest levels of cortisol and ACTH. The reason for this is that sleep causes inhibition of the release of ACTH; sleep is a regenerative time so there is little need for stress hormone release in the initial part of sleep, and this suppression can help maintain a person's sleepiness until a burst of cortisol signals the need to awaken in the morning. When we are sleep deprived, we experience a decrease in the total amount of cortisol that is secreted over the 24-hour period [7, 11].

Thyroid-Stimulating Hormone

Secreted by the pituitary, thyroid- stimulating hormone (TSH) stimulates the thyroid gland to release thyroid hormones. During the daytime, TSH levels are relatively low. They gradually increase during the early evening hours, and their maximal release is around the third sleep cycle of the evening. The later part of sleep manifests as a progressive decline of TSH. This is under circadian control. As our sleep stages deepen, suppression of TSH release increases and is greatest during N3 sleep [4].

Reproductive Hormones/Gonadal Axis

Secretion of these reproductive hormones differ during adolescence and adulthood. During prepubescence, luteinizing hormone (LH) and follicular-stimulating hormone (FSH) are responsible for initiating sexual maturation. There is increased release of both LH and FSH during prepubescence for both boys and girls, following a circadian rhythm. During puberty, the night-time release of gonadotropins (testosterone and estradiol) become pronounced in boys and girls, respectively. This circadian rhythm is not present during adulthood. While there may be an increase in testosterone release during the first REM cycle for men, this effect is not as pronounced as it was during puberty. For women, LH, FSH, and estradiol release are controlled by the menstrual cycle [3, 4].

Insulin Release/Glucose Levels

Blood glucose levels and insulin secretion are higher during early sleep and decrease during later sleep. This initial increase is driven by the greater proportion of N3 during early sleep, and the later decrease is due to increased REM during alter sleep, as well as eventual awakening. When we are sleep deprived and then have daytime recovery sleep during a nap, we experience increased slow wave (N3) sleep and an earlier peak in glucose levels. However, in this case the normal decrease in glucose would not be as robust, and we experience higher plasma levels of glucose. This is why people have less glucose tolerance if they are sleep deprived, which also increases evening levels of cortisol, which drives the activity of the sympathetic nervous system. Thus, when people are chronically sleep deprived, or if they are shift-workers (working a night shift over the long-term), they have a greater likelihood of developing diabetes and obesity, which also drives development of CV disease [12].

THE GASTROENTEROLOGY SYSTEM

Even though we do not consume food during sleep (although see the section on nocturnal eating disorder), the gastroenterology system continues to work. In other words, it is a myth that we stop digesting food when we go to sleep. Digestion starts with chewing, leading to the propagation of food along the esophagus. Once food enters the stomach, there is acidification of the ingested food, as well as forward propulsion of food into the duodenum [13].

The gastroenterology system is both controlled by circadian factors and influenced by REM and NREM sleep.

The secretion of gastric acid has a circadian pattern, with peak secretion between 10 PM and 2 AM [13].

The migrating motor complex (MMC) cause contractility of the gastrointestinal tract in a regular cycle. The duration of the MMC cycle decreases when we are asleep, and the motility of the small intestine diminishes. Although there isn't any synchronization of the NREM/REM cycle with the distribution of the MMC, amplitude of the gastric cycle declines in NREM and returns in REM [1–3]. NREM sleep is associated with decreased colonic contractions; therefore, there is increased water absorption and containment of the intestinal material. There is increased colonic pressure during REM sleep, and this is what maintains fecal continence during sleep [13].

We are at much higher risk of developing gastroesophageal reflux disease (GERD) during sleep. Given the decrease in intestinal motility, as well as the

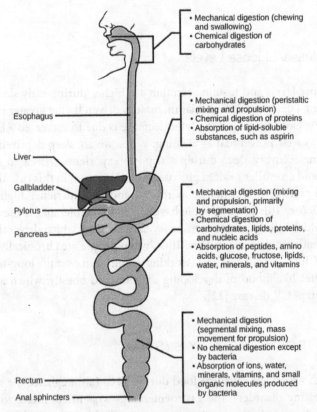

Figure 3.8 The gastrointestinal system. Problems with the pylorus (in particular with its ability to relax) is the underlying physiology behind gastroesophageal reflux disease (GERD).
SOURCE: Openstax, BiologyE.

increase in acid secretion, reflux and erosive esophageal changes are more common at night. OSA also predisposes patients to GERD; up to 60% of patients with OSA have GERD. When there is intermittent airway obstruction, as during OSA, this reduces the ability of the esophagus to empty appropriately, predisposing the OSA patient to developing GERD (Figure 3.8) [1–3].

THE IMMUNE SYSTEM

Proper sleep/wake cycles are the foundation on which proper cytokine release is based. Cytokines are small proteins (~5–20 kDa) that are important for cell signaling [14]. Leukocytes (or white blood cells) secrete important cytokines that help promote and rein in the immune system, as physiologically needed. These cytokines include interleukins (IL) and interferons. Sleep facilitates the healing process and regulates the release of these cytokines, which protect us against infections. Sleep deprivations can not only weaken immunity, which makes us more prone to infections, but improper secretion of these cytokines can also ramp up the immune system to pathologic levels by increasing pro-inflammatory cytokines like IL-6 and tumor necrosis factor alpha. This makes us more prone to developing autoimmune disorders like lupus and rheumatoid arthritis [1–4].

Cytokines, including IL1 and tumor necrosis factor alpha, are also involved in the regulation of sleep. They are an important aspect of the molecular network (including adenosine and nuclear factor kappa B) that comprises the sleep homeostat [14].

RENAL SYSTEM

The kidneys are important for maintaining water and sodium homeostasis in the body. Among its multitude functions, the renal system also filters out the body's waste byproducts. On average, the body produces about 1 to 2 liters of urine each day. This is all under the control of specific renal hormones (antidiuretic hormone, renin, aldosterone, and atrial natriuretic peptide) (Figure 3.9) [1–3].

Release of some of these hormones is dictated by the different sleep stages, while others are independent of sleep stage. Antidiuretic hormone is secreted in bursts and is independent of sleep stage. This results in the resorption of water.

Renin is secreted by specific juxtaglomerular cells of the kidneys. Through specific pathways, it eventually produces angiotensin II, which is a vasoconstrictor (causes tightening of the blood vessels) that stimulates the production of aldosterone from the adrenal glands (which sit on top of the kidneys). Aldosterone causes the absorption of sodium and water. Plasma renin activity (PRA) and aldosterone levels are affected by different sleep cycles. However, this is related to sleep itself rather than circadian factors. PRA increases during NREM sleep and decreases during REM. Aldosterone levels follow the PRA and correspondingly elevate during sleep in relation to the REM cycle [3, 4].

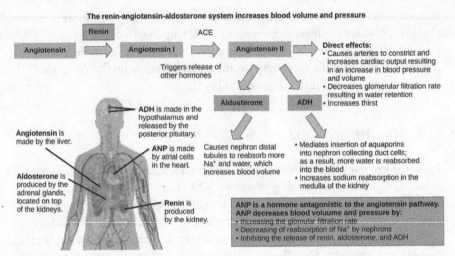

Figure 3.9 The effect of hormones on the balance of electrolytes and fluid in the body.
SOURCE: Openstax, BiologyE.

Renal blood flow changes very little during NREM but increases during REM through the dilation of blood vessels. Both sleep stages are associated with decreased urine flow and increased osmolality. This explains why we can normally sleep through the night without needing to use the bathroom. It also explains another clinical implication of untreated OSA. Patients with OSA that is not well controlled often urinate more at night because they have elevated levels of atrial natriuretic peptide compared to those without OSA. Due to the impact of OSA on the heart, more atrial natriuretic peptide is secreted by the heart cells and tries to respond appropriately to fluid overload by forcing the kidneys to excrete more fluids and electrolytes [15].

RESPIRATORY SYSTEM

The central controllers of breathing are in the medulla, the lowest part of the brainstem. Dorsally, or in the back region of the medulla, are the respiratory groups that promote inspiration. Ventrally, or in the front of the medulla, are in the respiratory pacing centers. Here too are the μ-opioid receptors, the opioid system which controls pain and is a crucial player in reward/addiction behaviors. This system is stimulated by recreational drugs such as heroin, prescription pain medications like morphine, and self-produced substances. Not only do these drugs dull pain, when the opioid system is stimulated the respiratory centers are also dulled. Therefore, recreational drugs like heroin are extremely dangerous for breathing, which is why overdose can have devastating effects [1–3].

The respiratory network receives input from three areas: (i) the forebrain, which sends electrical information regarding the sleep/wave state and other physiologic stages; (ii) chemical input from peripheral and central chemoreceptors (sensory

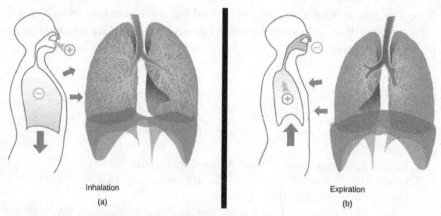

Figure 3.10 Lungs, diaphragm, and thoracic bellows involved in respiration.
SOURCE: Openstax, BiologyE.

cells or organ that responds to chemical stimuli) regarding acidity of the blood and amounts of oxygen and carbon dioxide; and (iii) vagus nerve with information from mechanoreceptors (sensory cells or organ that respond to mechanical stimulation like stretch) in the lungs and airways [1–4].

Correspondingly, output from these central controllers is to the phrenic and hypoglossal nerves, which control the diaphragm and swallowing, respectively. This information is then transferred to the thoracic bellows (muscles in the thorax controlling respiration) and lungs. These three components are all intertwined and necessary for the maintenance of normal respiration (Figure 3.10) [4, 7].

During NREM, respiratory rates decrease. The minute ventilation (volume of gas inhaled/exhaled per minute) progressively decreases across each NREM stage. Clinically, the transition from wakefulness to sleep is particularly associated with irregular breathing patterns, such as periodic breathing (pauses in breathing followed by a series of rapid and shallow breaths) and sleep-onset apnea [1–4].

These changes are even more profound during REM, during which respiration is relatively irregular. Minute ventilation during REM is about 40% lower than during wakefulness. There are a variety of reasons for this, including less metabolic demand on the body and increased airway resistance due to hypotonia of the upper airways. This irregularity in ventilation during REM sleep can be dangerous, especially for older patients with cardiopulmonary issues. Sleep itself leads to increased airway resistance and decreased tidal volume (volume of a normal breath of air). The upper airway is also far more collapsible during sleep, contributing to OSA [1–4, 7].

CONCLUSION

Changes to each system of our physiology during sleep are active and more complex than most people expect. Sleep is not a passive time; rather, it plays a very important role in the maintenance of life and the proper working of each of our organ systems. This is why disturbances to our sleep may cause significant impacts on our overall health.

REFERENCES

1. Berry RB. *Fundamentals of Sleep Medicine*. Philadelphia, PA: Elsevier/ Saunders; 2012.
2. Kushida CA. *Encyclopedia of Sleep*. Amsterdam: Elsevier; 2013.
3. Kryger MH, Avidan AY, Berry RB. *Atlas of Clinical Sleep Medicine*. Philadelphia, PA: Elsevier/Saunders; 2014.
4. Avidan AY, Barkoukis TJ. *Review of Sleep Medicine*. Philadelphia, PA: Elsevier/ Saunders; 2012.
5. Mullington J. Metabolic and endocrine changes during sleep. In: Wiley DC, Cory AC, eds. *Encyclopedia of Sleep*. Thousand Oaks, CA: SAGE; 2013:230–234.
6. Cold GE. Mean arterial pressure and intracranial pressure. *Anesthesiology*. 2003;99:1028.
7. Kryger MH, Roth T, Dement WC. *Principles and Practice of Sleep Medicine*. Philadelphia, PA: Elsevier; 2017.
8. Zambotti MD, Willoughby AR, Franzen PL, Clark DB, Baker FC, Colrain IM. K-complexes: interaction between the central and autonomic nervous systems during sleep. *Sleep*. 2016;39:1129–1137.
9. Montano N. Acute and chronic effects of sleep deprivation on autonomic nervous system in humans. *Auton Neurosci*. 2015;192:24.
10. Butler M, Kriegsfeld L, Silver R. Circadian regulation of endocrine functions. In: *Hormones, Brain and Behavior*. 2nd ed. Amsterdam, The Netherland: Academic Press/Elsevier; 2009:473–507.
11. Mak-Mccully RA, Rolland M, Sargsyan A, et al. Coordination of cortical and thalamic activity during non-REM sleep in humans. *Nat Comm*.2017;8:15499.
12. Potter GDM, Skene DJ, Arendt J, Cade JE, Grant PJ, Hardie LJ. Circadian rhythm and sleep disruption: causes, metabolic consequences, and countermeasures. *Endo Rev*. 2016;37:584–608.
13. Estep M, Orr W. The gut and sleep. In: Chokroverty S, Billiard M, eds. *Sleep Medicine*. New York, NY: Springer; 2015:451–456.
14. Imeri L, Opp MR. How (and why) the immune system makes us sleep. *Nat Rev Neurosci*. 2009;10:199–210.
15. Shantha GPS, Pancholy SB. Effect of renal sympathetic denervation on apnea-hypopnea index in patients with obstructive sleep apnea: a systematic review and meta-analysis. *Sleep Breath*. 2014;19:29–34.

4

Circadian Rhythmicity

JEANNE F. DUFFY AND JACOB E. MEDINA ■

INTRODUCTION

The circadian system regulates the timing of events across the 24-hour day in our cells, tissues, and organs, ensuring that our physiologic systems function optimally in response to regular changes in our behavior and our external environment. Over the past three decades, tremendous strides have been made in understanding how these internal clocks work at the genetic, molecular, and cellular level to create 24-hour rhythms, and the role that the circadian timing system plays in human sleep. In this chapter we will introduce the concept of the two-process model of human sleep–wake regulation; describe the anatomical features of the circadian timing system in humans and other mammals; explain how cellular feedback loops create near-24-hour rhythms in nearly all our cells; present some of the key features of the circadian timing system and how they impact our sleep and waking functions; and describe how many aspects of modern life impact the circadian system leading to mistimed or disrupted sleep.

THE TWO-PROCESS MODEL FOR HUMAN
SLEEP REGULATION

The two-process model for human sleep regulation, proposed by Borbély in the early 1980s, consists of two interacting physiologic processes: a sleep–wake homeostatic process and a circadian rhythm of sleep–wake propensity [1, 2]. The sleep–wake homeostat refers to a process by which sleep pressure builds up during wakefulness and is then dissipated during subsequent sleep (see Figure 4.1). The buildup of sleep pressure is modeled as a saturating exponential function and the dissipation as a decaying exponential function. When sleep duration and quality are sufficient, sleep pressure is fully dissipated during sleep and is at a basal level upon awakening. In cases where wake duration is extended and/or

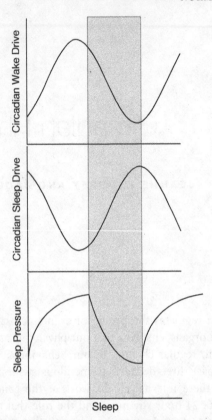

Figure 4.1 This figure depicts the two-process model for human sleep regulation, originally proposed by Dr. Borbély. Time is along the horizontal axis, which is approximately 40-hour long. The usual ~16-hour wake episode is followed by a usual ~8-hour nighttime sleep episode (shaded area), and a second ~16-hour wake episode. The bottom panel illustrates the build-up of a homeostatic sleep drive during wakefulness, which is subsequently dissipated during sleep and begins to rise again upon waking. The middle and upper panels illustrate rhythmic influences on sleep–wake propensity generated by the circadian timing system. The middle panel illustrates a circadian drive for sleep, which is lowest just prior to usual bedtime and is greatest just prior to usual wake time, while the top panel illustrates a circadian wake-promoting drive, which is greatest just before usual bedtime and at its nadir just prior to usual bedtime.

sleep duration/quality is reduced, the next day begins at a higher level on the sleep pressure curve.

The circadian process in the two-process model refers to a cyclic variation in sleep–wake propensity originating from the circadian timing system (see Figure 4.1). The rhythmic process from the circadian timing system promotes wake strongly at some circadian times while it strongly promotes sleep at other times. The precisely timed interaction of these two processes allows adult humans to do something that few other animals regularly do—have a long, consolidated wake bout each day and a long and consolidated sleep episode each night. There is compelling experimental evidence in support of this model, much of it from "forced desynchrony" experiments carried out in the 1990s by Drs. Czeisler and Dijk and colleagues. In those experiments, healthy adults were scheduled to live on an imposed rest-activity schedule that was shorter or longer than 24 hours, so that their circadian timing system could not entrain (synchronize) to the imposed day length. The imposed day lengths were typically 28 [3–5] or 20 [6] hours (i.e., 4 hours longer or shorter than usual). These experimental conditions resulted in the circadian timing system following its intrinsic near-24-hour cycle length throughout the month-long experiments [5], during which the sleep was scheduled every 20 or 28 hours. Thus, the circadian phase at which each sleep episode occurred was different, and the scheduled sleep opportunities moved from occurring during the biological night-time to the daytime and back again. At the end of the experiments, each epoch of sleep could be assigned both a circadian phase and a "time since lights out"; because the circadian time of sleep varied across the experiment the influences of circadian phase and time within sleep on sleep latency, depth, and continuity could be separated and quantified. These studies added additional support to existing evidence [7–14] that the circadian timing system has a strong influence on sleep latency, REM sleep, and sleep consolidation. In contrast, the same studies showed that slow-wave sleep and sleep consolidation are strongly influenced by time within the sleep episode.

CIRCADIAN RHYTHMS PROVIDE
AN ADAPTIVE ADVANTAGE

The term "circadian" comes from circa (approximately) and dies or dian (day) and refers to periodic changes in behavior or physiology that occur approximately daily. Circadian rhythms are hypothesized to have arisen early in evolutionary history, in response to the strong environmental cycles of light–dark, temperature, and humidity. Because an organism with a circadian clock can "predict" and be prepared for regularly occurring events, an organism with a circadian clock should have an adaptive advantage. Indeed, there is experimental evidence from both plants and insects to support this notion [15–18].

The advantage of having a functional circadian pacemaker has also been demonstrated in mammals [19, 20]. In one early such study, DeCoursey [21] captured wild chipmunks and subjected some of them to surgery; she lesioned their suprachiasmatic nucleus (SCN; the central circadian pacemaker; see the following discussion), while other animals had either sham surgery or none. All animals were given a radio transmitting device and after recovery from surgery were relocated back to where they had been captured. The animals were followed regularly for up to 2 years, and those with a functioning circadian clock were significantly more likely to survive. The animals with SCN lesions were more likely to be the victims of predation, likely because they were often found outside their burrows at night.

CIRCADIAN RHYTHM CRITERIA

For any biological rhythm to be considered circadian, that rhythm must meet all three of the following criteria: (i) it must be endogenous (self-sustaining in constant conditions), and exhibit a near 24-hour period (cycle length) under constant conditions; (ii) it must be able to be entrained (synchronized) by an external stimulus, such as light; and (iii) it must persist with the same period despite changes in physiological temperature, an effect known as temperature compensation [22].

There is specific terminology associated with circadian biology, and knowledge of this will be helpful for understanding the following sections and, indeed, most of the subsequent chapters of this book! Figure 4.2 illustrates some of these terms. First, the near 24-hour cycle length of a circadian system is called the *period*. When comparing the timing of a rhythm from one day to another, or between one individual and another, a convenient reference point along the rhythm is used and called the *phase*. The phase reference point may be the peak of the rhythm, the trough (or nadir), the onset, or the offset. The most commonly studied human circadian rhythms are core body temperature, in which the nadir is typically used as the phase reference, and melatonin secretion, for which the onset of secretion is typically used as the phase reference (see Figure 4.3). Another feature of a circadian rhythm is the amplitude, or peak-to-trough excursion.

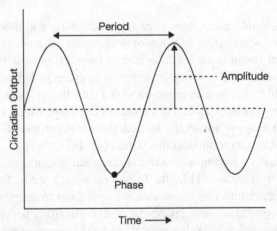

Figure 4.2 This figure illustrates features of a hypothetical circadian rhythm. The horizontal axis represents time, while the vertical axis represents the magnitude of the rhythm. The period of the rhythm is the amount of time it takes for the rhythm to complete one cycle, approximately 24 hours. The phase of the rhythm is a point of reference along the rhythm. In this example, the phase reference point is the nadir of the hypothetical rhythm. The amplitude of the rhythm is the magnitude of oscillation in the circadian signal, typically half the distance from peak to nadir, or the distance from mean to peak (as illustrated here) or mean to nadir.

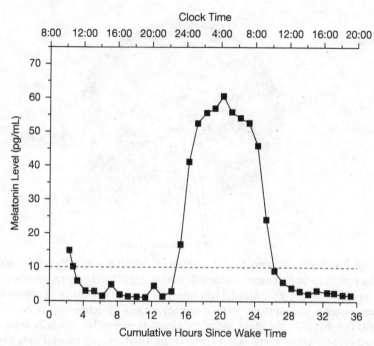

Figure 4.3 This figure shows the rhythm in plasma melatonin levels from a healthy 24-year-old woman who remained awake for 36 hours under constant dim light conditions. The lower *x* axis indicates when each sample was collected with respect to wake time, while the upper *x* axis represents the actual clock time of each sample. Blood samples were collected hourly from an IV placed in a vein in her forearm. The samples were processed and frozen until assay after the study was complete. Each filled square symbol represents the melatonin level in one of the hourly blood samples. The dashed horizontal line represents a 10 pg/mL threshold, which is sometimes used as a circadian phase marker. Linear interpolation between adjacent points is used to determine the exact point at which melatonin levels rise to 10 pg/mL (encircled X), referred to as DLMO (dim light melatonin onset).

ANATOMY OF THE CIRCADIAN TIMING SYSTEM

The mammalian circadian timing system is synchronized by a central pacemaker located in the SCN of the hypothalamus [23]. The SCN was recognized as the central pacemaker in mammals in the 1970s based on surgical lesion studies in rodents, which demonstrated that ablation of the SCN disrupted the pattern of rest–activity rhythms [24, 25]. Subsequent studies have demonstrated that there are circadian rhythms of metabolic [26] and electrical activity in the SCN [27] and that this is not a network property but occurs in individual SCN neurons [28]. Final evidence that the SCN is a central pacemaker was established after the discovery of a spontaneous mutation in hamsters that reduced the circadian period to 20 hours in the homozygous mutant animals [29]. Ablation of the SCN in these animals followed by transplantation of fetal SCN tissue from mutant to wild-type

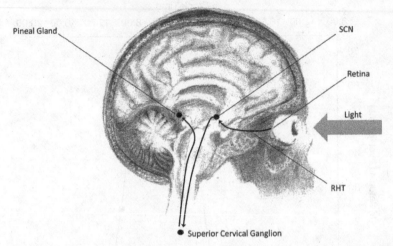

Figure 4.4 This figure illustrates the neuronal circuit which transmits light information from the environment to the suprachiasmatic nucleus (SCN) and, in turn, to the pineal gland, where melatonin is produced. Light enters the eye and stimulates photoreceptors in the retina; those photoreceptors send information along the retino-hypothalamic tract (RHT) to the SCN, the site of the central circadian pacemaker. The SCN sends information to the pineal gland via the spinal column and superior cervical ganglion. Melatonin production is acutely suppressed by exposure to light.

(or the reverse) showed that the rest–activity rhythm could be restored and that the period of the restored activity rhythm was that of the donor SCN; transplantation of any other brain tissue did not restore the rhythm [30].

SCN activity communicates a circadian signal to coordinate physiological and behavioral activity throughout the body, in anticipation of events in the external environment. Because the intrinsic circadian period is not exactly 24 hours, the circadian system needs to be entrained (reset) to remain synchronized to the external environment. Exposure to the light–dark cycle is the primary means by which the circadian timing system of many organisms, including humans, is entrained. When exposed to light, intrinsically photosensitive retinal ganglion cells, located in the retina, send a signal to the SCN via the retinohypothalamic tract (Figure 4.4) [31, 32].

The timing within the SCN can thus be adjusted slightly to maintain synchrony with the external environment, which is then transmitted to the rest of the body. One means by which this occurs is regulating the synthesis of melatonin, a night-active hormone produced by the pineal gland. The SCN innervates the pineal gland via an indirect pathway, which leads through the spinal cord [33]. The SCN sends a projection to preganglionic neurons in the intermediolateral cell column of the spinal cord, which then connects to cells in the superior cervical ganglion. From there, cells project directly to the pineal gland (see Figure 4.4). Using this pathway, the SCN can regulate the synthesis of melatonin by controlling the production of its rate-limiting enzyme, aralkylamine N-acetyltransferase. This system contains a feedback mechanism by the presence of melatonin receptors on the SCN, which inhibit its activity [34]. Essentially, the production of melatonin is suppressed by exposure to light. The SCN is also interconnected with a major sleep-promoting region of the hypothalamus, the ventrolateral preoptic nucleus. Neuronal activity in the ventrolateral preoptic nucleus inhibits activity of several structures in the arousal system, which facilitates sleep [35].

TRANSCRIPTIONAL–TRANSLATIONAL FEEDBACK LOOPS

Almost every cell in the human body contains its own oscillator with a self-sustaining near-24-hour rhythm that contributes to the daily rhythmicity of a large variety of physiological and metabolic activities, including immune responses and drug detoxification as well as renal, hepatic, pancreatic, endocrine, reproductive, respiratory, and cardiovascular functions [36]. The master circadian pacemaker in the SCN is not responsible for generating each cell's rhythm; rather, it is responsible for synchronizing the existing intrinsic rhythms. The rhythmicity of each cell is maintained by autoregulatory transcriptional–translational feedback loops. The mammalian clock mechanism consists of a core positive and core negative feedback loop to generate the clock's circadian output [37]. In the primary positive feedback loop, transcription factors CLOCK and BMAL1 heterodimerize to create a complex in the cytoplasm that initiates the transcription of PER and CRY genes. The primary negative feedback loop consists of PER and CRY heterodimers which re-enter the nucleus to suppress the activity of the CLOCK and BMAL1 complex [38, 39].

PHASE-RESPONSE CURVE

One very interesting feature of the circadian timing system is that it responds to many perturbations in a phase-dependent manner. This means that stimuli that can shift the timing of the system have different effects depending on the circadian time at which they are applied. One example of this is the response of the circadian system to light. As previously outlined, the period (cycle length) of the circadian system averages 24.2 hours in humans (ranging from about 23.5–24.7 in healthy, sighted adults [5, 40]). Because most individuals do not have an internal circadian period of exactly 24.0 hours, their circadian system must be reset each day to remain synchronized to the external environment. This process of daily resetting is called "entrainment." In humans and many other mammals, entrainment is largely achieved by exposure to the light–dark cycle. The phase-dependent response to light by the circadian timing system means that a light exposure of the exact same duration, intensity, and wavelength will have different effects depending on the time within the circadian cycle when that light exposure is applied. In general, light exposure at night causes larger effects than does light exposure during the day. Light exposure during the evening and early night causes phase delay shifts (shifts of the rhythms later), light exposure during the late night and morning cause phase advance shifts (shifts of the rhythms earlier), and light exposure during the middle of the day causes little or no change in rhythm timing [41–44]. The relationship between the phase when a light stimulus is given and the shift in timing of the circadian system in response to the light stimulus can be summarized and plotted as a phase-response curve (PRC; Figure 5.5).

IMPACT OF ARTIFICIAL LIGHT ON CIRCADIAN RHYTHMS AND SLEEP

Light exposure is the primary signal from the environment by which our internal rhythms are entrained. As previously described, circadian systems are believed to be so ubiquitous because life evolved on our strongly periodic planet. However, over the past hundred or so years, humans, through our use of artificial light, have markedly altered our light–dark environments. In fact, people living in modern societies are overwhelmed with artificial light, with most exposed to fewer than 2 hours of

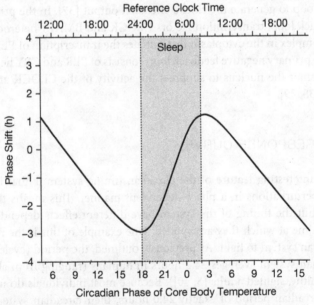

Figure 4.5 This figure shows a hypothetical phase response curve to a stimulus. The circadian system typically does not respond to stimuli the same way at different times of the circadian cycle but responds in a phase-dependent manner. In other words, a stimulus will have varying effects on the rhythm depending on the timing of that stimulus within the circadian cycle. A phase-response curve shows the magnitude of change in phase on the y axis with respect to the phase at which the stimulus was presented on the x axis. By convention, phase advances (shifts to an earlier hour) are presented as positive shifts while phase delays (shifts to a later hour) are presented as negative shifts.

outdoor levels of light each day [45–47]. Exposure to artificial light has also changed the duration of daily light exposure [48–50]. Rather than varying by season [51–53], modern humans live in a world beyond the natural day–night cycle of Earth's rotation—in a permanent summertime of extended light each day. In addition to altering the intensity and duration of light exposure, artificial light has also altered the spectral composition of light to which modern people are exposed. This latter change arises not only from sources of ambient lighting but from the recent increase in use of small, portable, light-emitting devices for work and entertainment.

This altered exposure to light, especially during the evening and night-time, may negatively impact our daytime performance and health. Evening exposure to light suppresses the release of melatonin, increases alertness, and shifts the circadian clock [54, 55]. Blue wavelength light in particular, which is prevalent in energy-efficient lighting and electronic devices, appears to have the greatest effect on the suppression of melatonin [56]. A recent study showed that night-time use of light emitting e-readers leads to a phase delay in the dim light melatonin onset of more than 1.5 hours the following evening [57]. This combination of melatonin suppression and circadian phase-shifting can delay the decision to go to sleep, delay the onset of sleep, and alter the structure of sleep [57, 58]. By delaying the timing of the circadian system, evening light exposure can also then delay wake time, or if wake time is fixed (using an alarm to wake for school or work), it can shorten sleep. Short and/or misaligned sleep is implicated in a myriad of social and health problems including absenteeism, poor academic performance, obesity, diabetes, metabolic syndrome, cardiovascular disease, cancer, and various psychiatric and mood disorders [59–65] (see Chapter 14 of this volume).

CONSEQUENCES OF SLEEP AT ADVERSE CIRCADIAN PHASE

As previously outlined, alignment between the sleep–wake homeostatic process and the circadian rhythm of sleep–wake propensity is critical for allowing a long, consolidated wake episode and long, consolidated sleep [3, 4]. However, there are situations in which modern humans experience a misalignment between these two sleep regulatory processes; these cause significant sleep disruption because the circadian timing system, while it can be reset to a new light–dark cycle, takes several days to do so.

Rapid travel across time zones is example of this disruption. Travel from the east coast of the United States to Europe crosses six time zones eastward, so upon landing the traveler's internal clock is set 6 hours too late and must reset 6 hours earlier to be in synch with the new time zone. When usual evening bedtime according to the clock in the new time zone occurs (e.g., 11 PM), the traveler's internal biological clock is not at all ready for sleep but is set to get ready for dinner (still set to 5 PM in their home time zone). Consequently, the traveler will have great difficulty falling asleep, and the next morning instead of being ready for sightseeing or a business meeting at 9 AM, their internal clock (still set at 3 AM in the home time zone) wants nothing more than to remain in bed. Eventually, with regular exposure to the light–dark cycle in the new time zone the traveler will adjust, but it will take days to a week or more before they are completely adjusted (depending on the exact timing and strength of their light–dark exposure).

Night shift workers also experience the negative consequences of trying to remain awake for work during their biological night-time and trying to sleep after returning home from work during their biological daytime. Sleep in night workers is significantly shorter and more disrupted than that of day or evening workers [66–71], and as a consequence, they are prone to medical problems related to shortened sleep [72–76]. While most travelers will adjust to their new time zone if they remain there long enough, even permanent night shift workers are unlikely to adapt to their inverted schedules [77, 78]. This is due to exposure to the natural light–dark cycle on the morning commute home or during the daytime, and because most night workers adopt a night–sleep/day–wake schedule on weekends or days off so they can interact with family and friends. Thus, unlike with jet lag, where the signals from the external environment are promoting resetting/adaptation to the new time zone, signals from the environment are interfering with adaptation for night workers are [79–81]. More about these issues and ways that they are treated are in Chapter 15 of this volume.

CONCLUSIONS

The circadian system plays a critical role in human sleep–wake regulation by producing a daily variation in sleep–wake propensity. This overall rhythm interacts with a sleep–wake homeostatic process and, when optimally aligned, allows humans to have long, consolidated wakefulness during the day and a long, consolidated sleep episode at night. The circadian timing system also plays an important role in REM sleep timing. While most cells contain autonomous circadian clocks, under normal conditions the cellular clocks are synchronized internally by signals from a master circadian pacemaker in the hypothalamus (the SCN) and rhythmic behaviors. The master clock itself is synchronized to the external environment by regular exposure to light and darkness. When sleep–wake behavior is not in proper alignment with the timing of the internal circadian system (such as what occurs after travel to another time zone or when working the night shift), sleep is fragmented and shortened, and it is difficult to maintain an extended episode of alert wakefulness.

ACKNOWLEDGMENTS

The authors wish to thank Dr. Cheryl M. Isherwood for preparing Figure 4.4 and John Wise for assistance with the references. The authors are supported in part by NIH grants P01 AG09975 and R01 AG044416, and ONR grant N00014-19-2239.

REFERENCES

1. Borbély AA. A two process model of sleep regulation. *Hum Neurobio.* 1982;1: 195–204.
2. Daan S, Beersma DGM, Borbély AA. Timing of human sleep: recovery process gated by a circadian pacemaker. *Am J Physiol.* 1984;246:R161–R183.
3. Dijk DJ, Czeisler CA. Paradoxical timing of the circadian rhythm of sleep propensity serves to consolidate sleep and wakefulness in humans. *Neurosci Lett.* 1994;166:63–68.
4. Dijk DJ, Czeisler CA. Contribution of the circadian pacemaker and the sleep homeostat to sleep propensity, sleep structure, electroencephalographic slow waves, and sleep spindle activity in humans. *J Neurosci.* 1995;15:3526–3538.
5. Czeisler CA, Duffy JF, Shanahan TL, et al. Stability, precision, and near-24-hour period of the human circadian pacemaker. *Science.* 1999;284:2177–2181.
6. Wyatt JK, Ritz-De Cecco A, Czeisler CA, Dijk DJ. Circadian temperature and melatonin rhythms, sleep, and neurobehavioral function in humans living on a 20-h day. *Am J Physiol.* 1999;277:R1152–R1163.
7. Carskadon MA, Dement WC. Sleep studies on a 90-minute day. *Electroen Clin Neuro.* 1975;39:145–155.
8. Carskadon MA, Dement WC. Distribution of REM sleep on a 90 minute sleep–wake schedule. *Sleep.* 1980;2:309–317.
9. Lavie P, Zomer J. Ultrashort sleep-waking schedule. II. Relationship between ultradian rhythms in sleepability and the REM-NON-REM cycles and effects of the circadian phase. *Electroen Clin Neuro.* 1984;57:35–42.
10. Lavie P. Ultrashort sleep-waking schedule III. "Gates" and "forbidden zones" for sleep. *Electroen Clin Neuro.* 1986;63:414–425.
11. Lavie P. Ultrashort sleep–wake cycle: timing of REM sleep. Evidence for sleep-dependent and sleep-independent components of the REM cycle. *Sleep.* 1987;10:62–68.
12. Strogatz SH, Kronauer RE, Czeisler CA. Circadian regulation dominates homeostatic control of sleep length and prior wake length in humans. *Sleep* 1986;9:353–364.
13. Strogatz SH, Kronauer RE, Czeisler CA. Circadian pacemaker interferes with sleep onset at specific times each day: role in insomnia. *Am J Physiol.* 1987;253:R172–R178.
14. Czeisler CA, Weitzman ED, Moore-Ede MC, Zimmerman JC, Knauer RS. Human sleep: its duration and organization depend on its circadian phase. *Science.* 1980;210:1264–1267.
15. Green RM, Tingay S, Wang ZY, Tobin EM. Circadian rhythms confer a higher level of fitness to Arabidopsis plants. *Plant Physiol.* 2002;129:576–584.
16. Klarsfeld A, Rouyer F. Effects of circadian mutations and LD periodicity on the life span of Drosophila melanogaster. *J Biol Rhythm.* 1998;13:471–478.
17. Rosato E, Kyriacou CP. The role of natural selection in circadian behaviour: a molecular-genetic approach. *Essays Biochem.* 2011;49:71–85.
18. Rosato E, Kyriacou CP. Flies, clocks and evolution. *Philos T Roy Soc B.* 2001;356: 1769–1778.
19. DeCoursey PJ. Survival value of suprachiasmatic nuclei (SCN) in four wild sciurid rodents. *Behav Neurosci.* 2014;128:240–249.

20. Spoelstra K, Wikelski M, Daan S, Loudon AS, Hau M. Natural selection against a circadian clock gene mutation in mice. *P Natl Acad Sci USA.* 2016;113:686–691.

21. DeCoursey PJ, Krulas JR. Behavior of SCN-lesioned chipmunks in natural habitat: a pilot study. *J Biol Rhythm.* 1998;13:229–244.

22. Pittendrigh CS. Circadian rhythms and the circadian organization of living systems. *Cold Spring Harb Sym.* 1960;25:159–184.

23. Weaver DR. The suprachiasmatic nucleus: a 25-year retrospective. *J Biol Rhythm.* 1998;13:100–112.

24. Moore RY, Eichler VB. Loss of a circadian adrenal corticosterone rhythm following suprachiasmatic lesions in the rat. *Brain Res.* 1972;42:201–206.

25. Stephan FK, Zucker I. Circadian rhythms in drinking behavior and locomotor activity of rats are eliminated by hypothalamic lesions. *P Natl Acad Sci USA.* 1972;69:1583–1586.

26. Schwartz WJ, Gainer H. Suprachiasmatic nucleus: use of (14)C-labeled deoxyglucose uptake as a functional marker. *Science.* 1977;197:1089–1091.

27. Inouye ST, Kawamura H. Persistence of circadian rhythmicity in a mammalian hypothalamic "island" containing the suprachiasmatic nucleus. *P Natl Acad Sci USA.* 1979;76:5962–5966.

28. Welsh DK, Logothetis DE, Meister M, Reppert SM. Individual neurons dissociated from rat suprachiasmatic nucleus express independently phased circadian firing rhythms. *Neuron.* 1995;14:697–706.

29. Ralph MR, Menaker M. A mutation of the circadian system in golden hamsters. *Science.* 1988;241:1225–1257.

30. Ralph MR, Foster RG, Davis FC, Menaker M. Transplanted suprachiasmatic nucleus determines circadian period. *Science.* 1990;247:975–978.

31. Moore RY, Lenn NJ. A retinohypothalamic projection in the rat. *J Comp Neurol.* 1972;146:1–14.

32. Gooley JJ, Lu J, Chou TC, Scammell TE, Saper CB. Melanopsin in cells of origin of the retinohypothalamic tract. *Nat Neurosci.* 2001;4:1165.

33. Teclemariam-Mesbah R, Ter Horst GJ, Postema F, Wortel J, Buijs RM. Anatomical demonstration of the suprachiasmatic nucleus-pineal pathway. *J Comp Neurol.* 1999;406:171–182.

34. Liu C, Weaver DR, Jin X, et al. Molecular dissection of two distinct actions of melatonin on the suprachiasmatic circadian clock. *Neuron.* 1997;19:91–102.

35. Sherin JE, Shiromani PJ, McCarley RW, Saper CB. Activation of ventrolateral preoptic neurons during sleep. *Science.* 1996;271:216–219.

36. Mohawk JA, Green CB, Takahashi JS. Central and peripheral circadian clocks in mammals. *Annu RevNeurosci.* 2012;35:445–462.

37. Ko CH, Takahashi JS. Molecular components of the mammalian circadian clock. *Hum Mol Genet.* 2006;15:R271–R277.

38. Bell-Pedersen D, Cassone VM, Earnest DJ, et al. Circadian rhythms from multiple oscillators: lessons from diverse organisms. *Nat Rev Genet.* 2005;6:544–556.

39. Honma S. The mammalian circadian system: a hierarchical multi-oscillator structure for generating circadian rhythm. *J Physiol Sci.* 2018;68:207–219.

40. Duffy JF, Cain SW, Chang AM, et al. Sex difference in the near-24-hour intrinsic period of the human circadian timing system. *P Natl Acad Sci USA.* 2011;108:15602–15608.

41. Daan S, Pittendrigh CS. A functional analysis of circadian pacemakers in nocturnal rodents. II. The variability of phase response curves. *J Comp Physiol A.* 1976;106:253–266.

42. Czeisler CA, Kronauer RE, Allan JS, et al. Bright light induction of strong (type 0) resetting of the human circadian pacemaker. *Science.* 1989;244: 1328–1333.

43. Khalsa SBS, Jewett ME, Cajochen C, Czeisler CA. A phase response curve to single bright light pulses in human subjects. *J Physiol (Lond).* 2003;549:945–952.

44. Rahman SA, St Hilaire MA, Chang AM, et al. Circadian phase resetting by a single short-duration light exposure. *JCI Insight.* 2017;2:e89494.

45. Cole RJ, Kripke DF, Wisbey J, et al. Seasonal variation in human illumination exposure at two different latitudes. *J Biol Rhythm.* 1995;10:324–334.

46. Kawinska A, Dumont M, Selmaoui B, Paquet J, Carrier J. Are modifications of melatonin circadian rhythm in the middle years of life related to habitual patterns of light exposure? *J Biol Rhythm.* 2005;20:451–460.

47. Scheuermaier K, Laffan AM, Duffy JF. Light exposure patterns in healthy older and young adults. *J Biol Rhythm.* 2010;25:113–122.

48. de la Iglesia HO, Fernandez-Duque E, Golombek DA, et al. Access to electric light is associated with shorter sleep duration in a traditionally hunter-gatherer community. *J Biol Rhythm.* 2015;30:342–350.

49. Wright KP Jr., McHill AW, Birks BR, Griffin BR, Rusterholz T, Chinoy ED. Entrainment of the human circadian clock to the natural light-dark cycle. *Curr Biol.* 2013;23:1554–1558.

50. Vondrasová D, Hájek I, Illnerová H. Exposure to long summer days affects the human melatonin and cortisol rhythms. *Brain Res.* 1997;759:166–170.

51. Yetish G, Kaplan H, Gurven M, et al. Natural sleep and its seasonal variations in three pre-industrial societies. *Curr Biol.* 2015;25:2862–2868.

52. Stothard ER, McHill AW, Depner CM, et al. Circadian entrainment to the natural light-dark cycle across seasons and the weekend. *Curr Biol.* 2017;27:1–6.

53. Illnerová H, Zvolsky P, Vanecek J. The circadian rhythm in plasma melatonin concentration of the urbanized man: the effect of summer and winter time. *Brain Res.* 1985;328:186–189.

54. Green A, Cohen-Zion M, Haim A, Dagan Y. Evening light exposure to computer screens disrupts human sleep, biological rhythms, and attention abilities. *Chronobiol Int.* 2017;34:855–865.

55. Cajochen C, Frey S, Anders D, et al. Evening exposure to a light-emitting diodes (LED)-backlit computer screen affects circadian physiology and cognitive performance. *J Appl Physiol* 2011;110:1432–1438.

56. West KE, Jablonski MR, Warfield B, et al. Blue light from light-emitting diodes elicits a dose-dependent suppression of melatonin in humans. *J Appl Physiol.* 2011;110:619–626.

57. Chang AM, Aeschbach D, Duffy JF, Czeisler CA. Evening use of light-emitting eReaders negatively affects sleep, circadian timing, and next-morning alertness. *P Natl Acad Sci USA.* 2015;112:1232–1237.

58. Chinoy ED, Duffy JF, Czeisler CA. Unrestricted evening use of light-emitting tablet computers delays self-selected bedtime and disrupts circadian timing and alertness. *Physiol Rep.* 2018;6:e13692.

59. Stevens RG, Blask DE, Brainard GC, et al. Meeting report: the role of environ-mental lighting and circadian disruption in cancer and other diseases. *Environ Health Persp.* 2007;115:1357–1362.

60. Arora T, Hussain S, Lam KBH, Yao GL, Thomas GN, Taheri S. Exploring the com-plex pathways among specific types of technology, self-reported sleep duration and body mass index in UK adolescents. *Int J Obes (Lond).* 2013;37:1254–1260.

61. Arora T, Broglia E, Thomas GN, Taheri S. Associations between specific technologies and adolescent sleep quantity, sleep quality, and parasomnias. *Sleep Med.* 2014;15:240–247.

62. Cain N, Gradisar M. Electronic media use and sleep in school-aged children and adolescents: a review. *Sleep Med.* 2010;11:735–742.

63. Gradisar M, Wolfson AR, Harvey AG, Hale L, Rosenberg R, Czeisler CA. The sleep and technology use of Americans: findings from the National Sleep Foundation's 2011 Sleep in America poll. *J Clin Sleep Med.* 2013;9:1291–1299.

64. Roenneberg T, Allebrandt KV, Merrow M, Vetter C. Social jetlag and obesity. *Curr Biol.* 2012;22:939–943.

65. Baron KG, Reid KJ. Circadian misalignment and health. *Int Rev Psychiatr.* 2014;26:139–154.

66. Åkerstedt T, Wright KP. Sleep loss and fatigue in shift work and shift work disorder. *Sleep Med Clin.* 2009;4:257–271.

67. Bonnefond A, Harma M, Hakola T, Sallinen M, Kandolin I, Virkkala J. Interaction of age with shift-related sleep–wakefulness, sleepiness, performance, and social life. *Exp Aging Res.* 2006;32:185–208.

68. Drake CL, Roehrs T, Richardson G, Walsh JK, Roth T. Shift work sleep dis-order: prevalence and consequences beyond that of symptomatic day workers. *Sleep.* 2004;27:1453–1462.

69. Vetter C, Fischer D, Matera JL, Roenneberg T. Aligning work and circadian time in shift workers improves sleep and reduces circadian disruption. *Curr Biol.* 2015;25:907–911.

70. Czeisler CA, Johnson MP, Duffy JF, Brown EN, Ronda JM, Kronauer RE. Exposure to bright light and darkness to treat physiologic maladaptation to night work. *New Engl J Med.* 1990;322:1253–1259.

71. Chinoy ED, Harris MP, Kim MJ, Wang W, Duffy JF. Scheduled evening sleep and enhanced lighting improve adaptation to night shift work in older adults. *Occup Environ Med.* 2016;73:869–876.

72. Cheng P, Drake C. Shift work disorder. *Neurol Clin.* 2019;37:563–577.

73. Wickwire EM, Geiger-Brown J, Scharf SM, Drake CL. Shift work and shift work sleep disorder: clinical and organizational perspectives. *Chest.* 2017;151:1156–1172.

74. Knutsson A. Health disorders of shift workers. *Occup Med (Lond).* 2003;53:103–108.

75. Lin X, Chen W, Wei F, Ying M, Wei W, Xie X. Night-shift work increases morbidity of breast cancer and all-cause mortality: a meta-analysis of 16 prospective cohort studies. *Sleep Med.* 2015;16:1381–1387.

76. Gu F, Han J, Laden F, et al. Total and cause-specific mortality of U.S. nurses working rotating night shifts. *Am J Prevent Med.* 2015;48:241–252.

77. Boivin DB, James FO. Circadian adaptation to night-shift work by judicious light and darkness exposure. *J Biol Rhythm.* 2002;17:556–567.

78. Dumont M, Benhaberou-Brun D, Paquet J. Profile of 24-h light exposure and circadian phase of melatonin secretion in night workers. *J Biol Rhythm.* 2001;16:502–511.

79. Bjorvatn B, Kecklund G, Åkerstedt T. Rapid adaptation to night work at an oil platform, but slow readaptation after returning home. *J Occup Environ Med.* 1998;40:601–608.

80. Bjorvatn B, Kecklund G, Åkerstedt T. Bright light treatment used for adaptation to night work and re-adaptation back to day life: a field study at an oil platform in the North Sea. *J Sleep Res.* 1999;8:105–112.

81. Smith MR, Fogg LF, Eastman CI. Practical interventions to promote circadian adaptation to permanent night shift work: Study 4. *J Biol Rhythm.* 2009;24:161–172.

5

Culture and Sleep—Focus on Infancy

KRISTIN P. TULLY AND JAMES J. MCKENNA ■

INTRODUCTION

The ways we think about and experience sleep are significantly shaped by our culture. One way to uncover our values and ideologies is by how we define a "good night's sleep." Perspectives vary. An excellent example of this is our expectations for infant sleep and night-time parenting practices, which differ dramatically. This is because cultural practices reflect cultural understandings. The generally perceived worldwide norm for how infants sleep actually reflects behavior typical of formula-fed infants who are put to sleep in their own rooms. This is because that is how babies have primarily been studied; the result is that we often think the patterns associated with that context—such as early consolidation of bouts of sleep—are appropriate, achievable, and desirable for infants. Yet programs of research, clinical guidance, and individual conversations are increasing expanding the information that shapes how we determine where we sleep, the structure of the sleep environment, with whom we sleep, how healthful we consider our sleep patterns to be, and the ways we support each other with sleep. This is important, because for all people sleep is critical to health. The varying ideas in this scientific field are also opportunities to listen, grow, and more deeply care for each other. This contextual area will form the main focus of our chapter—but first, let's turn to a more general understanding of individual differences.

INDIVIDUAL DIFFERENCES

Like most behaviors, sleep is a biocultural process. This means that human biology, including one's psychological status and developmental needs, intersect.

Our functioning is in constant transaction with daily life. For example, how you evaluate your sleep matters to your health. If you think that you have not been getting enough sleep, your worry can elevate cortisol levels and your general feelings of stress. Further, as individuals, with our unique metabolisms, temperaments, and energetic needs, we differ on how much sleep each of us actually needs. There is no single "right way" to sleep. As is true for all aspects of our biological and behavioral functioning, we experience genomic-based individual differences. These person-to-person variations include sleep latency (how quickly we fall asleep), our movement patterns, the positions we assume during sleep, the length of time we spend in each stage of sleep, and how many times we awaken briefly, without knowing it. Such individual differences remain relevant across the life span.

Each of us exhibits what some call a unique "sleep personality" from infancy up to and throughout old age. Our uniqueness reflects the shape and size (i.e., the weight) of our bodies and impacts aspects of self-care needs. For example, your thermoregulation influences how many blankets you need to stay warm (or cool) and how much bed clothing you like to wear while sleeping. Whether you sleep prone, supine, spread out, curled up, thrash around, or stay still can all vary enormously amongst us. Such variability understandably makes it difficult for sleep recommendations made by national organizations to account for what is optimal for each individual. The National Sleep Foundation offers age-based recommendations (for and against specific ranges) for the total number of hours of sleep per day, with the caveat of "may be appropriate" in between these positive and negative categories, to acknowledge individual variability [1]. But still, it is important to understand and validate the range of these human sleep experiences, to avoid unnecessary intervention, frustration, or suffering and to remember that sleep-related changes appropriate for one person might undermine another. When it comes to sleep patterns, one size does not fit all.

SLEEP PLASTICITY

Sleep is a fascinating topic, in part because of the many different ways humans practice it and how our diverse cultures determine how we evaluate its quality, it such as answering the question posed above: what constitutes a "good night's sleep"? Moreover, although adhering to a sleep routine has its advantages for most adults, that schedule also depends on what is going on in our day-to-day lives; we can and need to structure our sleep to accommodate our schedules and specific activities. Sleep is "plastic." We can stay awake longer than we otherwise would by changing the tempo, degree, and the amount of physical activity in which we engage or by changing dietary practices such as when and what we choose to eat. For example, some of us consume stimulating substances like caffeine or depressive substances like alcohol, impacting our sleep physiology. Many of us also experience artificial lights around bedtime such as with cell phones and or computers, again altering sleep behaviors. In addition to changes in when and how we fall asleep, we can also make ourselves wake up even when we may prefer to sleep (i.e., with an alarm clock when we are tired).

CULTURAL ASSUMPTIONS

A starting point for exploring cultural aspects of sleep is examination of the language that we use to describe it. What is considered in our own culture to be a "sleep problem"? What does it mean to be someone who has "trouble sleeping"? What should we do about sleep difficulties? These perspectives about what's typical, concerning, and requiring intervention are influenced by the ways we have been socialized to think about sleep in our respective cultures. The questions are certainly not neutral, nor are the ways in which we seek to answer them. Many cultures, for example, are not concerned about the concept of "not getting enough sleep." Our Western knowledge about sleep and ideas of what is normal and desirable emerge within a specific and highly *scientized* Western industrialized context, without even realizing how differently we think about sleep outside of a broader comparative cross-cultural perspective. The evidence base (i.e., what is considered to be known) and gaps in our understanding (i.e., what is considered to be unknown) reflect the particular cultural assumptions within which empirical questions are raised and what researchers operating within this cultural framework think to ask, chose to prioritize, and can get funding awarded to advance. The American Academy of Pediatrics acknowledges that there is insufficient good-quality patient-oriented evidence [2, 3]. Further, efforts to document and assess infant sleep reflect the culture in which such investigation is conducted and the methods adopted. Field [4] reviewed the infant sleep literature and found almost exclusive use of parental report. Yet, when Tully and her colleagues compared multiple methods of infant sleep assessment, they found discrepancies in epoch-by-epoch (codes every 30 seconds from overnight video recordings) and overall outcomes [5]. Using parental report of infant sleep along with actigraphy (recording of small movements; see Chapter 22 of this volume) versus overnight filming during the same observation period showed different outcomes. Actigraphy and sleep diaries significantly overestimate sleep period duration and underestimate the number of night waking episodes, compared with video observation [5]. It would benefit both the field of infant sleep and families if more precise, objective measures were used; this would reduce bias about what constitutes healthful and appropriate infant sleep. Until then, health recommendations should be interpreted with an understanding that they are based on limited and potentially biased data.

PUBLIC HEALTH

Even how and what information is disseminated about sleep by medical authorities reflect powerful underlying cultural values. Public health education campaigns are targeted to selected stakeholders, with intentional tones and takeaway messages to achieve specific aims. Further, economic motivations are a real factor in many attempts to solve adult or infant "sleep problems." For example, there exists, in the United States and other countries, a whole field of so-called sleep consultants, who lack any core training curriculum or certification. Some of these individuals falsely liken an infant's unwillingness to fall asleep alone and/or sleep continuously through the night, for example, as signs of a developmental pathology—their solution to which is "sleep training." Others market products to "naturally" sleep train, as if that were the goal instead of optimally supporting infant health and development while helping adults cope with the inherent challenge of infant caregiving.

This gap between cultural ideals and human needs is an opportunity for more authentic engagement. We tend to understand and "buy into" narratives that fit with our personal, but also culturally influenced, views. How we reconcile information as individuals, parents, healthcare leaders (i.e., those who develop health messages)—and how strategies are implemented (through patient–provider communication, adopted in family life, and covered through insurance programs) is not consistent worldwide. Recognizing this insofar as how knowledge about sleep and other health topics is generated is necessary to comprehensively understand human health and offer effective support. Likewise, recognizing one's cultural influences and the motivations of others can help give us a balanced perspective as information and health care consumers. It is important to critically assess what is being presented and the potential impacts on our trajectories of health.

THE CASE OF INFANT SLEEP

The field of pediatric sleep science offers enormous opportunity for advancement. Recognition of multidirectional influences on health is an important part of understanding what it means to be human. Currently, the mainstream expectation is for infants to sleep without sensing a caregiver, having minimal awakenings, and to not solicit adults if (when) they do awaken. One of the conversations we have with new parents is "Is he or she a good sleeper?" without realizing what it really means to "sleep like a baby." It is clear that alternative perspectives are not only desirable but necessary to becoming more realistic and inclusive.

Sleep environment guidance can reflect the variety of arrangements infants can and do experience—the sleep surface should be firm, free from soft bedding, pillows, and toys, and responsive parenting should not be undermined by pharmacological substances or alcohol. Families live in diverse conditions with varying infant needs and responses to particular parenting approaches. Caregivers adopt infant sleep practices for a variety of reasons, which may differ from original plans and reflect considerations more central to their daily lives than other factors [6, 7]. McKenna and Gettler [8] have argued:

Only where sweeping public health recommendations acknowledge and respect maternal capacities and biologically-appropriate emotions and motivations for mothers to sleep close to their infants will there be any hope that these recommendations can be adopted and implemented in ways which promote the survival and well being of the greatest number of mother-infant dyads. (p. 272)

These authors [8] further point out that ways of reading and interpreting evidence "not only assume incorrectly that powerful factors that motivate forms of co-sleeping can always be denied, but that they should be" (p. 272). We are equipped to meaningfully advance these conversations.

SAFER INFANT SLEEP

The relevance of culture with sleep is clear when we consider infant safety. Messaging to parents to never bed share has largely not been accompanied by conversations about why arrangements might confer risk. At the least, context is missing. Even further away from shared decision-making, however, is the use scare tactics as a driver of U.S. public education campaigns. An explicit example is http://city.milwaukee.gov/Safe-Sleep-Campaign. These attempts to inform families of the potential for hazardous arrangements contribute instead to concepts of "bad mothering" and fear. It is no wonder that some mothers may intentionally withhold or otherwise misrepresent information about their infant sleep practices [9]. Yet this driving of parents' nighttime behavior under-ground, as articulated by Kendall-Tacket and colleagues [10, 11], contributes to sofa/recliner co-sleeping, which is much more hazardous for infants than other sleep arrangements [2, 3]. The "letter of the law" gets mixed up with the "spirit" [7].

An appreciation of such nuanced circumstances and contexts, and human biology itself, enables a more holistic picture about sleep. Throughout the last century, however, the scientific study of infant sleep has consisted almost exclusively of studying infants who are fed formula and/or cows' milk while they sleep in a room on their own; this is done to produce models of allegedly "normal, healthy" (i.e., universal, normal) human infant sleep. It is therefore necessary in the United States to critically examine the extraordinary way that Western cultural values concerning how infants *should* sleep became one and the same with the science that studies it, mistaking social ideology for empirically established scientific truths. (Figure 5.1)

The stakes are high. From the moment we are born, and then throughout our lifespans, sleep is a significant aspect of our lives. We all sleep to survive. Yet, the ways that many of us institute or interpret infant sleep is reflective of our Western culture that fosters independence. These expectations could not be further from what most humans do globally and what our ancestors experienced. Indeed, cultural values are embedded in and reflective of ideas about how we *want* babies to sleep, or the way our values dictate that they *should* sleep.

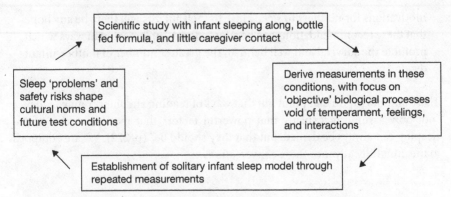

Figure 5.1 A cycle of solitary infant sleep as "normal" and best practice.
SOURCE: Adapted from McKenna JJ, McDade T. Why babies should never sleep alone: a review of the co-sleeping controversy in relation to SIDS, bedsharing and breast feeding. *Paediatr Respir Rev.* 2005;6:134–152; Tully KP, Ball HL. Misrecognition of need: women's experiences of and explanations for undergoing cesarean delivery. *Soc Sci Med.* 2013;85:103–111.

CONSIDERING BIOLOGICAL NORMS

Cultural dismantling the evolved components of biologically appropriate infant sleep can easily occur in the absence of centering our focus on the lactating mother and her breastfed infant. What does a mother need at night? What does the baby need? Where is the overlap and where are the tensions? Considering the interrelated functioning of breastfeeding mother–baby dyads can transform how we consider infant sleep. For example, if an infant is going to nurse with a mother in a side-lying position (see Figure 5.2), the baby needs to be on her back (supine) and within sensory range (co-sleeping) for access. When night-time breastfeeding in bed is not a part of families' stories, then potentially dangerous infant positioning on the stomach (prone) and solitary sleep (separate room) become options. An infant on his or her own is thought of as an individual, instead of part of a mutually regulating dyad. In contrast, does it not make sense for a caregiver sharing a surface with a baby or otherwise in close proximity to repeatedly reposition him or her to have access to the mother's breast (such as going from stomach- to back-sleeping). When you are breastfeeding every few hours in bed, then infants would most likely remain in a position to readily do so.

One of your chapter authors (Dr. James McKenna) has often suggested that the biological norm for night-time infant sleep and care should be breast-sleeping [12]. This term refers to the infant on a shared surface with the breastfeeding mother and that the baby-mom pair are positioned relative to each other. Breastfeeding women have been observed to characteristically turns toward their infants during shared sleep, curling up around them [13]. However, the American Academy of Pediatrics currently recommends room-sharing without bedsharing [2], despite the strong positive relationship with bedsharing and breastfeeding promotion (more feeds per night [14]) and breastfeeding throughout the first year [15, 16].

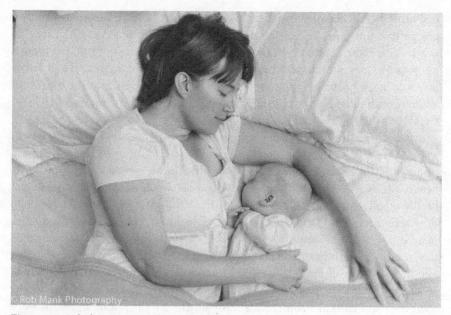

Figure 5.2 Side-lying nursing/breastsleeping.
SOURCE: Image courtesy of Rob Mank through the Baby Sleep Information Source website https://www.basisonline.org.uk/co-sleeping-image-archive/

For those who do not intend to bedshare, the arrangement often still occurs because of maternal tiredness and the hormones associated with breastfeeding often lead to unintentional shared sleep after night-time feeding [7].

Lack of exclusive and continued breastfeeding, prone positioning, and lack of room-sharing are each risk factors of sudden infant death syndrome [2, 3]. Obviously, with such outcomes, especially for infants born with only 25% of their adult brain volume, the topic is important not only because of how rested and energetic we adults feel and how we evaluate our sleep, but also for the impact of sleep on our children's mortality, morbidity, and developmental trajectories. Culture and sleep matter on every level and, as has been shown, are inseparable.

SLEEP IN THE IMMEDIATE POSTPARTUM PERIOD

Let's focus further attention to the perinatal period. From the moment infants are born, the way they are treated and cared for reflect bio-social understanding of their biomedical needs. The global standard of healthcare services in birthing facilities is currently to have healthy infants physically close to their caregivers, including through early and prolonged skin-to-skin contact. This aspect of the World Health Organization and UNICEF best practices [17] impacts every infant outcome measured—such as heart rate, temperature, weight gain, crying, sleep, and breastfeeding outcomes [18]. Less attention is paid to women's experience of their postpartum care and the ways in which health services impact their sleep and other needs. Inpatient postnatal facilities, such as birth centers or hospital postpartum units, follow nursing protocols structured protect infant safety. The way that care is structured varies according to understandings of risk. But there is a substantial gap in understanding how the frequency of clinical staff and visitor presence in the postnatal unit room impacts maternal and infant sleep outcomes. We may be inhibited in transitioning from the birth facility to home as well as we could have otherwise.

Especially in the United States with our rapid patient turnover, which occurs as early as 24 to 48 hours following vaginal birth and 48 to 96 hours following cesarean birth, limits time for clinical staff to educate families fully on priority health issues. The high volume, relatively short stays, need for mother–infant health monitoring, and multiple administrative tasks to be completed prior to discharge mean that many staff members are in and out of postnatal unit rooms, in addition to "traffic" from family visitors. Previous research has demonstrated that routine maternity care experiences include frequent interruptions for new families following childbirth. In fact, Morrison and Ludington-Hoe [19] found an average of 53 entrances to each postnatal unit room in a U.S. sample of healthy mother–infant pairs at a community hospital. This number of in-and-outs over a day or two translates as a nearly constant stream of activity. Mother–infant pairs do not receive enough protected time to sleep, recover, and prepare for the transition to home. Mothers also perceive this "traffic" as negatively interfering with breastfeeding [19]. Further investigation of the journey through the postnatal unit and discharge might indicate unmet needs and opportunities for change.

Although maternal sleep is a core part of functioning and recovery from the childbirth process, it is not currently promoted on postnatal units beyond a 2-hour period of daytime "quiet hours." Additionally, little is understood about fathers' sleep, or that of other partners, or the impact on these individuals transitioning to new family dynamics and the ways in which their degree of exhaustion may influence maternal and infant care. For infants, harms of excess parental sleep fragmentation at the birthing facility include separation from rooming-in and supplementation with formula. A mom may feel it is necessary to have her baby looked after by nursing staff so she has an opportunity for adequate rest. Efforts to satiate newborns, prolong the time between feedings, or consolidate sleep may contribute to early postnatal formula use. For mothers, harms include fatigue, deviation from personal breastfeeding goals, and increased risk for mental health concerns such as postpartum depression. Parents may be unprepared for the strains caused by postpartum sleep fragmentation; thus, there are opportunities for the health care system to better support healthy family sleep during the perinatal period.

SLEEP DURING THE FOURTH TRIMESTER

The anthropological concept of the "fourth trimester" of pregnancy [20] draws attention to the pre- and postnatal continuum of maternal–infant development and interaction. A component of this ever-evolving relationship is that the umbilical cord and placenta are replaced by breasts in delivering calories, antibodies, bioactives, immune factors, macro and micronutrients, minerals, proteins, stem cells, and fatty acids. The human infant is born the least mature, neurologically, of all primate mammals, and the most dependent on physiological and behavioral regulation by the caregiver for the longest period of time; Donald Winnecot thus once aptly said, "There is no such thing as a baby, there is a baby and someone." Another way to think about this is to consider that nothing an infant can or cannot do makes sense except in light of contact with their mother's body, the only environment to which the infant is adapted. Sarah Hrdy put it this way: "For species such as primates the mother is the environment" [21]. Altogether, the cumulative evidence justifies Kitzinger calling this critical phase of infant development the fourth trimester, with a warning that "we neglect it at our peril" [20]. New families in Western cultures unnecessary suffer from (i) societal failure to recognize the mutual regulation of infants and their caregivers; (ii) misrecognition of infant cues; and (iii) misattribution of maternal challenges with the transition to motherhood as personal failings. A fourth trimester perspective centers on the interrelated needs of the mother–infant dyad to establish the care they need after birth, which is just as intense and important as during pregnancy [9, 22].

The fourth trimester concept makes two primary contributions to issues around culture and sleep. First, while maternal–infant biology and behavior are different before and after birth, the mechanisms by which they interact are actually similar. In the words of Ashley Montagu, human infants are "external gestates" [23]. Humans are mammals (primates) with highly dependent offspring, who keep those offspring within close proximity both day and night. Caregiver responsiveness to their babies is necessary not only for keeping infants safe and warm, but this model of infant care also reflects lactation physiology [24]. Full breastfeeding necessitates frequent removal of milk from the breasts; if lactating mothers of infants sleep through the night and do not breastfeed or express (remove milk manually or using a pump for this purpose), they would awaken with breasts painfully engorged with milk. This negative feedback would cue their bodies to make less milk over time, which is fine if they desire to wean their infant. However, relatively infrequent infant feeding can lead to producing less milk than the baby needs and subsequently deviation from personal breastfeeding goals.

This leads to the second contribution focusing the fourth trimester lens on the culture of health around parent–infant sleep: the intersection of postpartum needs including sleep, infant feeding, maternal recovery, and mood intersect (see Figure 5.3). In other words, the way mothers sleep impacts infant feeding, reflecting and contributing to maternal physical and emotional well-being. Tully and Ball [25] have suggested that mothers continually perform "balancing acts" with infant feeding and other aspects of infant- and self-care. They explain that frequent breastfeeding is biologically appropriate for infants due to their small stomachs and low solute composition of human milk. However, optimal infant feeding is challenging to realize and maintain because it is associated with fragmented maternal sleep [26], which is a major concern for many parents [27].

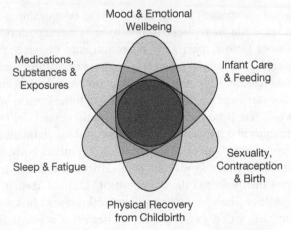

Figure 5.3 Interrelatedness of maternal fourth trimester health domains.
SOURCE: Adapted from Tully KP, Stuebe AM, Verbiest SB. The 4th trimester:
A critical transition period with unmet maternal health needs. *Am J Obstet
Gynecol.* 2017;217(1):37–41.

Feeding occupies a large proportion of the infant's waking time and much
of early mother–infant interaction. Therefore, the feeding experience has
consequences for the dyad's overall relationship [28]. Similarly, mother–infant
and family interactions have consequences for the feeding experience, such as
assessment of and response to infant cues regarding hunger and satiety. Further,
Montgomery-Downs and colleagues have demonstrated that women's reported
sleep patterns in the weeks following childbirth drive maternal fatigue levels,
with more fragmented sleep being associated with higher levels of fatigue [29].
Fragmented sleep is also associated with increased maternal anxiety, stress, and
depressive symptoms [30, 31]. An inherent fourth trimester challenge is that the
infant's needs necessitate fragmented caregiver sleep or use of multi-caregiver
strategies. An approach that can be used to mitigate sleep challenges is "sleeping
in shifts." This means that one caregiver (i.e., the mother) is the primary respondent to the infant's needs during the first half of the night and another caregiver tends to the needs of both the baby and mother during the second half of
the night. If the mother and infant are breastfeeding but not bedsharing, then the
nonmaternal shift might entail bringing the infant to the mother to nurse in the
side-lying position, while she primarily remains asleep. The infant can then be
placed back into the crib or other sleep location.

CURRENT CONTROVERSIES

Many U.S. parents experience a cycle of unrealistic expectations, due in large
part to culturally specific information perpetuated about sleep. In addition to
complete omission the evolved biology of human infant sleep, there is inadequate support for family-centered desires, insufficient recognition of different

infant temperaments, and lack of awareness of or respect for circumstances, including what parents really want and why. Both frustration and fatigue can result from this context. In the nationally representative Listening to Mothers III survey, sleep disruption was the most prevalent concern of U.S. mothers during their first 2 postpartum months [32]. Whereas infants usually awaken every few hours, adults generally benefit from periods of more prolonged bouts of sleep. Overall, people react to this patent–infant sleep mismatch in one of two ways. Some strive for solitary infant sleep (meaning the baby sleeps on a different surface than the caregiver and perhaps in his or her own room) and independent infant settling (known as "self-soothing" often leading to "sleep training," motivated by thinking that this is in the best interest of both parents *and* infants). Sleep training can take many forms, although these practices are all intended to "teach" infants to be self-sufficient. However, infants are not little adults. Their sleep architecture, feeding patterns, and emotional needs are unique to their developmental phase. Yet, culturally based frameworks engineered for what adults want infants to do are prevalent. Infant night waking is not pathological, despite the scientific literature being rampant with infant "sleep problems" defined as infant "night waking" or the infant being awake at night for a certain periods (e.g., see [33]). Fragmented infant sleep is not a regulatory problem; it is the biological norm, even when it is personally challenging and not socially accepted.

Careful reading of scientific papers also provides insight into their authors' biases. In the journal *Pediatrics*, Paul and colleagues [34] refer to "unnecessary parental responses to infant night wakings" (p. 7). Judgment-based statements like this masquerading as scientific objectivity is pervasive in the field of infant sleep [35]. This lack of clarity creates stigma that, in turn, impedes shared understanding. What and who determines which parental responses are appropriate? Both basic human infant biology (including infant needs) and parental biology are critical here and outweigh a culture of relatively arbitrary judgment and/or personal preferences expressed by some researchers or clinicians. There is not an opportunity for authentic patient–provider engagement surrounding sleep practices when either side of the conversation is ill-equipped to be open-minded, or when assumptions are faulty.

Tully and colleagues [7] found that parents often report an intent to adhere to national-level infant sleep guidance (e.g., to sleep on separate surfaces), but then bed share for a variety of reasons, including ease of night-time parenting and for emotional connection. Currently, when women know they are not meeting healthcare provider expectations of some health behaviors, they feel like they must be dishonest [9]. Women may choose not to disclose the truth about issues such as infant sleep locations because they feel that the subsequent exchanges would be less than helpful [9]. Tully and colleagues [7] found when participants reported not bed sharing, probing led to their report of some co-sleeping in other circumstances. One participant said that she would feed her baby in the reclining armchair in the living room at night, fall asleep, and then wake up for the next feed there. The mother described it as not an ideal situation. But, when we have that growth spurt issue, I don't get any rest. It has become a bad habit [that] I'm going to start breaking him of and myself of. I heard about squashing him, [but] if I thought he were in any danger of that I would lay him back down [in his bassinet]. [7]

This example makes it clear that there are rampant missed opportunities for risk reduction and wellness promotion.

Just because something is difficult does not mean that the source (in this case, the infant) is a problem. We might reconsider the need to validate how challenging infant-, family-, and self-care can all be. Our society expects adults to operate as they did before becoming parents. This does not reflect reality, so we should not pretend that it does. One way that parents and infants navigate their overlapping and divergent sleep needs is by determining infant sleep locations. Parent–infant room sharing and the particular sleep arrangements families experience at home are complex, reflecting family preferences, needs, and constraints, and often also reflecting lack of access to resources or dangerous external environments [35].

CONCLUSION

Some of our understandings of infant sleep and parenting have been too narrowly defined. Expectations of our babies and ourselves—and the environments in which we navigate these—often differ from our needs. Shifting narratives is not easy. However, whether we recognize it or not, infant sleep is intricately tied to cultural understandings, and specifically to infant feeding methods.

Since breastfeeding is one of the most impactful health behaviors for both children and women [36], models of infant sleep should not only accommodate lactation physiology and mother–infant dyadic relational needs, but also promote them. Models of infant sleep generated from formula-fed infants are inappropriate as the standard for all. The field of sleep science, clinical counseling, and inclusive (and holistic) maternal–infant support requires a revolutionary transformation. We should respectfully yet boldly challenge the foundational assumptions on which the field of infant sleep research has been based. Sleep is a dynamic process and recognition of multidirectional influences is an important part of understanding what it means to be human.

Biological anthropologists have challenged the traditional paradigm by integrating human evolutionary, cross-cultural, and cross-species data to produce new studies with new assumptions about how to study what truly amounts of more normal and healthy human infant sleep. Indeed, new data and biological knowledge and understandings are proving remarkably relevant (see [6, 37]) to Winnicott's statement, "There is no such thing as a baby, there is a baby and someone" [38]—meaning that rather than two biological entities present, a mother and her infant are but one highly integrated biobehavioral dyadic system.

ACKNOWLEDGMENTS

We thank the individuals and families who have contributed their time and thoughts to research studies to advance understanding and support for all.

REFERENCES

1. Hirshkowitz M, Whiton K, Albert SM, et al. National Sleep Foundation's updated sleep duration recommendations: final report. *Sleep Health.* 2015;1(4):233–243.
2. Moon RY, Darnall RA, Feldman-Winter L, Goodstein MH, Hauck FR; Task Force on Sudden Infant Death Syndrome. SIDS and other sleep-related infant deaths: evidence base for 2016 updated recommendations for a safe infant sleeping environment. *Pediatrics,* 2016;138(5):e20162940.
3. Moon RY, Darnall RA, Feldman-Winter L, Goodstein MH, Hauck FR; Task Force on Sudden Infant Death Syndrome. SIDS and other sleep-related infant deaths: updated 2016 recommendations for a safe infant sleeping environment. *Pediatrics.* 2016;138(5):e20162938.
4. Field T. Infant sleep problems and interventions: a review. *Infant Behav Dev.* 2017;47:40–53.
5. Camerota M, Tully KP, Grimes M, Gueron-Sela N, Propper CB. Assessment of infant sleep: how well do multiple methods compare? *Sleep.* 2018;41(10):zsy146.
6. Ball HL, Tomori C, McKenna JJ. Toward an integrated anthropology of infant sleep. *Am Anthropol.* 2019;121(3):595–612.
7. Tully KP, Holditch-Davis D, Brandon D. The relationship between planned and reported home infant sleep locations among mothers of late preterm and term infants. *Matern Child Health J.* 2015;19(7):1616–1623.
8. McKenna JJ, Gettler LT. Mother-infant cosleeping with breastfeeding in the Western industrialized context: A bio-cultural perspective. In: Hale TW, Hartmann PE, eds. *Textbook of Human Lactation.* Amarillo, TX: Hale; 2007:271–302.
9. Tully KP, Stuebe AM, Verbiest SB. The 4th trimester: A critical transition period with unmet maternal health needs. *Am J Obstet Gynecol.* 2017;217(1):37–41.
10. Kendall-Tackett KC, Cong Z, Hale TW. Mother–infant sleep locations and nighttime feeding behavior. *Clin Lactat.* 2010;1(1):27–31.
11. Kendall-Tackett KC, Cong Z, Hale TW. Factors that influence where babies sleep in the United States: the impact of feeding method, mother's race/ethnicity, partner status, employment, education, and income. *Clin Lactat.* 2016;7(1):18–29.
12. McKenna JJ, Gettler LT. There is no such thing as infant sleep, there is no such thing as breastfeeding, there is only breastsleeping. *Acta Paediatr.* 2016;105(1):17–21.
13. Ball HL. Parent-infant bed-sharing behavior: effects of feeding type and presence of father. *Hum Nat,* 2006;17(3):301–318.
14. McKenna JJ, Mosko SS, Richard CA. Bedsharing promotes breastfeeding. *Pediatrics.* 1997;100(2 Pt 1):214–249.
15. Ball HL, Howel D, Bryant A, Best E, Russell C, Ward-Platt M. Bed-sharing by breastfeeding mothers: who bed-shares and what is the relationship with breastfeeding duration? *Acta Paediatr.* 2016;105(6):628–634.

16. Baddock SA, Purnell MT, Blair PS, Pease AS, Elder DE, Galland BC. The influence of bed-sharing on infant physiology, breastfeeding and behavior: a systematic review. *Sleep Med Rev.* 2019;43:106–117.

17. World Health Organization. Ten steps to successful breastfeeding. https://www.who.int/nutrition/bfhi/ten-steps/en/. Revised 2018. Retrieved August 2, 2019.

18. Moore ER, Bergman N, Anderson GC, Medley N. Early skin-to-skin contact for mothers and their healthy newborn infants. *Cochrane Db Syst Rev,* 2016;11:CD003519.

19. Morrison B, Luddington-Hoe S. Interruptions to breastfeeding dyads in an DRP unit. *MCH Am J Matern Child Nur.* 2012;37(1):36–41.

20. Kitzinger S. The fourth trimester? *Midwife Health Visit Comm Nurs.* 1975;11(4):118–121.

21. Hrdy SB. *Mother Nature: Maternal Instincts and How They Shape the Human Species.* 1st Ballantine Books ed. New York, NY: Ballantine Books; 2000.

22. Verbiest SB, Tully KP, Simpson M, Stuebe AM. Elevating mothers' voices: recommendations for improved patient-centered postpartum care. *J Behav Med.* 2018;41(5):577–590.

23. Montagu A. *Touching: The human significance of the skin.* 3rd ed. New York, NY: Harper & Row; 1986.

24. Ball HL, Klingaman KP. Breastfeeding and mother–infant sleep proximity: Implications for infant care. In: Trevathan WR, Smith EO, McKenna JJ, eds. *Evolutionary Medicine and Health: New Perspectives.* New York, NY: Oxford University Press: Oxford; 2008:226–241.

25. Tully KP, Ball HL. Trade-offs underlying maternal breastfeeding decisions: a conceptual model. *Matern Child Nutr.* 2013;9(1):90–98.

26. Tikotzky L, De Marcas G, Har-Toov J, Dollberg S, Bar-Haim Y, Sadeh A. Sleep and physical grown in infants during the first 6 months. *J Sleep Res.* 2010;19:103–111.

27. Sadeh A. The role and validity of actigraphy in sleep medicine: an update. *Sleep Med Rev.* 2011;15(4):259–267.

28. Pearson RM, Lightman SL, Evans J. The impact of breastfeeding on mothers' attentional sensitivity towards infant distress. *Infant Behav Dev.* 2011;34:200–205.

29. Montgomery-Downs HE, Insana SP, Clegg-Kraynok MM, Mancini LM. Normative longitudinal maternal sleep: the first 4 postpartum months. *Am J Obstet Gynecol.* 2010;203(5):465.e1–7.

30. McBean AL, Montgomery-Downs HE. Diurnal fatigue patterns, sleep timing, and mental health outcomes among healthy postpartum women. *Biol Res Nurs.* 2015;17(1):29–39.

31. Park EM, Meltzer-Brody S, Stickgold R. Poor sleep maintenance and subjective sleep quality are associated with postpartum maternal depression symptom severity. *Arch Womens Ment Health.* 2013;16(6):539–547.

32. Declercq ER, Sakala C, Corry MP, Applebaum S, Herrlich A. *Listening to Mothers III: New Mothers Speak Out.* New York: Childbirth Connection; 2013.

33. Schmied V, Beake S, Sheehan A, McCourt C, Dykes F. Women's perceptions and experiences of breastfeeding support: a metasynthesis. *Birth,* 2011;38(1):49–60.

34. Paul IM, Hohman EE, Loken E, et al. Mother–infant room-sharing and sleep outcomes in the INSIGHT Study. *Pediatrics.* 2017;140(1):e20170122.

35. Tully KP, Sullivan CS. Parent–infant room-sharing is complex and important for breastfeeding. *Evid Based Nurs*. 2018;21(1):18.
36. Bartick MC, Schwarz EB, Green BD, et al. Suboptimal breastfeeding in the United States: maternal and pediatric health outcomes and costs. *Matern Child Nutr*. 2017;13(1):12366.
37. Marinelli KA, Ball HL, McKenna JJ, Blair PS. An integrated analysis of maternal–infant sleep, breastfeeding, and sudden infant death syndrome research supporting a balanced discourse. *J Hum Lact*. 2019;35(3):510–520.
38. Winnicot DW. The theory of the parent–infant relationship. *Int J Psycho-Anal*. 1960;41:585–595.

6

History of Dreaming

CHIARA BARTOLACCI, SERENA SCARPELLI,
ANASTASIA MANGIARUGA, AND LUIGI DE GENNARO ■

INTRODUCTION

As passionate researchers in sleep psychophysiology, we all remember the first
time we stepped into the sleep laboratory.

At first, the perspective of staring at a screen for at least 8 hours did not seem
that much of a fun. Looking for waves and events you at first could not even define
by word scared us, but at the end, it somehow became our comfort zone: during
the night most of the faculties are empty spaces, where quietness accompanies not
only participant's sleep, but also your own peace of mind.

As a trainee, you are forced to grow up since the first experimental night: you
start wondering how a rapid eye movement (REM) sleep would look like, but then
you find yourself lost between electrodes cables, experimental procedures, electroencephalogram (EEG) monitoring, K-complexes, and sleep spindles—all those
words did not sound like what Freud was telling you from the books they made
you study during the bachelor. So, is there something else behind dream interpretation at the end? As psychologists and sleep experts, we all came up with the
same answer: well, yes! There is brain activity! And every new discover relating
sleep brainwaves and dream patterns still sound impressive to us.

I (CB) had the opportunity to work together with SS and AM since the very
first day of my experience in DG's sleep laboratory. Together we discovered that
the experimental nights sometimes feel never-ending, and frustration comes out
when you cannot observe what needed to complete the sample for your study.

Nonetheless, you can also experience rather peculiar events that "make your
night." When the aim of your study is to wake up the unfortunate participant many
times, with the purpose to ask if he or she was dreaming something, observing the
EEG activity and passage of stages will certainly not help you resist to the strong
sleep pressure. And you recognize all the signs of sleepiness because you are the
expert of that!

Sometimes, instead of the nice "yes/no" answer to the magic question "Can you please tell me what was passing through your mind?" the participant just stares at you from the camera (that is supposed to record any movement and sound coming from the recording room) and you get a disgruntled "Is that really necessary that you wake me up all of these times?" Eventually, you've had to reassure the nice elderly woman who loaned her brainwaves to science that, no, electrodes were not there to read her thoughts or show us her dreams. But often you can see their curiosity in taking part in something so exciting such as a sleep study. Some others just ask you if they can come back, because they never sleep that nicely at home! Things like these were our reward for every moment of boredom and frustration.

As the authors of this chapter, we all worked together on different perspectives and features of dreaming. When you study the oneiric activity the most frequent question is "Why do we dream? Why should we create absurd stories or relive trivial moments of our existence while we are sleeping?" We know we still have to work hard to answer to these questions, but finally we can provide some fascinating answers in a way that has nothing to envy from the romanticism of poetry and art.

Science makes it compelling: long debates, great puzzles, and increasingly advanced technologies are the protagonists of this story. When you come into this world, you learn that many other researchers have ventured into this same path before you, maybe asking your same questions. We are sure each one of them felt that spark and that thrill that hits you in the stomach and leads you onto this path. From that moment on, you have the opportunity to live your dreams and those of other people.

In this chapter, we draw a historical excursus of dream studies. We want to explain the main steps of the important contributions to the study of dreaming, its links with memory and with emotions, and its changes in the lifespan. Here we illustrate how research techniques and new experimental horizons have evolved, and we focus on the main theoretical models of dreaming, trying to give an overall view of this complex and fascinating phenomenon.

BIRTH OF THE PSYCHOPHYSIOLOGY OF DREAMING

In the late 1920s, psychiatrist Hans Berger introduced a new technique to detect cortical activity from the scalp of a human being. In 1929, he showed the first registration of cortical electric activity obtained by means of an electroencephalography machine, from which it was possible to get an EEG printed on paper (Figure 6.1) [1]. In subsequent years, this technique was also adopted for sleep recordings [2], revealing that the electrical activity was not homogeneous, but changed from night to night.

For several decades, ocular movements observed during sleep were considered casual and insignificant. However, Eugene Aserinsky, a physiology student at the University of Chicago under the supervision of Nathaniel Kleitman (Figure 1.1)

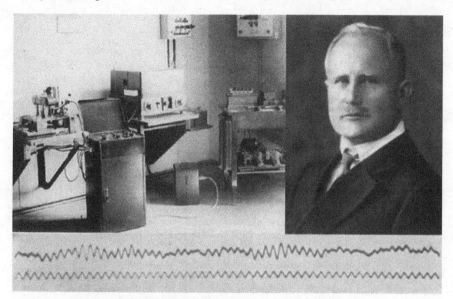

Figure 6.1 Hans Berger and his EEG machine.

revolutionized sleep science by using electrooculography (EOG) to measure cerebral activity and ocular movements simultaneously.

Although previously described by two Russian pediatricians working at the Infant Department of the Leningrad Pedological Institute [3], the lack of EEG recordings limited their observation in newborns to a phenomenological description. Aserinsky and Kleitman [4] discovered specific intervals with rapid and recurrent eye movement and bursts of alpha activity comparable to those that occur during wakefulness [4]. They named this particular kind of sleep REM, which, because of its features (i.e., desynchronized EEG activity, muscular atonia, and REMs), is also known as "paradoxical sleep." On the other hand, non-REM (NREM) sleep consists of two lighter sleep stages (stages 1 and 2—also now known as N1 and N2) and two deeper sleep stages (stages 3 and 4—also now known as combined N3), and exhibits slow, synchronized EEG activity. Essentially, 1953 marks the birth of the psychophysiology of sleep (Figure 6.2).

Until then, psychoanalysis held primacy in the study of dreams. Freudian theories about their interpretation considered oneiric (i.e., relating to dreams or dreaming) activity as a doorway to access the unconscious functions of the mind in neurosis care [5]. Since 1953, enthusiasm over the discovery of REM sleep considerably influenced dreaming research in several critical ways, including development of the idea that the specific physiology of REM sleep would generate oneiric activity, since it was observed that the highest probability of subjects recalling their dreams occurred upon awakening from this stage [6].

For several years thereafter, almost all studies were based on the biunivocal correspondence "REM = dreaming" [7–12]. In fact, because of the specific physiological differences between sleep stages, many researchers considered REM sleep

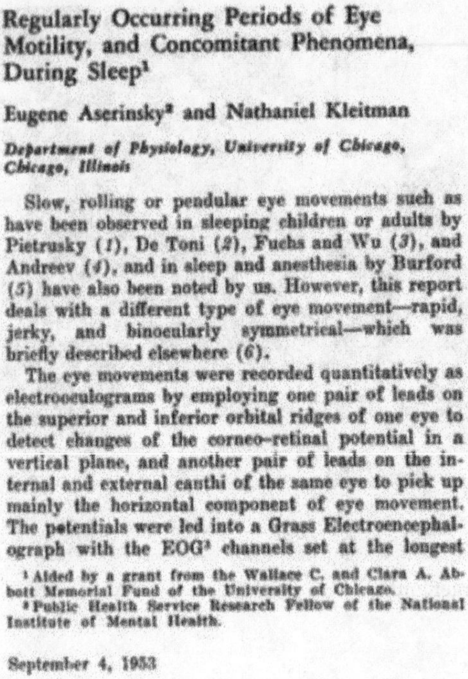

Regularly Occurring Periods of Eye Motility, and Concomitant Phenomena, During Sleep[1]

Eugene Aserinsky[2] and Nathaniel Kleitman

Department of Physiology, University of Chicago, Chicago, Illinois

Slow, rolling or pendular eye movements such as have been observed in sleeping children or adults by Pietrusky (1), De Toni (2), Fuchs and Wu (3), and Andreev (4), and in sleep and anesthesia by Burford (5) have also been noted by us. However, this report deals with a different type of eye movement—rapid, jerky, and binocularly symmetrical—which was briefly described elsewhere (6).

The eye movements were recorded quantitatively as electrooculograms by employing one pair of leads on the superior and inferior orbital ridges of one eye to detect changes of the corneo-retinal potential in a vertical plane, and another pair of leads on the internal and external canthi of the same eye to pick up mainly the horizontal component of eye movement. The potentials were led into a Grass Electroencephalograph with the EOG[3] channels set at the longest

[1] Aided by a grant from the Wallace C. and Clara A. Abbott Memorial Fund of the University of Chicago.
[2] Public Health Service Research Fellow of the National Institute of Mental Health.

September 4, 1953

Figure 6.2 The discovery of REM sleep.

to be the neural correlate of dreaming. Researchers asked subjects if they were dreaming something before they had awakened, and thus influenced the answers they received. Indeed, any individual could have a different subjective interpretation to the word *dream*. Bearing this consideration in mind, in 1962 the psychologist David Foulkes realized that it was also possible to obtain oneiric reports after awakenings from NREM sleep simply by modifying the question and using more liberal criteria; Foulkes asked the participants about "anything passing through your mind" [13, 14].

After several in-depth analyses in this direction, two fundamental studies questioned the correspondence of REM = dreaming. Antrobus [15] and Foulkes and Schmidt [16] reported that sleep mentation occurred for the whole night, without any qualitative or quantitative difference between REM and NREM sleep. Indeed, dreams occurred in any sleep stage, during slow-wave activity and sleep onset or relaxed wakefulness (e.g., hypnagogic and hypnopompic hallucinations) [17]; sometimes, they were even longer in NREM than in REM sleep [16, 18].

Currently, the correspondence "REM sleep = dreaming" is still present, but it has transformed in the context of a long debate about the different mechanisms of dream generation [19]. According to many neuropsychological, neuroimaging, and EEG studies, it can now be stated that mental activity occurs for the entire sleep period [13, 20], although with some differences regarding *dreamlike* features (e.g., multiple characters, vivid images, structured and bizarre plot) [15, 16, 20–24] versus *thought-like* features (e.g., vague and few images) [20].

In this context, some researchers have hypothesized that dreams produced during REM sleep would be more *dreamlike* and that dreams generated during NREM sleep would be more *thought-like*. Thus, they proposed the so-called two-generation model [12, 19]. However, this hypothesis has yet to be demonstrated [15, 25]. Indeed, many vivid and hallucinatory dreams also occur in NREM sleep, such as *pavor nocturnus* from stages 3 and 4 [19, 26–28] or hypnagogic and hypnopompic hallucinations in transient states of sleep–wakefulness [29]. For these reasons, assuming the homogeneity of mental activity during sleep, the one-generation model has been proposed [13, 20, 30] and is discussed more in detail later in the chapter.

METHODOLOGICAL ISSUES IN DREAMING RESEARCH

Dreaming is a peculiar form of mental activity: because it occurs during sleep, it cannot be observed directly, but only after awakenings, through narration of contents that can be recalled. We can study oneiric activity using different approaches: phenomenological, neuropsychological, and psychophysiological [31]. The phenomenological approach is based on self-reported questionnaires about dreams and is particularly useful in psychotherapeutic settings where dream content might be analyzed. The neuropsychological approach investigates the relationships between dream reports and cerebral features through neuro-imaging or lesion techniques. Finally, the psychophysiological approach is based on polysomnographic recordings of one or more nights of sleep in a laboratory. Usually, participants are awakened to verify the presence of dream recall and to compare the presence/absence of dreams [25, 32–39] or the report's features [36], correlating them with the specific EEG activity preceding the awakening. Data can also be collected after a whole night of undisturbed sleep, observing the features of the dream content upon awakening, or by means of experimental manipulations of the dream experience to observe whether such manipulations are incorporated in oneiric activity (e.g., providing different sensorial stimuli while the person is sleeping or monitoring incorporation of emotional waking-life experiences into dreams) [6, 21, 40–43].

All three approaches are characterized by the same methodological limitation: the impossibility of directly observing what is happening in our minds while we are sleeping [44, 45]. Therefore, scientists must consider the difficulty of defining the time-coupling between the sleep stages and the occurrence of dream experience [46]. Also, the dream report collection upon awakening is an indirect method influenced both by the physiological background of waking-life and by individual variables, such as personality, cognitive functions, and sociocultural features [12, 47]. Moreover, some individuals can show a major propensity to consider their inner life experiences, such as their oneiric activity, and this is an aspect that affects the dream recall frequency. For this reason, high-recall individuals have been differentiated from low-recall ones [48, 49].

Overall, dream features can vary, leading to quantitative and qualitative differences. We can observe differences in the reports' length, narrative style, degree of emotion, bizarreness or vividness, or the preponderance of dreamlike compared to thought-like mental activity [12, 13,15, 16, 20–24, 50–63].

On the other hand, some effects—due to the unusual sleeping location—that interfere with both sleep quality and oneiric features often occur in laboratory studies [12]. We should also consider that dream recall must first be retrieved from memory storage and then communicated to the interlocutor through language, in a structured narration. For these reasons, the modalities of retrieving memories, of their cognitive representation and their grammar, the lexical and morphosyntactic organization into coherent speech must also be considered. At any level in each of these processes, casual events could occur (e.g., physiological and/or psychological effects), which can influence the final narration [25].

Finally, the dream report must also be processed by the researcher. To obtain the most impartial elaboration possible, rating scales such as the Hall and Van de Castle [64] scale have been developed, which allow the researcher to implement an objective analysis of the presence of positive and negative emotions as well as degree of bizarreness and vividness in dream content. Other tools consider the number of words produced in oneiric narration (e.g., report length) [15] or the presence of possible incorporations from the environment [21]. Therefore, in studies of dreaming, it is important to bear all these aspects in mind, as they could elude experimental control and influence the dream itself.

In the final section of this chapter, parasomnias will be presented as a new frontier in dream studies that allow us to overcome some of these limitations and offering a more direct way to gain access to the oneiric trace. For now, one need only consider that in the history of dreaming, several methodological issues have stimulated reflections on amnestic consolidation mechanisms during sleep and lability of dream recall upon awakening. Next, we will describe in depth which brain areas are activated during oneiric activity and which predict subsequent dream recall.

EVOLUTION OF DREAM NEUROPSYCHOLOGY

As previously mentioned, David Foulkes was the psychologist who changed the way we approach the study of dreams, by defining dreams not just as narrative content but as "anything passing through your mind" [13]. In this way, he discovered the presence of sleep mentation in NREM sleep. Indeed, he rejected the two-generation model, which hypothesizes two distinct sources of dream generation—one in REM and one in NREM sleep—and determining qualitative and quantitative differences in respective oneiric activities. Consequently, he proposed the one-generation model, according to which mental activity during sleep is always the same across REM and NREM sleep [15, 16, 65].

The one-generation model was substantially confirmed by neuropsychological findings, which corroborate the dissociation between REM sleep and dreaming

[30, 66]. Mark Solms was the first scientist to examine a large number of cerebral lesion studies, integrating data from 332 patients with data from previous literature, to create a neuropsychology of dreams [6, 30, 66]. One of his substantial contributions was the identification of two cortical systems that activate during sleep: a posterior system that involves the temporal–parietal–occipital junction (TPJ) [30, 66], and an anterior system that includes the ventromedial prefrontal cortex (vmPFC) and the white matter surrounding the anterior horns of the lateral ventricles [30, 66, 67]. In fact, an alteration in mental imagery during both waking and sleep resulted from a TPJ lesion, and total dream loss resulted from an anterior system lesion [30, 66, 67]. Both forms of damage were associated with anoneria, the global or partial cessation of dreaming subsequent to a brain lesion [30, 66], independent of REM sleep.

What is the role of these regions in waking life? The TPJ is an associative area involved in the generation of visual imagery [68], which assembles information from different sensorial inputs into a single representation [69, 70] and deals with attention positioning, episodic memory, and language [71]. On the other hand, the vmPFC appears to be involved in mental representation and in situational evaluation [71]. Moreover, it has extent dopaminergic connections with the limbic structures, making up the mesocorticolimbic circuit which, if stimulated, can induce hallucinatory psychotic symptomatology, nightmares, and very vivid dreams [71, 72]. Therefore, it seems likely that lesions in such areas also provoke dream cessation, although these studies have never considered dream recall ability prior to cerebral damage, which represents an undoubted limitation [47].

In the late 1990s, researchers began studying brain activity during sleep, thanks to new neuroimaging techniques, which were particularly useful in demonstrating which brain areas are activated during different stages of sleep. In this way, measurements by positron emission tomography and functional magnetic resonance imaging showed an increased regional brain activity in the limbic and paralimbic structures, pontine tegmentum, thalamus, and basal forebrain during REM sleep, as compared to wakefulness [10, 11, 73, 74] and NREM sleep [10, 73, 75]. Moreover, one of the first neuroimaging studies collecting dream reports [9] found a bilateral activation of the amygdala in subjects reporting a dream experience upon awakenings only from REM sleep. How can these results be interpreted? Today, it is well known that dreaming is not restricted to REM sleep and that the correspondence "REM = dreaming" is outdated. Nevertheless, some REM sleep features make it an optimal background for dream experiences, particularly regarding emotional load, high vividness, and bizarreness [76]. In fact, most of the regions involved in emotional memory processes [77, 78] are more active during REM sleep than NREM or wakefulness (e.g., amygdaloid complexes, hippocampal formation, and anterior cingulate cortex) [9–11, 79, 80], which are probably charged with reprocessing emotional events during REM sleep [81–83].

Finally, neuroimaging studies have identified some brain areas that deal with thought functions in waking life but are hypoactive during REM sleep, such as the dorsolateral PFC, precuneus, orbitofrontal cortex, and posterior cingulate gyrus

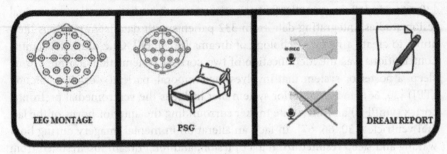

Figure 6.3 Experimental dream research procedure.

[9–11]. These results may explain why superior functions, such as executive function, insight, and time perception are altered in our dreams [79].

EEG STUDIES ON DREAMING

Polysomnographic techniques (also see Chapter 22 of this chapter) are the pivotal method of investigating oneiric activity. They consist of contemporary registration of EEG, EOG, and muscular activity (electromyography). In this way, it is possible to study both dreams and specific EEG patterns of activity that precede the presence or absence of dream recall upon awakening from a particular sleep stage (Figure 6.3). It should be noted that EEGs show that brain activity during sleep is not homogeneous; several differences in various cerebral areas can be observed [84–86]. In fact, brain regions would not be "asleep" in the same way, and it is possible to pinpoint areas with slower EEG activity (i.e., the deepest sleep that generally involves regions mainly utilized when we are awake) alongside areas with more rapid activity [44]. For this reason, it is possible to talk about "local sleep" [87], which allows researchers to hypothesize that states of consciousness in wakefulness and sleep are not always clearly distinguishable, but rather depend on contiguous mechanisms that also share some aspects of cognitive functioning.

Activation and Continuity Models

Dreaming could be defined as a peculiar kind of cognitive activity that occurs during sleep and can be retrieved from memory upon awakening. Nevertheless, this retrieval is not always simple to obtain, and the cerebral mechanisms that allow people to do so are still largely unknown.

In 1976, Koulack and Goodenough showed that the brain could not memorize ongoing mental activity during sleep. The authors proposed the arousal–retrieval model, hypothesizing that mnestic (i.e., relating to memory) encoding and consolidation could happen in conjunction with an activation episode, either during sleep or after a proper awakening. The model states that the impossibility of dream recall is associated with lower arousal and a smaller number of awakenings during the night, which determine a reduced consolidation in long-term memory storage [88].

Some years later, Hobson and McCarley [7] assumed the mind–brain iso-morphism and proposed the activation/synthesis model, suggesting that oneiric features depend on the physiological background of the specific sleep stage. In this respect, the dream is considered the product of neuronal volleys. Such neural volleys are transmitted from the brainstem to the forebrain and limbic system and handle the elaboration and organization of oneiric imagery [12].

In 1991, John Antrobus introduced the so-called activation model by pub-lishing a review that presented dreaming in association with local and periodic activations during sleep of the same cerebral structures designated for perception, motor, and cognitive information processing in a waking state [89]. In support of these hypotheses, more recent studies have found lower dream recall rates [90] and the absence of lucid dream experiences [36] in association with slow wave activity without awakenings. Moreover, such models find confirmation in studies that hypothesize that the frequency of dream recall is linked to specific EEG char-acteristics [36, 39, 49, 88, 89, 91–95] and in studies investigating the presence of intrasleep activations [49, 71] (e.g., on patients with insomnia [96]).

Many studies have also confirmed the activation models, pinpointing dream recall in association with a consistent drop of slow-wave activity in the frontal and posterior regions [37], in the left frontal and temporoparietal areas [39], and in the centro-parietal regions [34] upon awakening from NREM sleep, but also in the TPJ upon awakening both from REM and NREM sleep, as demonstrated by high-density EEG techniques [36]. Interestingly, Siclari and colleagues [36] observed that dream experience is related to delta activity decrease in the TPJ, both when participants were able to evoke the dream content, and when they were unable to do so. In this regard, the authors suggested that dream experience would be strongly associated with a higher level of awareness, due to a permissive physiological background (e.g., a decrease in slower EEG activity and increasing cortical arousal).

In light of this, the TPJ would play a pivotal role in oneiric imagery formation. The finding of faster EEG activity during dream generation suggests this area as a possible neural correlate of consciousness in dreaming [36]. Furthermore, studies of lucid dreams (i.e., oneiric activity during which the person is aware that they are dreaming [97]), show other aspects. In fact, it is highly probable that slow-wave activity increase does not permit dream recall or lucid dreaming, though the rapid activity increase (specifically, gamma activity) in relation to dream experiences has been associated with lucid dream production [94]. Indeed, Voss and colleagues demonstrated that induction of gamma oscillations in the frontal regions increases self-awareness levels in dreaming during REM sleep, using transcranial alternating current stimulation.

In addition to the activation hypothesis, another perspective that seeks to ex-plain oneiric mechanisms is the continuity hypothesis proposed by Hall and Norby [98], who stated for the first time that behaviors, thoughts, fantasies, and emotions would have their own continuity in sleep [99, 100]. Many studies were successfully carried out to verify this assumption, taking into account several aspects of mental activity during sleep. In the following paragraphs, we will consider neurocognitive studies that support this hypothesis.

Dream recall upon awakening could considered a peculiar form of declarative memory—specifically, episodic memory, which permits us to retrieve oneiric elements and to structure a complex narration after awakening [35]. Such retrieval can occur only when the mnestic trace was previously consolidated.

At the beginning of the 21st century, several studies investigated EEG activity preceding the dream recall, with the aim of identifying specific patterns of activity that could predict the presence of dream recall [32-39]. In this regard, it was shown that dream recall in REM sleep is associated with frontal [33-35] and temporoparietal [33] alpha activity decrease, delta activity decrease, occipital alpha and beta power increase [32, 34], and frontal theta activity increase [35, 38]. Conversely, delta activity decrease [34, 36, 37, 39], occipital gamma activity increase [36], and alpha power decrease [33, 35] have been found in NREM sleep.

What might these results show? First, it is necessary to consider that EEG studies investigating mnestic neural processes in waking life link information retrieval to the frontal theta activity increase [101-104]. In contrast, other cases reveal an association between decreased alpha activity and cognitive activity in temporoparietal areas [105]. This decrease predicts successful performance in episodic declarative memory tasks [102, 106], that is, the ability to remember past experiences and events [107]. Moreover, the alpha and theta activity seem to show opposite and complementary mechanisms during cognitive elaboration, which is associated with a higher alpha frequency decrease and a lower theta power increase [106].

However, without probing complex EEG studies that investigate the cognitive processes of the waking state, it is only necessary to consider that various studies have pinpointed similar scenarios between sleep and wakefulness. Therefore, it could be hypothesized that the alpha activity decrease and the theta activity increase can be associated with cognitive elaboration in both sleep and waking life, indicating that the coding and retrieval processes of episodic memories are the same across different states of consciousness [35, 105].

Emotions in oneiric activity represent a very important issue for both the current study of dreaming and the continuity hypothesis (for a review, see [46]). Considering that most regions of the brain that process emotional information in the waking state also exhibit high EEG activity during REM sleep [9, 49, 108-110], this particular stage of sleep—and the theta activity specifically—probably process mnestic emotional contents occurring during waking life [111]. REM sleep would thus also have a pivotal role in the processing and consolidation of emotional experiences [46]. Since is not rare for dreams to contain negative emotions [112-115] and waking-life elements [42, 116-118], it is reasonable to suppose that the limbic system activation [108] and the reward dopaminergic mesolimbic system activation [119] during dream experiences can contribute to emotional processing and learning [108, 120]. On the other hand, experimental deprivation of REM sleep compromises emotional memory consolidation [121-124], without suppressing the presence of dreaming [125, 126]. This represents further evidence that the correspondence "REM = dreaming" has been disproven and is not empirically grounded [25, 127].

Moreover, recent neuroimaging studies have shown interesting results. On the one hand, qualitative and quantitative interindividual differences in dream reports are correlated with the structural parameters of limbic areas [72, 109]; on the other hand, people experiencing fearful emotions in their dream experience also show more frequent activation of the medial prefrontal cortex (mPFC) and deactivations of the insula, amygdala, and cingulate cortex when they are exposed to aversive stimuli [128]. In other words, the mPFC carries out inhibitory control over fearful expressions, regulating amygdala activity, as in wakefulness [129]. In addition, the TPJ—a crucial area for dreaming [30]—has been implicated in information processing linked to the theory of mind, a model used to explain the attributions and inferences mechanisms of others' emotional states [130–132], empathy, and social cognition in the waking state [133–137]. However, studies of people suffering from posttraumatic stress disorder) show that grave trauma—such as sexual abuse, kidnapping or war experiences—influence dream content for many years afterwards. In this regard, the strong emotional intensity influences the rate of incorporating waking events in oneiric activity [138, 139].

The default mode network (DMN) also seems to play a role in dreaming. The DMN is a system located in the mPFC and medial temporal lobe [140] that deals with the elaboration of mental imagery and daydreaming [71, 79, 141]. Since daydreaming consists of thoughts, sensations, and imaginative elements [142], dream contents during sleep also have these features [141]. For this reason, it has been proposed that both phenomena are an expression of the same cognitive process, because they share some neural correlates with dreaming (i.e., DMN) [108, 143, 144].

In conclusion, dream research using EEG and neuroimaging techniques has developed considerably over the last 20 years. However, different experimental protocols and the necessity of carrying out multiple study objectives have often led to conflicting or partially coherent results. The two main dreaming models—activation and continuity—have been assumed to be in conflict with one another; only recently have researchers begun to consider the two hypotheses as complementary [25, 39, 145]. Presenting both models herein is intended to underline the important contributions made by each, and to show how they allow us to better comprehend the neural correlates of a phenomenon as common, fascinating, and complex as dreaming.

State-Like and Trait-Like Variables

We need to clarify that most studies have tried to pinpoint the possible relations between electrical activity patterns in certain cerebral areas and the presence of dream recall, without responding to a very important question: are these patterns state-like or trait-like phenomena? State-like phenomena consist of recognizable, specific EEG activations that are associated with an electrophysiological background, thus determining or predicting successful dream recall (state-like hypothesis). In contrast, trait-like phenomena suggest that dream recall ability upon awakening depends on specific EEG features. In this regard, the trait-like hypothesis refers to the particular individual electrophysiology that permanently allows dream recall [127]. These same stable features have been suggested as determining the dream recall frequency (i.e. differentiating high-recallers and low-recallers, as previously described) [49].

However, we also need to consider that dream experience can vary because of chronobiological phenomena (e.g., homeostatic and circadian variables, which can play a fundamental role in the specific scenario of physiological activity during sleep [146, 147]; also see Chapter 4 of this volume). Goodenough and colleagues [148] first observed that the length of an oneiric report showed a predictable trend. They found longer dream reports (i.e., reports involving a greater number of words) followed NREM sleep, in the process of transitioning to REM [148]. More recently, remarkable differences have been observed between the first third and the last part of the night [146, 147]: for example, dream contents become longer, more subjectively realistic and engaging in later sleep cycles, than early periods of sleep [146]. Until now, few studies have investigated these aspects. A greater number of EEG and neuroimaging studies are based on between-subject studies that do not allow researchers to determine whether the patterns observed are attributable to state-like or trait-like phenomena. In fact, only within-subject studies provide useful information on this issue [36, 38, 39, 91, 95, 127]. Moreover, to obtain a better control of chronobiological variables, protocols based on multiple awakenings during the night are needed to observe how circadian and homeostatic biological trends influence the presence or absence of dream recall. Through multiple awakenings, within-subject studies can assess both state- and trait-like variables and their interactions with chronobiological variables [25, 38]. Currently, few studies have been conducted in this direction without providing univocal results [38]. However, it needs to be specified that these findings represent only a partial attempt at studying this phenomenon [35], while other studies have exclusively investigated interindividual [72, 109] or intraindividual features [49]. Others have utilized nap protocols [127, 145], which could yield discordant results compared to whole-night investigations, due to the instability of naps compared to consolidated nocturnal sleep.

In conclusion, despite the evident signs of progress made in dreaming research in the last decades, empirical data on EEG patterns of dream recall are still scarce and have not determined whether the presence of dream recall depends on state-like or trait-like factors.

DREAMING ACROSS THE LIFESPAN

In the last few decades, some authors have hypothesized that mental activity during sleep plays a role in the development of cognitive processes [149–155].

Some researchers have found that the kind of mental activity in dreams changes across the lifespan. From this perspective, mental processes during sleep could help us better understand the mechanisms of human cognitive and emotional development [156].

Very few studies have investigated dream production during childhood in healthy subjects; Foulkes was one of the pioneers in this field [151, 152] who explored, for the first time, the hypothesis that dream recall may directly reflect cognitive maturation. Until then, dream studies focused on parasomnias and psychiatric conditions [157, 158]. It also needs to be considered that it is not possible to investigate the presence of dreams in subjects below the age of 3 years, because of the presence of infantile amnesia, which does not permit very young children to recall and organize memories, such as dream reports [159, 160]. Foulkes [161] pointed out a general limitation in language production and emotional comprehension in infancy, in association with oneiric production and its successful recall. In children younger than seven years, he reported a dream frequency rate of 20%, compared to 80% to 90% in adults [151]. However, when specific associations between language development and oneiric characteristics were investigated, no correlation was found [151, 152]. Correlations were indeed reported using a subtest of the Wechsler Intelligence Scale for Children [162], the Block Design Test, which assessed specific visuospatial and organization abilities [156, 162, 163]. To a certain extent, sleep mentation and mental imagery are linked to dream recall in childhood [151, 153, 154, 164].

More recently, some studies have found an association between executive function and dream features [155]. However, and in contrast to Foulkes's studies [150–152], these authors did not find any correlation between visuospatial abilities and the number of recalled dreams [162, 163]. Moreover, Sàndor et al. [155] found a correlation between dream bizarreness and some neuropsychological measures, and Colace [165] showed an association between dream bizarreness and long-term memory in children aged 3 to 5 years.

It has been noted that dream content during ages 2 to 5 years lacks characteristics such people, events, and objects; thus these reports are of static scenes with a single character. We find longer reports from children ages of 5 to 7 years, when they begin to represent themselves in their dreams, in a narrative structure with emotional content (for a review, see [156]). In other words, the period in which children begin to narrate their dreams is associated with their cognitive maturation [108]. Some studies show that at four years of age, children begin to distinguish dream from reality and that age nine years, when their cognitive abilities have matured, they gain a complete understanding of these differences [108, 151, 164, 166–167].

Nevertheless, thorough comprehension of these phenomena is not yet possible, nor is it possible to carry out a direct comparison with dreams in adulthood. At this point, the only available data focus on the relations between brain maturation and changes in the alpha and theta EEG activity across the lifespan [105]. Brain maturation has been associated to a progressive increase in alpha activity from infancy to adolescence, with a parallel reduction in delta and theta power [29].

Specifically, the alpha rhythm in children shows a posterior–anterior gradient in wakefulness [105], and the shift from resting states to cognitive activities during wakefulness is characterized by alpha suppression and theta increase [105]. On the other hand, the theta activity shows a medial frontal gradient (i.e., the frontal midline theta), which is involved in memory processes and is predictive of cognitive performance in successful wakefulness [168, 169]. Theta activity is also implicated in hippocampus–prefrontal cortex connectivity [170], and we can observe that topographical changes of cortical oscillatory activity in sleep involves the cerebral areas that also process memory encoding during wakefulness [111].

This relationship between sleep and memory functioning [171, 172] also characterizes aging with cognitive deterioration and changes in dream recall rates [156] (also see Chapter 12 of this volume). Sleep in the elderly shows altered structure and features, such as sleep architecture and homeostatic and circadian characteristics [10]. These include a lower total sleep time, lower slow wave activity with more time spent in stages N1 and N2, a reduction in REM sleep, more intrasleep awakenings, and more daily naps [173]. Moreover, it should be noted that K-complexes [174, 175] and sleep spindles [175–177] decrease with age. Specifically, these elements are associated with the early stages of cognitive deterioration conditions, such as Alzheimer's disease [178–180]. These features may be related to different aspects of dream recall; in fact, in the elderly we can observe a general reduction in dream recall frequency [159, 181–184]. This may be due to age-related decline and/or a lower interest in their own oneiric activity [182, 185]. Furthermore, there is also a strong association between visual memory measures and dream length, without any correlation with recall frequency [181].

To some extent, older adults show some changes in their oneiric activity, and, more generally, this may support the parallel development of cognitive performance and features of dream reports across the lifespan, although this relationship needs to be clarified through longitudinal investigations [156].

DREAM-ENACTING BEHAVIOR: A NEW FRONTIER IN DREAM EXPERIENCE STUDIES

It is understandable that dreaming has historically been studied from many points of view, focusing on different aspects of the phenomenon. Indeed, dreaming is a multicomponent phenomenon of sleep that is characterized by sensory imagery, emotional arousal, and apparent speech and motor activity [186]. We have already described the difficulties with investigating this phenomenon, insofar as dreams are not directly observable. From a scientific point of view, the dream report is certainly indispensable, but, at the same time, it is not very reliable because biases that affect its narration after awakening. For these reasons, promising future directions in dream studies are represented by dream-enacting behaviors (DEBs), namely, the behavioral enactment during sleep of the emotional, verbal, or motor components of complex dreams [108, 186] that may allow us to directly observe dream content while the dreamer is still asleep. In fact, DEBs are considered a viable way to access dreams [187, 188]. Specifically, DEBs occur in some types of parasomnias, such as REM behavior disorders (RBDs; also see Chapter 19 of this volume). This type of REM sleep parasomnia was identified in 1986 by Carlos Schenck and Mark Mahowald [189], who observed patients with violent and often high emotionally loaded behaviors (i.e., aggressive and negative emotions) [46] in the absence of normal REM sleep atonia, and dream reports congruent with such behaviors [187]. Arnulf and colleagues [190] assessed the so-called scanning perception in RBD patients by assessing their REMs of mental oneiric images to find a strong agreement (90%) between the direction of REMs and the body movements of patients who suffer from RBD.

Assuming facial expressions during sleep to be DEBs, Rivera-García and colleagues [191] investigated the activations of facial musculature during REM sleep in healthy subjects as an index of emotional dreams. In fact, the literature shows that DEBs are more frequent during highly emotional dreams, like nightmares [186, 191]. They found an activation of corrugator and zygomatic facial muscles associated with a higher incidence of negative emotional dream experiences during REM sleep.

Other NREM parasomnias also provide potentially useful information, such as somnambulism and *pavor nocturnus*, which are part of the so-called disorders of arousal. In this regard, recent studies of disorders of arousals have asked subjects to report any mental element that they could remember from the night just passed; in this way, researchers have found different mental content, with perceptual and cognitive elements and a high emotional load [192].

Finally, the phenomenon of sleep talking (ST) has been suggested as an additional way to investigate the qualitative and quantitative features of dreaming, since observing vocal activation during sleep could be considered a direct way to access dreams [188]. In this respect, different studies have analyzed the relationship between oneiric activity and ST, for the purpose of establishing whether the words expressed could be considered a verbal component of dream production [193, 194]. MacNeilage et al. [195] reported an association between the propensity to talk during sleep and dream recall frequency upon awakening. Other authors have found a specific EEG activity during "dream speech," namely, the presence of verbal production within oneiric activity, which seems to be associated with cortical EEG patterns of linguistic production in wakefulness [36, 196]. In a single-case study, Noreika and colleagues [197] showed a theta and alpha activity decrease during hypnagogic (i.e., at sleep onset) hallucinations, specifically linguistic hallucinations. Interestingly, these studies were carried out in subjects who did not suffer from parasomnias, overcoming the issue of generalizing the results to the normal population. Finally, further studies into the relationship between dream activity and ST have found that dream recall frequency is positively related to ST propensity [195], suggesting a close association between these two manifestations of sleep mentation.

Sleep verbalizations could be the result of complex and abrupt movement-arousal episodes, namely, motor activations that involve specific verbal neural circuits [193, 198]. As indicated by Alfonsi et al. [188], studies of ST and dream contents are based on two different hypotheses: (i) there is no degree of correspondence between ST and sleep mentation, due to the absence of any obvious relationship between them or to a complete amnesia [199], and (ii) there are different degrees of correspondence between ST and sleep mentation [193, 200, 201]. Supporting the latter, Arkin [193] reported different orders of concordance between sleep speech and later dream reports and, specifically, that the degree of concordance may occur on a continuum that varies from a perfect match with dream content, to a certain degree of emotional or conceptual linkage, to a total lack of concordance.

In summary, several studies agree on the hypothesis that ST is consistent with the content of dreams because of its high level of concordance with subsequent dream reports [188].

CONCLUSIONS

From the beginning of the 20th century to present day, empirical studies of dream recall have increased and improved considerably. After a long debate about the generation of dreams and the possible differences between dreams occurring during REM and NREM sleep, research is now focused on which areas are more active during a dream experience. The use of neuroimaging and EEG techniques allow us to study the sleeping brain and, in parallel, the cognitive activity that occurs while sleeping. In this way, it is possible to access the oneiric world and to better understand brain mechanisms of the states of consciousness, along with how they change from waking life to sleep. However, neural correlates of dreams are still not completely elucidated, because many studies have utilized different protocols without homogeneous results. Thus, it is still unclear how specific variables affect oneiric production (e.g., oscillatory activity, homeostatic and circadian effects, state-/trait-like features), and insufficient studies have been conducted in these directions. Moreover, the impossibility of investigating the phenomenon directly represents a basic limitation requiring specific considerations. To partially overcome this issue, DEBs are now being used as a model to observe dream content directly. In this respect, some parasomnias may represent a new frontier for investigating the neural correlates of mental activity during sleep.

Given all of that, dreaming research is an important way of examining cognitive activity during conditions of reduced self-awareness. As such, establishing uniform scientific protocols with the aim of identifying the neural correlates underlying consciousness processes across different physiological states is a top goal in this field.

ACKNOWLEDGMENTS

This work was funded by the BIAL Foundation.

REFERENCES

1. Millett D. Hans Berger: From psychic energy to the EEG. *Perspect Biol Med.* 2001;44:522–542.

2. Loomis B, Harvey EN, Hobart GA. Cerebral states during sleep, as studied by human brain potentials. *J Exp Psychol* 1937;21:127–144.

3. Denisova MP, Figurin NL. Periodic phenomena in the sleep of children. *Nov Refl Fiziol Nerv Syst.* 1926;2:338–345.

4. Aserinsky E, Kleitman N. Regularly occurring periods of eye motility, and concomitant phenomena, during sleep. *Science.* 1953;118:273–274.

5. Freud S. The interpretation of dreams. In: Strachey J, trans. and ed. *The Standard Edition of the Complete Psychological Works of Sigmund Freud.* Vols. IV and V. London, UK: Hogarth Press; 1953. (Originally published 1900)

6. Eiser AS. Physiology and psychology of dreams. *Semin Neurol.* 2005;25(1):97–105.

7. Hobson JA, McCarley RW. The brain as a dream state generator: an activation-synthesis hypothesis of the dream process. *Am J Psychiat.* 1977;134:1335–1348.

8. Hobson JA. *The Dreaming Brain.* New York, NY: Basic Books; 1988.

9. Maquet P, Peters JM, Aerts J, Delfiore G, Degueldre C, Luxen A, Franck G. Functional neuroanatomy of human rapid-eye-movement sleep and dreaming. *Nature.* 1996;383:163–166.

10. Braun AR, Balkin TJ, Wesenten NJ, et al. Regional cerebral blood flow throughout the sleep-wake cycle: an H2 (15) O PET study. *Brain.* 1997;120:1173–1197.

11. Nofzinger EA, Mintun MA, Wiseman M, Kupfer DJ, Moore RY. Forebrain activation in REM sleep: an FDG PET study. *Brain Res.* 1997;770:192–201.

12. Hobson JA, Pace-Schott EF, Stickgold R. Dreaming and the brain: toward a cognitive neuroscience of conscious states. *Behav Brain Sci.* 2000;23:793–842.

13. Foulkes D. Dream reports from different stages of sleep. *J Abnorm Soc Psychol.* 1962;65:14–25.

14. Horne J. *Why We Sleep: The Functions of Sleep in Humans and Other Mammals.* Oxford, UK: Oxford Medical Publications; 1988.

15. Antrobus J. REM and NREM sleep reports: comparison of word frequencies by cognitive classes. *Psychophysiology.* 1983;20:562–568.

16. Foulkes D, Schmidt M. Temporal sequence and unit composition in dream reports from different stages of sleep. *Sleep.* 1983;6:265–280.

17. Cavallero C. REM sleep = dreaming: the never-ending story. *Behav Brain Sci.* 2000;23:916–917.

18. Cavallero C, Foulkes D, Hollifield M, Terri R. Memory sources of REM and NREM dreams. *Sleep.* 1990;13:449–455.

19. Nielsen TA. A review of mentation in REM and NREM sleep: "covert" REM sleep as a possible reconciliation of two opposing models. *Behav Brain Sci.* 2000;23:851–866.

20. Foulkes D. Dreams of the male child: four case studies. *J Child Psychol Psychiatr.* 1967;8:81–97.

21. Foulkes D, Rechtschaffen A. Presleep determinants of dream content: effects of two films. *Percept Motor Skills.* 1964;19:983–1005.

22. Casagrande M, Violani C, Lucidi F, Buttinelli E, Bertini M. Variations in sleep mentation as a function of time of night. *Int J Neurosci.* 1996;85:19–30.

23. Stickgold R, Pace-Schott E, Hobson JA. A new paradigm for dream research: mentation reports following spontaneous arousal from REM and NREM sleep recorded in a home setting. *Conscious Cogn.* 1994;3:16–29.

24. Waterman D, Elton M, Kenemans JL. Methodological issues affecting the collection of dreams. *J Sleep Res.* 1993;2:8–12.

25. Bartolacci C, Scarpelli S, De Gennaro L. L'attività elettrica cerebrale (EEG) predice la presenza del ricordo dei sogni? [Does electric brain activity (EEG) predict the presence of dream recall?] *Rivista Sperimentale di Freniatria* 2017;141:79–99.

26. Fisher C, Byrne JV, Edwards A, Kahn E. A psychophysiological study of nightmares. *J Am Psychoanal Ass.* 1970;18:747–782.

27. Fisher C, Byrne JV, Edwards A, Kahn E. REM and NREM nightmares. *Int Psychiatr Clin.* 1970;7:183–187.

28. Kahn E, Fisher C, Edwards A. Night terrors and anxiety dreams. In: Ellman SJ, Antrobus JS. *The Mind in Sleep: Psychology and Psychophysiology.* New York, NY: Wiley, 1991;437–447.

29. Nielsen T. Microdream neurophenomenology. *Neurosci Conscious.* 2017; 2017:1–17.

30. Solms M. Dreaming and REM sleep are controlled by different brain mechanisms. *Behav Brain Sci.* 2000;2:843–850.

31. Fagioli I. Mental activity during sleep. *Sleep Med Rev.* 2002;6:307–320.

32. Takeuchi T, Ogilvie RD, Murphy TI, Ferrelli AV. EEG activities during elicited sleep onset REM and NREM periods reflect different mechanisms of dream generation. *Clin Neurophysiol.* 2003;114:210–220.

33. Esposito MJ, Nielsen TA, Paquette T. Reduced alpha power associated with the recall of mentation from Stage 2 and Stage REM sleep. *Psychophysiology.* 2004;41:288–297.

34. Chellappa SL, Frey S, Knoblauch V, Cajochen C. Cortical activation patterns herald successful dream recall after NREM and REM sleep. *Biol Psychol.* 2011;87: 251–256.

35. Marzano C, Ferrara M, Mauro F, et al. Recalling and forgetting dreams: theta and alpha oscillations during sleep predict subsequent dream recall. *J Neurosci.* 2011;31:6674–6683.

36. Siclari F, Baird B, Perogamvros L, et al. The neural correlates of dreaming. *Nat Neurosci.* 2017;20:872–878.

37. Siclari F, Bernardi G, Cataldi J, Tononi G. Dreaming in NREM sleep: a high-density EEG study of slow waves and spindles. *J Neurosci.* 2018;38:9175–9185.

38. Scarpelli S, Marzano C, D'Atri A, Gorgoni M, Ferrara M, De Gennaro L. State-or trait-like individual differences in dream recall: preliminary findings from a within-subjects study of multiple nap REM sleep awakenings. *Front Psychol.* 2015;6:928.

39. Scarpelli S, D'Atri A, Mangiaruga A, et al. Predicting dream recall: EEG activation during NREM sleep or shared mechanism with wakefulness? *Brain Topogr.* 2017;30:629–638.

40. Dement W, Wolpert EA. The relation of eye movements, body motility, and external stimuli to dream content. *J Exp Psychol.* 1958;55:543–553.

41. Solomonova E, Carr M. Incorporation of external stimuli into dream content. In: Valli K, Hoss R, eds. *Dreams: Understanding Biology, Psychology and Culture.* Valli K, Hoss R, eds. Westport, CT: Greenwood, 2019:213–218.

42. Vallat R, Chatard B, Blagrove M, Ruby P. Characteristics of the memory sources of dreams: a new version of the content-matching paradigm to take mundane and remote memories into account. *PLOS ONE* 2017;12:e0185262.

43. Eichenlaub JB, van Rijn E, Gaskell MG, et al. Incorporation of recent waking-life experiences in dreams correlates with frontal theta activity in REM sleep. *Soc Cogn Affect Neurosci.* 2018;13:637–647.

44. De Gennaro L, Marzano C, Cipolli C, Ferrara M. How we remember the stuff that dreams are made of: neurobiological approaches to the brain mechanisms of dream recall. *Behav Brain Res.* 2012;226:592e6.

45. Cipolli C, Ferrara M, De Gennaro L, Plazzi G. Beyond the neuropsychology of dreaming: insights into the neural basis of dreaming with new techniques of sleep recording and analysis. *Sleep Med Rev.* 2017;35:8–20.

46. Scarpelli S, Bartolacci C, D'Atri A, Gorgoni M, De Gennaro L. The functional role of dreaming in emotional processes. *Front Psychol.* 2019;10:459.

47. Schwartz S, Maquet P. Sleep imaging and the neuropsychological assessment of dreams. *Trends Cogn Sci.* 2002;6:23–30.

48. Blagrove M, Pace-Schott E. Trait and neurobiological correlates of individual differences in dream recall and dream content. *Int Rev Neurobiol.* 2010;92:155–180.

49. Eichenlaub JB, Bertrand O, Morlet D, Ruby P. Brain reactivity differentiates subjects with high and low dream recall frequencies during both sleep and wakefulness. *Cereb Cortex.* 2014;24:1206–1215.

50. Rechtschaffen A, Verdone P, Wheaton J. Reports of mental activity during sleep. *Can Psychiat Assoc J* 1963;8:409–414.

51. Monroe L, Rechtschaffen A, Foulkes D, Jensen J. The discriminability of REM and NREM reports. *J Person Soc Psychol.* 1965;2:456–460.

52. Pivik T, Foulkes D. NREM mentation: relation to personality, orientation time, and time of night. *J Consul Clin Psychol.* 1968;32:144–151.

53. Herman J, Ellman S, Roffwarg H. The problem of NREM dream recall reexamined. In: Arkin A, Antrobus JS, Ellman S, eds. *The Mind in Sleep: Psychology and Psychophysiology.* Hillsdale, NJ: Erlbaum, 1978; 59–62.

54. McCarley RW, Hoffman E. REM sleep dreams and the activation-synthesis hypothesis. *Am J Psychiatr.* 1981;138:904–912.

55. Antrobus JS, Hartwig P, Rosa D, Reinsel R, Fein G. Brightness and clarity of REM and NREM imagery: photo response scale. *Sleep Res.* 1987;16:240.

56. LaBerge S. Lucid dreaming: psychophysiological studies of consciousness during REM sleep. In: Bootsen R, Kihlstrom JF, Schacter DL, eds. *Sleep and Cognition.* Washington, DC: American Psychological Association Press; 1990:109–126.

57. LaBerge S. Physiological studies of lucid dreaming. In: Antrobus, JS, Bertini, M, eds. *The neuropsychology of sleep and dreaming.* Hillsdale, NJ: Erlbaum; 1992:289–304.

58. Reinsel R, Antrobus JS, Wollman M. Bizarreness in dreams and waking fantasy. In: Antrobus JS, Bertini M, eds. *The Neuropsychology of Sleep and Dreaming.* Mahwah, NJ: Erlbaum; 1992:157–183.

59. Cavallero C, Cicogna P, Natale V, Occhionero M, Zito A. Slow wave sleep dreaming: dream research. *Sleep.* 1992;15:562–566.

60. Williams J, Merritt J, Rittenhouse C, Hobson JA. Bizarreness in dreams and fantasies: implications for the activation-synthesis hypothesis. *Conscious Cogn.* 1992;1:172–185.

61. Revonsuo A, Salmivalli C. A content analysis of bizarre elements in dreams. *Dreaming.* 1995;5:169–187.

62. Hobson JA. Dreaming as delirium: a mental status analysis of our nightly madness. *Sem Neurol.* 1997;17:121–128.

63. Nielsen T, Mentation during sleep: the NREM/REM distinction. In: Lydic R, Baghdoyan HA, eds. *Handbook of Behavioral State Control: Cellular and Molecular Mechanisms.* Boca Raton, FL: CRC; 1999:101–128.

64. Schredl M. Characteristics and contents of dreams. *Int Rev Neurobiol.* 2010;92:135–154.

65. Foulkes D. *Dreaming: A Cognitive-Psychological Analysis.* Hillsdale, NJ: Erlbaum; 1985.

66. Solms M. *The Neuropsychology of Dreams: A Clinico-Anatomical Study.* Hillsdale, NJ: Erlbaum; 1997.

67. Solms, M. Neurobiology and the neurological basis of dreaming. *Handb Clin Neurol* 2011;98:519–544.

68. Kosslyn SM, Alpert NM, Thompson WL, Chabris CF, Rauch SL, Anderson AK. Identifying objects seen from different viewpoints: a PET investigation. *Brain.* 1994;117:1055–1071.

69. Rhawn J. *Cingulate Girus: Neuropsychiatry, Neuropsychology, Clinical Neuroscience.* 3rd ed. New York, NY: Academic Press; 2000.

70. Von Stein A, Rappelsberger P, Sarnthein J, Petsche H. Synchronization between temporal and parietal cortex during multimodal object processing in man. *Cereb Cortex.* 1999;9:137–150.

71. Eichenlaub JB, Nicolas A, Daltrozzo J, Redouté J, Costes N, Ruby P. Resting brain activity varies with dream recall frequency between subjects. *Neuropsychopharmacology.* 2014;39:1594–1602.

72. De Gennaro L, Lanteri O, Piras F, et al. Dopaminergic system and dream recall: an MRI study in Parkinson's disease patients. *Hum Brain Map.* 2016;37:1136–1147.

73. Braun AR, Balkin TJ, Wesensten NJ, et al. Dissociated pattern of activity in visual cortices and their projections during human rapid eye movement sleep. *Science.* 1998;279:91–95.

74. Maquet P. Functional neuroimaging of normal human sleep by positron emission tomography. *J Sleep Res.* 2000;9:207–232.

75. Maquet P, Ruby P, Maudoux A, et al. Human cognition during REM sleep and the activity profile within frontal and parietal cortices: a reappraisal of functional neuroimaging data. *Prog Brain Res.* 2005;150:219–227.

76. Carr M, Solomonova E. Dream recall and content in different stages of sleep and time-of-night effect. In: Valli K, Hoss R, Gongloff R, eds. *Dreams: Biology, Psychology and Culture.* Santa Barbara, CA: Greenwood; 2018:167–172.

77. Armony JL. Current emotion research in behavioral neuroscience: the role(s) of the amygdala. *Emot Rev.* 2013;7:280–293.

78. Phelps EA, LeDoux JE. Contributions of the amygdala to emotion processing: from animal models to human behavior. *Neuron.* 2005;48:175–187.

79. Desseilles M, Dang-Vu TT, Sterpenich V, Schwartz S. Cognitive and emotional processes during dreaming: a neuroimaging view. *Conscious Cogn.* 2011;20:998–1008.

80. Corsi-Cabrera M, Velasco F, Río-Portilla Y, et al. Human amygdala activation during rapid eye movements of rapid eye movement sleep: an intracranial study. *J Sleep Res.* 2016;25:576–582.

81. Deliens G, Gilson M, Peigneux P. Sleep and the processing of emotions. *P Exp Brain Res.* 2014;232:1403–1414.

82. Hobson JA, Pace-Schott EF. The cognitive neuroscience of sleep: neuronal system, consciousness and learning. *Nat Rev Neurosci.* 2002;3:679–693.

83. van der Helm E, Yao J, Dutt S, Rao V, Saletin JM, Walker MP. REM sleep depotentiates amygdala activity to previous emotional experiences. *Curr Biol,* 2002;21:2029–2032.

84. Finelli LA, Borbelyn AA, Achermann P. Functional topography of the human nonREM sleep electroencephalogram. *Eur J Neurosci.* 2001;13:2282–2290.

85. Ferrara M., De Gennaro L, Curcio G, Cristiani R, Corvasce C, Bertini M. Regional differences of the human sleep electroencephalogram in response to selective slow-wave sleep deprivation. *Cereb Cortex.* 2002;12:737–748.

86. Marzano C, Ferrara M, Curcio G, De Gennaro L. The effects of sleep deprivation in humans: topographical electroencephalogram changes in non-rapid eye movement (NREM) sleep versus REM sleep. *J Sleep Res.* 2010;19:260–268.

87. Ferrara M, De Gennaro L. Going local: insights from EEG and stereo-EEG studies of the human sleep–wake cycle. *Curr Top Med Chem.* 2011;11:2423–2537.

88. Koulack D, Goodenough DR. Dream recall and dream recall failure: an arousal–retrieval model. *Psychol Bull.* 1976;83:975–984.

89. Antrobus JS. Dreaming: cognitive processes during cortical activation and high afferent thresholds. *Psychol Rev.* 1991;98:96–121.

90. De Gennaro L, Marzano C, Moroni F, Curcio G, Ferrara M, Cipolli C. Recovery sleep after sleep deprivation almost completely abolishes dream recall. *Behav Brain Res.* 2010;206:293–298.

91. Siclari F, LaRocque JJ, Bernardi G, Postle BR, Tononi G. The neural correlates of consciousness in sleep: a no-task, within-state paradigm. *Nat Neurosci.* 2017;20:872–878.

92. Zimmerman WB. Sleep mentation and auditory awakening thresholds. *Psychophysiology.* 1970;6:540–549.

93. Rosenblatt SI, Antrobus JS, Zimler JP. The effect of post-awakening differences in activation on the REM–NREM report effect and recall of information from films. In: Antrobus JS, Bertini M, eds. *The Neuropsychology of Sleep and Dreaming.* London, UK: Psychology Press; 2016:215–224.

94. Voss U, Holzmann R, Hobson A, et al. Induction of self-awareness in dreams through frontal low current stimulation of gamma activity. *Nat Neurosci.* 2014;17:810–812.

95. D'Atri A, Scarpelli S, Schiappa C, et al. Cortical activation during sleep predicts dream experience in narcolepsy. *Ann Clin Transl Neurol.* 2019;6(3):445–455.

96. Schredl M, Schäfer G, Weber B, Heuser I. Dreaming and insomnia: dream recall and dream content of patients with insomnia. *J Sleep Res.* 1998;7:191–198.

97. LaBerge S, Levitan L, Dement WC. Lucid dreaming: physiological correlates of consciousness during REM sleep. *J Mind Behav.* 1986;7(2–3):251–258.

98. Hall CS, Nordby V. *The Individual and His Dreams.* New York, NY: New American Library; 1972.

99. Schredl M. The continuity between waking and dreaming: empirical research and clinical implications. In: Kramer M, Glucksman M, eds. *Dream Research*. New York, NY: Routledge, 2015:41–51.

100. Domhoff GW. The invasion of the concept snatchers: the origins, distortions, and future of the continuity hypothesis. *Dreaming.* 2017;27:14–39.

101. Hsieh LT, Ranganath C. Frontal midline theta oscillations during working memory maintenance and episodic encoding and retrieval. *NeuroImage.* 2014;85:721–729.

102. Sederberg PB, Kahana MJ, Howard MW, Donner EJ, Madsen JR. Theta and gamma oscillations during encoding predict subsequent recall. *J Neurosci.* 2003;23:10809–10814.

103. Burgess AP, Gruzelier JH. Short duration synchronization of human theta rhythm during recognition memory. *NeuroReport* 1997;8:1039–1042.

104. Klimesch W, Doppelmayr T, Schimke H, Ripper B. Theta synchronization in a memory task. *Psychophysiology.* 1997;34:169–176.

105. Klimesch W. EEG alpha and theta oscillations reflect cognitive and memory performance: a review and analysis. *Brain Res Rev.* 1999;29:169–195.

106. Mölle M, Marshall L, Gais S, Born J. Grouping of spindle activity during slow oscillations in human non-rapid eye movement sleep. *J Neurosci.* 2002;22:10941–10947.

107. Tulving E. Episodic memory: From mind to brain. *Rev Neurol.* 2002;160:S9–S23.

108. Nir Y, Tononi G. Dreaming and the brain: from phenomenology to neurophysiology. *Trends Cogn Sci.* 2010;14:88–100.

109. De Gennaro L, Cipolli C, Cherubini A, et al. Amygdala and hippocampus volumetry and diffusivity in relation to dreaming. *Hum Brain Mapp.* 2011;32:1458–1470.

110. Vallat R, Eichenlaub JB, Nicolas A, Ruby P. Dream recall frequency is associated with medial prefrontal cortex white-matter density. *Front Psychol.* 2018;9:1856.

111. Nishida M, Pearsall J, Buckner RL, Walker MP. REM sleep, prefrontal theta, and the consolidation of human emotional memory. *Cereb Cortex.* 2009;19:1158–1166.

112. Foulkes D, Sullivan B, Kerr N, Brown L. Appropriateness of dream feelings to dreamed situations. *Cogn Emot.* 1988;2:29–39.

113. Merritt JM, Stickgold R, Pace-Schott E, Williams J, Hobson JA. Emotion profiles in the dreams of men and women. *Conscious Cogn.* 1994;3:46–60.

114. Nielsen TA, Deslauries D, Baylor GW. Emotions in dream and waking event reports. *Dreaming.* 1991;1:287–300.

115. Fosse R, Stickgold R, Hobson JA. Brain–mind states: reciprocal variation in thoughts and hallucinations. *Psychol Sci.* 2001;12:30–36.

116. Wamsley EJ, Tucker M, Payne JD, Benavides JA, Stickgold R. Dreaming of a learning task is associated with enhanced sleep-dependent memory consolidation. *Curr Biol.* 2010;20:850–855.

117. Stickgold R, Hobson JA, Fosse R, Fosse M. Sleep, learning, and dreams: off-line memory reprocessing. *Science.* 2001;294:1052–1057.

118. Eichenlaub JB, Cash SS, Blagrove M. Daily life experiences in dreams and sleep-dependent memory consolidation. In: Axmacher N, Rasch B, eds. *Cognitive Neuroscience of Memory Consolidation*. Cham, Switzerland: Springer; 2017: 161–172.

119. Perogamvros L, Schwartz S. The roles of the reward system in sleep and dreaming. *Neurosci. Biobehav Rev.* 2012;36:1934–1951.

120. Perogamvros L, Dang-Vu TT, Desseilles M, Schwartz S. Sleep and dreaming are for important matters. *Front Psychol.* 2013;4:474.

121. Cartwright R, Lloyd S, Butters L, Weiner L, McCarthy L, Hancock J. The effects of REM time on what is recalled. *Psychophysiology.* 1975;12:561–568.

122. Wagner U, Gais S, Born J. Emotional memory formation is enhanced across sleep intervals with high amounts of rapid eye movement sleep. *Learn Mem.* 2001;8:112–119.

123. Lara-Carrasco J, Nielsen TA, Solomonova E, Levrier K, Popova A. Overnight emotional adaptation to negative stimuli is altered by REM sleep deprivation and is correlated with intervening dream emotions. *J Sleep Res.* 2009;18:178–187.

124. Spoormaker VI, Gvozdanovic GA, Sämann PG, Czisch M. Ventromedial prefrontal cortex activity and rapid eye movement sleep are associated with subsequent fear expression in human subjects. *Exp Brain Res.* 2014;232:1547–1554.

125. Landolt HP, Raimo EB, Schnierow BJ, Kelsoe JR, Rapaport MH, Gillin JC. Sleep and sleep electroencephalogram in depressed patients treated with phenelzine. *Arch Gen Psychiatr.* 2001;58:268–276.

126. Oudiette D, Dealberto MJ, Uguccioni G, et al. Dreaming without REM sleep. *Conscious Cogn.* 2012;21:1129–1140.

127. Scarpelli S, Marzano C, D'Atri A, Gorgoni M, Ferrara M, De Gennaro L. State-or trait-like individual differences in dream recall: preliminary findings from a within-subjects study of multiple nap REM sleep awakenings. *Front Psychol.* 2015;6:928.

128. Sterpenich V, Perogamvros L, Tononi G, Schwartz S. Fear in dreams and in wakefulness: Evidence for day/night affective homeostasis. *Hum Brain Mapp.* 2019. doi:10.1002/hbm.24843 [Epub ahead of print]

129. Phelps EA, Delgado MR, Nearing KI, LeDoux JE. Extinction learning in humans: role of the amygdala and vmPFC. *Neuron.* 2004;43:897–905.

130. Donaldson PH, Rinehart NJ, Enticott PG. Noninvasive stimulation of the temporoparietal junction: a systematic review. *Neurosci Biobehav Rev.* 2015;55: 547–572.

131. Ye H, Chen S, Huang D, Zheng H, Jia Y, Luo J. Modulation of neural activity in the temporoparietal junction with transcranial direct current stimulation changes the role of beliefs in moral judgment. *Front Hum Neurosci.* 2015;9:659.

132. Biervoye A, Dricot L, Ivanoiu A, Samson D. Impaired spontaneous belief inference following acquired damage to the left posterior temporoparietal junction. *Soc Cogn Affect Neurosci.* 2016;11:1513–1520.

133. Saxe R, Kanwisher N. People thinking about thinking people: the role of the temporo-parietal junction in "theory of mind." *Neuroimage.* 2003;19:1835–1842.

134. Young L, Dodell-Feder D, Saxe R. What gets the attention of the temporo-parietal junction? An fMRI investigation of attention and theory of mind. *Neuropsychologia.* 2010;48:2658–2664.

135. Santiesteban I, White S, Cook J, Gilbert SJ, Heyes C, Bird G. Training social cognition: from imitation to theory of mind. *Cognition.* 2012;122:228–235.

136. Van Overwalle F, Vandekerckhove M. Implicit and explicit social mentalizing: dual processes driven by a shared neural network. *Front Hum Neurosci.* 2013;7:560.

137. Jeurissen D, Sack AT, Roebroeck A, Russ BE, Pascual-Leone A. TMS affects moral judgment, showing the role of DLPFC and TPJ in cognitive and emotional processing. *Front Neurosci.* 2014;8:18.

138. Schredl M. Dream content analysis: basic principles. *Int J Dream Res.* 2010; 3:65–73.
139. Schredl M, Göritz AS. Changes in dream recall frequency, nightmare frequency, and lucid dream frequency over a 3-year period. *Dreaming.* 2015;25:81–87.
140. Andrews-Hanna JR, Reidler JS, Sepulcre J, Poulin R, Buckner RL. Functional-anatomic fractionation of the brain's default network. *Neuron.* 2010;65:550–562.
141. Domhoff W. The neural substrate for dreaming: is it a subsystem of the default network? *Conscious Cogn.* 2010;20:1163–1174.
142. Smallwood J, Schooler JW. The restless mind. *Psychol Bull.* 2006;132:946.
143. Fosse R, Domhoff GW. Dreaming as non-executive orienting: A conceptual framework for consciousness during sleep. In: Barrett D, McNamara P, eds. *The New Science of Dreaming: Content, Recall, and Personality Correlates.* Westport, CT: Praeger; 2007:49–78.
144. Ioannides AA, Kostopoulos GK, Liu L, Fenwick PB. MEG identifies dorsal medial brain activations during sleep. *NeuroImage.* 2009;44:455–468.
145. Scarpelli S, De Gennaro L. Electrophysiological pattern of dream experience. *J Public Health Emerg.* 2017;20:872–878.
146. Nielsen T. Chronobiological features of dream production. *Sleep Med Rev.* 2004;8:403–424.
147. Nielsen TA. Dream analysis and classification: the reality simulation perspective. In: Kryeger M, Roth T, Dement WC, eds. *Principles and Practice of Sleep Medicine.* New York: Elsevier; 2010:595–603.
148. Goodenough DR, Lewis HB, Shapiro A, Jaret L, Sleser I. Dream reporting following abrupt and gradual awakenings from different types of sleep. *J Pers Soc Psychol.* 1965;2:170–179.
149. Butler SF, Watson R. Individual differences in memory for dreams: the role of cognitive skills. *Percep Mot Skills.* 1985;61:823–828.
150. Foulkes D. *Children's Dreams: Longitudinal Studies.* New York: Wiley; 1982.
151. Foulkes D. Dreaming and REM sleep. *J Sleep Res.* 1993;2:199–202.
152. Foulkes D, Hollifeld M, Sullivan B, Bradley L, Terry R. REM dreaming and cognitive skills at ages 5–8: a cross-sectional study. *Int J Behav Dev.* 1990;13:447–465.
153. Sándor P, Szakadát S, Bódizs R. Ontogeny of dreaming: a review of empirical studies. *Sleep Med Rev.* 2014;18:435–449.
154. Sándor P, Szakadát S, Kertész K, Bódizs R. Content analysis of 4 to 8 years-old children's dream reports. *Front Psychol.* 2015;6:534.
155. Sándor P, Szakadát S, Bódizs R. The development of cognitive and emotional processing as reflected in children's dreams: active self in an eventful dream signals better neuropsychological skills. *Dreaming.* 2016;26:58–78.
156. Mangiaruga A, Scarpelli S, Bartolacci C, De Gennaro L. Spotlight on dream recall: the ages of dreams. *Nat Sci Sleep.* 2018;10:1–12.
157. Wittmann L, Zehnder D, Schredl M, Jenni OG, Landolt MA. Posttraumatic nightmares and psychopathology in children after road traffic accidents. *J Trauma Stress.* 2010;23:232e9.
158. Germain A, Nielsen TA. Sleep pathophysiology in posttraumatic stress disorder and idiopathic nightmare sufferers. *Biol Psychiatr.* 2003;54:1092–1098.
159. Nielsen T. Variations in dream recall frequency and dream theme diversity by age and sex. *Front Neurol.* 2012;4:106.

160. Llewellyn S. Such stuff as dreams are made on? Elaborative encoding, the ancient art of memory, and the hippocampus. *Behav Brain Sci.* 2013;36:589–659.

161. Foulkes D. Home and laboratory dreams: four empirical studies and a conceptual reevaluation. *Sleep.* 1979;2:233e51.

162. Wechsler D. *Manual for the Wechsler Preschool and Primary Scale of Intelligence.* San Antonio, TX: Psychological Corporation; 1967.

163. Groth-Marnat G, Teal M. Block design as a measure of everyday spatial ability: a study of ecological validity. *Percept Mot Skills.* 2000;90:522–526.

164. Siegel AB. Children's dreams and nightmares: emerging trends in research. *Dreaming.* 2005;15:147–154.

165. Colace C. *Children's Dreams: From Freud's Observations to Modern Dream Research.* 1st ed. London, UK: Karnac Books; 2010.

166. Strauch I. REM dreaming in the transition from late childhood to adolescence: a longitudinal study. *Dreaming.* 2005;15:155e69.

167. Evans RC. Dream conception and reality testing in children. *J Am Acad Child Psychiatr.* 1973;12:73–92.

168. Nyhus E, Curran T. Functional role of gamma and theta oscillations in episodic memory. *Neurosci Biobehav Rev.* 2010;34:1023–1035.

169. Klimesch W, Doppelmayr M, Russegger H, Pachinger T. Theta band power in the human scalp EEG and the encoding of new information. *NeuroReport.* 1996;7:1235–1240.

170. Anderson KL, Rajagovindan R, Ghacibeh GA, Meador KJ, Ding M. Theta oscillations mediate interaction between prefrontal cortex and medial temporal lobe in human memory. *Cereb Cortex.* 2010;20:1604–1612.

171. Diekelmann S, Born J. The memory function of sleep. *Nat Rev Neurosci.* 2010;11:114–126.

172. Ellenbogen JM1, Payne JD, Stickgold R. The role of sleep in declarative memory consolidation: passive, permissive, active or none? *Curr Opin Neurobiol.* 2006;16:716–722.

173. Pace-Schott EF, Spencer RM. Sleep-dependent memory consolidation in healthy aging and mild cognitive impairment. *Curr Top Behav Neurosci.* 2015;25:307–330.

174. Schwarz JFA, Akerstedt T, Lindberg E, Gruber G, Fischer H, Theorell-Haglo WJ. Age affects sleep microstructure more than sleep macrostructure. *J Sleep Res.* 2017;26:277–287.

175. Crowley K, Trinder J, Kim Y, Carrington M, Colrain IM. The effects of normal aging on sleep spindle and K-complex production. *Clin Neurophysiol.* 2002;113:1615–1622.

176. Landolt HP, Dijk DJ, Achermann P, Borbély AA. Effect of age on the sleep EEG: slow-wave activity and spindle frequency activity in young and middle- aged men. *Brain Res* 1996;738:205–212.

177. Carrier J, Monk TH, Buysse DJ, Kupfer DJ. Sleep and morningness–eveningness in the "middle" years of life (20–59 y). *J Sleep Res.* 1997;6:230–237.

178. Gorgoni M, Lauri G, Truglia I, et al. Parietal fast sleep spindle density decrease in Alzheimer's disease and amnesic mild cognitive impairment. *Neural Plast.* 2016;2016:8376108.

179. De Gennaro L, Gorgoni M, Reda F, et al. The fall of sleep K-complex in Alzheimer disease. *Sci Rep.* 2017;7:39688.

180. Reda F, Gorgoni M, Lauri G, et al. In search of sleep biomarkers of Alzheimer's disease: K-complexes do not discriminate between patients with mild cognitive impairment and healthy controls. *Brain Sci.* 2017;7: e51.

181. Waterman D. Aging and memory for dreams. *Percept Mot Skills.* 1991;73:355–365.

182. Giambra LM, Jung RE, Grodsky A. Age changes in dream recall in adulthood. *Dreaming.* 1996;6:17–31.

183. Funkhouser AT, Hirsbrunner HP, Cornu C, Bahro M. Dreams and dreaming among the elderly: an overview. *Aging Ment Health.* 1999;3:10–20.

184. Zanasi M, De Persis S, Caporali M, Siracusano A. Dreams and age. *Percept Mot Skills.* 2005;100:925–938.

185. Cohen DB. Remembering and forgetting dreaming. In: Kihlstrom JF, Evans FJ, eds. *Functional Disorders of Memory.* New York, NY: Wiley; 1979:239–274.

186. Nielsen T, Svob C, Kuiken D. Dream-enacting behaviors in a normal population. *Sleep.* 2009;32:1629e36.

187. Arnulf I. REM sleep behavior disorder: motor manifestations and pathophysiology. *Movem Disord.* 2012;27:677–689.

188. Alfonsi V, D'Atri A, Scarpelli S, Mangiaruga A, De Gennaro L. Sleep talking: a viable access to mental processes during sleep. *Sleep Med Rev.* 2019;44:12–22.

189. Schenck CH, Bundlie SR, Ettinger MG, Mahowald MW. Chronic behavioral disorders of human REM sleep: a new category of parasomnia. *Sleep.* 1986;9:293–308.

190. Arnulf I. The "scanning hypothesis" of rapid eye movements during REM sleep: a review of the evidence. *Arch Ital Biol.* 2011;149:367–382.

191. Rivera-García AP, López Ruiz IE, Ramírez-Salado I, González Olvera J, Guerrero FA, Jiménez-Anguiano A. Emotional facial expressions during REM sleep dreams. *J Sleep Res.* 2018;28:e12716.

192. Cameron WB. Some observations and a hypothesis concerning sleep talking. *Psychiatry.* 1952;15:95–96.

193. Arkin AM, Toth MF, Baker J, Hastey JM. The degree of concordance between the content of sleep talking and mentation recalled in wakefulness. *J Nerv Ment Dis.* 1970;151:375–393.

194. Arkin AM, Antrobus JS, Toth MF, Baker J, Jackler F. A comparison of the content of mentation reports elicited after nonrapid eye movement (NREM) associated sleep utterance and NREM "silent" sleep. *J Nerv Ment Dis.* 1972;155:427–445.

195. MacNeilage PF, Cohen DB, MacNeilage LA. Subject's estimation of sleeptalking propensity and dream-recall frequency. *J Consult Clin Psychol.* 1972;39:341.

196. Hong CCH, Jin Y, Potkin SG, et al. Language in dreaming and regional EEG alpha power. *Sleep.* 1996;19:232–235.

197. Noreika V, Canales-johnson A, Koh J, Taylor M, Massey I. Intrusions of a drowsy mind: neural markers of phenomenological unpredictability. *Front Psychol.* 2015;6:1–10.

198. Chase RA, Cullen JK, Niedermeyer EFL, Stark RE, Blumer DP. Ictal speech automatisms and swearing: studies on the auditory feedback control of speech. *J Nerv Ment Dis.* 1967;144:406–20.

199. Kamiya J. Behavioral, subjective and physiological aspects of drowsiness and sleep. In: Fiske DW, Maddi SR, eds. *Functions of Varied Experience*. Homewood, IL: Dorsey Press; 1961:145–174.

200. Rechtschaffen A, DR G, Shapiro A. Patterns of sleep talking. *Arch Gen Psychiatr.* 1962;7:418e26.

201. Gastut H. A clinical and polygraphic study of episodic phenomena during sleep. *Recent Adv Biol Psychiatr.* 1965;7:197–221.

7

Cognition and Memory

ERIN J. WAMSLEY ■

INTRODUCTION

College students routinely pull "all-nighters" before an exam, hoping to improve grades by replacing otherwise "wasted" time asleep with long hours spent poring over course information. What these students fail to recognize is that, far from being a waste of time, sleep is actually essential to the formation and long-term retention of memory. For all kinds of learning and memory, from the memorization of words to the refinement of motor skills, sleep is a time when newly learned information is strengthened and reorganized in the brain. And beyond aiding in simple "memorization," sleep may also help us with related cognitive abilities (see Box 7.1) including problem-solving and creative insight. In this chapter, I will review some of the scientific evidence showing how important sleep is for these functions, as well as current theories on exactly how the sleeping brain accomplishes these feats.

THE BENEFITS OF SLEEP FOR MEMORY

Memory Consolidation: Behavioral Findings

Scientists first learned that sleep helps with memory retention over 100 years ago, before the stages of sleep had even been discovered. In the 1920s, psychologists Drs. Jenkins and Dallenbach showed that sleeping after you learn something leads to improved memory [1]. In their classic study, participants first learned a list of 10 "nonsense" syllables (like "shog" and "ched") and were then tested on how many of these words they could remember 1 hour, 2 hours, 4 hours, and 8 hours later. Not surprisingly, most of these hard-to-remember words were forgotten after an 8-hour day of wakefulness. But in contrast, when participants *slept* during these 8 hours, they still remembered the majority of the words.

Box 7.1

GLOSSARY

Cognition

Cognition is a catch-all term for the information processing functions of our mind and brain, including those that lead to thought, memory, decision-making, problem-solving, and creativity. Among the many types of scientists who study sleep, cognitive psychologists and cognitive neuroscientists have a special interest in the role of sleep in functions like memory and decision making.

Memory Encoding and Consolidation

The process of learning new information for the first time is often referred to as *encoding*. Following encoding, memories undergo a process of consolidation, during which new memory traces become increasingly stabilized against interference, and in some cases, even reorganized in the brain.

Memory Reactivation

One proposed mechanism of consolidation is the iterative reactivation of memory traces in the brain. In the 1990s, it was first demonstrated that after rats navigated through an environment, neuronal firing patterns in the hippocampus describing this experience were reactivated during subsequent sleep. It is now known that this neural-level reactivation of memory also occurs in diverse other regions of the brain.

Synaptic Strength

Synaptic strength can be thought of as a sort of "connection strength" between two neurons. The synapse is a point of communication between neurons, where the axon terminal of a presynaptic (sending) neuron interfaces with the dendrite of a postsynaptic (receiving) neuron. But not all synapses are created equal. A strong synapse is one through which an action potential fired by the presynaptic neuron has a large effect on the membrane potential of the postsynaptic neuron—for example, strongly pushing this receiving neuron closer to firing its own action potential. In contrast, a weaker synapse is less effective at allowing the activity of the presynaptic neuron to drive changes in the postsynaptic cell. Changes in synaptic strength are thought to be a crucial biological mechanism of memory—during encoding, patterns of synaptic strength change to encode new information into our neural networks. As discussed in the text, multiple theories propose ways that sleep affects memory by altering synaptic strength.

The basic observation that sleep boosts memory for recently learned information has been demonstrated time and again in contemporary studies. In fact, for
each of the many different forms of learning that have been studied—for example,
verbal, spatial, motor, perceptual, emotional—the consistent finding is that *sleep
after learning leads to improved memory later on.* For example, in studies using the
classic paired associates verbal learning task, participants memorize a list of arbitrary word pairs (e.g. alligator–cigar) and are later tested on their ability to recall
the second word (cigar), when prompted with the first (alligator–???). Relative to
an equivalent period of daytime wakefulness, both a night of sleep [2] and a short
daytime nap [3] after learning lead to superior memory later (Figure 7.1).

The effect of sleep on memory is not limited to the memorization of words,
however. The same effect holds true for procedural memory, a form of skill
memory that includes your memory for how to do things like riding a bike or
tying your shoe. When participants practice tricky motor skills like quickly typing
a sequence of numbers or tracing the outline of a shape while watching their hand
in a mirror, they improve their skill more after a period of sleep than after an equal
amount of time spent awake [4, 5].

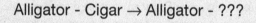

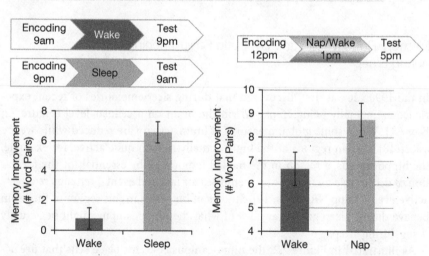

Figure 7.1 Sleep improves verbal memory. *Top:* The paired associates task is a classic
declarative memory test in which participants must memorize a list of word pairs and
are later tested on their ability to recall the second word of the pair when supplied with
the first. *Left:* Participants who learned a list of paired associates in the evening, just prior
to a night of sleep, showed superior memory when tested 12 hours later, compared to
participants who learned the same words in the morning and were tested after 12 hours
of wakefulness [2]. *Right:* A daytime nap is similarly beneficial for verbal learning. After
learning a list of paired associates, participants who were randomly assigned to take a 90-
minute nap showed significantly improved memory, compared to participants who did
not take a nap [3].

Mechanisms of Sleep's Effect on Consolidation

But exactly *how* does sleep lead to these memory improvements? When Drs. Jenkins and Dallenbach first discovered the effect of sleep on memory back in the 1920s, it was widely (and wrongly) believed that pretty much nothing was happening in the mind and brain during sleep. Because of this, it seemed that newly learned information was probably maintained during sleep simply due to a lack of new, interfering learning and activity. Meanwhile, it was reasoned, memory would naturally get worse across wakefulness due to the many experiences that you have during a typical day (consider all the talking, reading, and video watching you do during a typical 8-hour stretch of your day).

Today, most neuroscientists understand that the effect of sleep on memory is not due solely to a lack of interfering experiences during sleep. Instead, the evidence supports the notion that the effect of sleep on memory is caused by an active processing of recent memory occurring in the sleeping brain [6, 7]. This change in our understanding comes about because we now know that the sleeping brain is actually doing a lot, even though the body appears inactive. You have already learned in earlier chapters that sleep consists of a highly organized and complex set of brain states, cycling across the night in a predictable pattern. Beyond this, two lines of memory-related research suggest that specific memory-related processes are occurring in the sleeping brain, particularly during the nonrapid eye movement (NREM) stages.

Memory Reactivation and Synaptic Strengthening during Sleep

In the 1990s, it was first discovered that during sleep, memories of recent experience are actually being "replayed" in the brain on a cellular level (Figure 72; Box 7.1). While some global measures of brain activity are reduced while we are asleep [8], certain regions of the brain actually remain quite active; for example, the hippocampus, a region in the medial temporal lobe essential for the formation of declarative memory (e.g., memories for fact and events) remains relatively active even during NREM [9, 10]. Studies of how cells in this region of the brain behave during sleep give us an idea of what the hippocampus might be actually *doing* during sleep.

As illustrated in Figure 7.2, the hippocampus contains place cells that fire action potentials only when an organism is standing in a particular spot. As a consequence, while a rat runs down a track or through a maze, we can map this movement though space via the predictable firing of the place cells that represent each spot along that track (Figure 7.2, Top). Amazingly, when this rat falls asleep after running on such a track or maze, the same place cells fire again and in the same order, as if the rat were now "dreaming" that it was again running down the same track as it did while awake [11]! This has been referred to as the reactivation of memory during sleep, and we now know that it happens not just in the hippocampus, but in other brain regions as well.

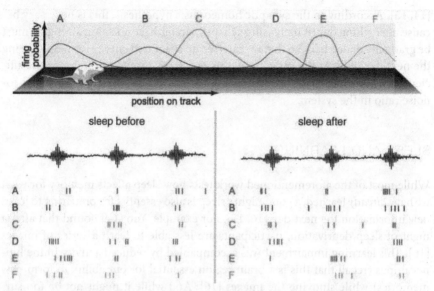

Figure 7.2 Cellular memory reactivation in sleep. When rats fall asleep after practicing running on a track, neurons in the hippocampus fire in the same order as they did during waking track-running. *Top:* As a rat runs down a linear track, hippocampal place cells A to F fire in order, representing the rat's current position on the track. Curves represent the probability that each cell will fire an action potential, as a function of where the animal is standing. *Bottom:* During sleep before track running, these cells were active, but fired in a random order. However, during sleep *after* running on the track, the cells repeatedly fire in the *same order* as during the rat's experience of track running (A•B•C•D•E•F).
SOURCE: O'Neill J, Pleydell-Bouverie B, Dupret D, Csicsvari J. Play it again: reactivation of waking experience and memory. *Trends Neurosci.* 2010;33:220–229. Reprinted with permission from Elsevier.

According to one model, this repeated cellular-level reactivation of recent experience during sleep strengthens synaptic connections between neurons representing a memory (see Box 7.1), accounting for sleep's beneficial effect on memory performance [12, 13].

The Synaptic Homeostasis Hypothesis

An alternate model proposes that sleep helps memory mainly by *reducing* the overall strength of synaptic connections between neurons (Box 7.1). Here's the logic: it is well known that learning new things while awake involves increasing synaptic strength in memory networks, as we forge new connections between neurons that encode a memory. But we cannot infinitely increase synaptic strength throughout the brain, as both space and energy are limited and will eventually run out. That's where sleep comes in—there is strong evidence suggesting that brain-wide, overall synaptic strength is reduced during sleep

[14, 15]. According to the synaptic homeostasis hypothesis, this is necessary because after a long day of increasing synaptic strength, connection strengths must be gradually dialed back so that we can free up space and energy for new learning the next day [14]. At the same time, this process is thought to increase the efficiency of networks that encode existing memories, by reducing the signal-to-noise ratio in the system.

SLEEP AND LEARNING

While most of the aforementioned work tests how sleep affects memory for what we have *already* learned, a good night's sleep is also essential for preparing to learn *new* information the next day [16, 17]. For example, Yoo et al. found that after a night of sleep deprivation, participants are less able to learn a series of images [16]. This learning impairment was accompanied by reduced activity in the hippocampus (recall that this is a brain region essential for our ability to form new memories) while studying the images [16]. And while it might not be too surprising that staying up all night would impair learning, other evidence suggests that missing out on even a few hours of sleep can similarly damage your ability to learn; participants who were allowed only 5 hours of sleep each night for 5 nights showed a similar level of impairment in their ability to learn [17]. So, while sleeping *after* learning is beneficial for the consolidation of memory, sleep *before* learning is important too. In other words, you need to get a good night's rest to process what you learned yesterday *and* to prepare your hippocampus to load up on new information the next day.

Can You Learn While Asleep?

Wouldn't it be great if you could play a recording of French vocabulary while you sleep and then ace the exam without even studying? While human imagination has long been gripped by the idea that we might be able to memorize new information during sleep (Figure 7.3), unfortunately, this type of "sleep learning" is more dream than reality. During sleep, the processing of sensory information from the outside world is greatly reduced compared to when we are awake, and we don't seem to be able to remember complicated information from audio and video recordings played while we are sleeping. So, you can forget about replacing studying with a recorded lecture played under your pillow the night before the exam; encoding complex new information is not one of the sleeping brain's cognitive abilities.

However, some specific types of very simple new learning might be possible during sleep. In sleep, we do retain some limited ability to process sensory information. For example, our sleeping brain responds to sounds by generating K-complexes in the electroencephalogram (also see Chapter 1 of this volume). And brain responses like this are even more readily generated to *meaningful* sounds,

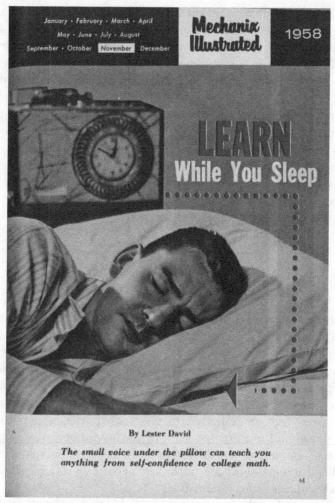

January · February · March · April
May · June · July · August
September · October · November · December

Mechanix Illustrated

1958

LEARN
While You Sleep

By Lester David

*The small voice under the pillow can teach you
anything from self-confidence to college math.*

61

Figure 7.3 Learn while you sleep? Contrary to the claim of this 1950s magazine cover, there is no evidence that we can learn complex new material like math or languages during sleep. Instead, sleep helps us process information that we already learned the previous day and to prepare us for new learning the following day.

such as the sound of our own name [18], showing that not only can our auditory system detect sounds while we are sleeping, but, to some degree, the meaning of sounds is still processed as well.

This rudimentary ability to continue detecting sounds and smells during sleep can be used to show that some learning *is* in fact possible during sleep. For example, a simple, nonconscious form of learning called classical conditioning can happen while sleep. In one study, researchers trained sleeping participants to sniff their nose in reaction to a neutral sound by repeatedly pairing the sound with the stinky smell of rotten fish, all while participants slept. In comparison, a different neutral sound was paired with a pleasant smell. After waking up, participants still "sniffed" more when they heard the sound that had been paired with the bad smell, even though they had no conscious memory of having learned this [19].

Consolidation of already-learned information can also be triggered by sounds and smells during sleep. In a technique called "targeted memory reactivation," sounds or smells present while participants learn something during wakefulness are again presented while they sleep [20, 21]. Presenting these learning-related sounds and smells during NREM sleep enhances memory, even though after waking up, participants don't recall having heard the sounds. How does it work? Scientists propose that when a sound that accompanied a learning task is playing during sleep, this triggers our sleeping brain to reactivate that particular memory (perhaps via the hippocampus), thus leading to synaptic strengthening and consolidation, as previously described [22]. There aren't yet any studies showing whether this technique can be used for practical applications like boosting grades—but stay tuned!

SLEEPING ON A PROBLEM

There may be some truth to the old adage that it pays to "sleep on a problem." You've probably heard stories to this effect, of famous scientists and inventors who were inspired with the solution to a problem during a dream. For example, sewing-machine inventor Elias Howe purportedly had a design breakthrough during sleep that led to his first sewing machine patent. After dreaming that he was being chased by cannibals wielding sharp spears with holes in the tips, Howe allegedly awoke with the realization that his sewing machine would work best with the thread hole in the point of the needle instead of the base [23]. While these sorts of anecdotes are impossible to verify, they have inspired sleep laboratory studies that show, in fact, sleep may help us come up with novel solutions to problems based on existing information.

Wagner and colleagues [24] were among the first to demonstrate this, using a clever test of mathematical problem solving. In their task, participants see a string of 8 numbers and are instructed to use a set of step-by-step rules to come up with a single-digit answer. This is a pretty boring test, because there is a total of 390 problems to solve, and each one takes around 9 seconds to figure out. But that's where the tricky part comes in—unbeknownst to the participants, there is actually a hidden shortcut method that allows you to instantly figure out the solution *without* going through the full step-by-step problem-solving process. The shortcut method reduces the time it takes to finish this boring task by about 75%, but it's tough to figure out and not everyone catches on. Sleep helps with this—participants who slept after their first try at the task were more than twice as likely to later figure out the shortcut when they did the test a second time.

Sleep appears to help with other types of problem-solving as well. For example, Beijamini and colleagues [25] used the video game Speedy Eggbert Mania to test sleep's effect on spatial reasoning problems, showing that taking a nap helps participants beat levels in this puzzle game on which they had previously been

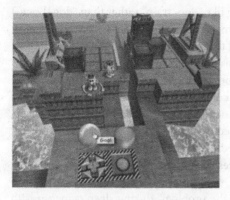
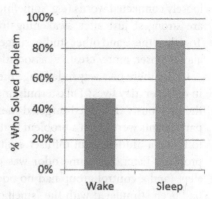

Figure 7.4 Solving problems during sleep. *Left:* In the game Speedy Eggbert Mania, players must clear a series of levels by figuring out how to arrange boxes in a particular way that allows escape. *Right:* Participants who napped after playing the game were nearly twice as likely to solve a level that they had been stuck on [25].

stuck (Figure 7.4). Together, these and other studies show that sleep is not simply *strengthening* memory (i.e., helping us memorize a few more words or type a little faster). Instead, sleep helps us use what we have learned in the past to make more effective decisions in the future.

SLEEP AND CREATIVITY

Sleep and dreaming have also been proposed to facilitate creativity, inspiring the creation of works of art throughout history. For example, the Beatles' famous song *Yesterday* and Stravinski's ballet *The Rite of Spring* were both purportedly written just after their authors awoke from a dream that inspired the work [23]. Are these just legends, or is sleep actually a more creative state of mind? While creativity of this artistic magnitude can be difficult to capture in the laboratory, researchers have devised methods of testing the effect of sleep on relatively minor expressions of creative thinking.

Sleep researcher Sara Mednick, for example, has used a classic test of creativity called the "remote associates test" to understand how sleep helps us come up with creative ideas. In this test, participants are shown word triplets and are challenged to think of a *fourth* word that is associated with the other three (e.g., when shown the words *Heart, Sixteen,* and *Cookies,* the correct response is *Sweet,* because it can pair with all three words in the problem: *Sweet*heart, *Sweet* sixteen, *Sweet* cookies). In a 2009 paper, Mednick showed that after working on this task, participants who obtained rapid eye movement (REM) sleep during an afternoon nap were better able to come up with these creative word associations during a later test [26]. This fits nicely with other evidence that REM sleep specifically (as opposed to NREM sleep) facilitates the ability to think of loosely associated information. For example, a related study used a word priming paradigm to show that associations between loosely connected words (e.g. something like "dog–train" rather than "dog–bone") are strongest just after awakening from REM, rather than NREM sleep [27]. Together, these and other studies suggest that REM sleep could be a brain state that allows looser, more "creative" associations between concepts to emerge.

Could there be a way to leverage the power of sleep to help us be more creative in our everyday lives? Dijksterhuis and colleagues asked just this question, using the previously described targeted memory reactivation technique. Before sleep, participants were given a problem that required a creative solution. Unbeknownst to them, a hidden scent diffuser emitted a specific odor while they studied this problem. Later, this same odor was presented to some participants while they slept (and a control group had no odor presented). After awakening, those who had been stimulated with the "smell of the problem" during sleep came up with solutions judged to be more creative than those of the control subjects [28]!

Admittedly, these laboratory studies might not exactly replicate the type of creativity that we attribute to Stravinsky and the Beatles. But they do suggest that, indeed, our minds are particularly able to come up with novel ideas during sleep, perhaps particularly during REM sleep.

CONCLUSION

While sleep probably has multiple important functions, at least one of these appears to be its role in supporting memory and related cognitive functions. Far from a waste of time, periods of sleep following learning help us to solidify what we have learned into a more permanent form of long-term storage, while also reorganizing information in the sleeping brain in a way that facilitates abilities like problem-solving and creativity. Moreover, without adequate sleep, we are ill-prepared to learn new information. So, while sleeping during class isn't going to be much help, sleeping *after* class could be an effective study strategy.

REFERENCES

1. Jenkins JG, Dallenbach KM. Oblivescence during sleep and waking. *Am J Psychol.* 1924;35:605–612.
2. Payne JD, Tucker MA, Ellenbogen JM, et al. Memory for semantically related and unrelated declarative information: the benefit of sleep, the cost of wake. *PLOS ONE* 2012;7:e33079.
3. Tucker MA, Hirota Y, Wamsley EJ, Lau H, Chaklader A, Fishbein W. A daytime nap containing solely non-REM sleep enhances declarative but not procedural memory. *Neurobiol Learn Mem.* 2006;86:241–247.
4. Walker MP, Brakefield T, Morgan A, Hobson JA, Stickgold R. Practice with sleep makes perfect: sleep-dependent motor skill learning. *Neuron.* 2002;35:205–211.

5. Backhaus J, Junghanns K. Daytime naps improve procedural motor memory. *Sleep Med.* 2006;7:508–512.

6. Diekelmann S, Born J. The memory function of sleep. *Nat Rev Neurosci.* 2010;11:114–126.

7. Stickgold R, Walker MP. Sleep-dependent memory triage: evolving generalization through selective processing. *Nat Neurosci.* 2013;16:139–145.

8. Braun AR, Balkin TJ, Wesenten NJ, et al. Regional cerebral blood flow throughout the sleep-wake cycle: An H2 (15) O PET study. *Brain.* 1997;120:1173–1197.

9. Peigneux P, Laureys S, Fuchs S, et al. Are spatial memories strengthened in the human hippocampus during slow wave sleep? *Neuron.* 2004;44:535–545.

10. Nofzinger EA, Buysse DJ, Miewald JM, et al. Human regional cerebral glucose metabolism during non-rapid eye movement sleep in relation to waking. *Brain J Neurol.* 2002;125:1105–1115.

11. Lee AK, Wilson MA. Memory of sequential experience in the hippocampus during slow wave sleep. *Neuron.* 2002;36:1183–1194.

12. O'Neill J, Pleydell-Bouverie B, Dupret D, Csicsvari J. Play it again: reactivation of waking experience and memory. *Trends Neurosci.* 2010;33:220–229.

13. Marshall L, Born J. The contribution of sleep to hippocampus-dependent memory consolidation. *Trends Cogn Sci.* 2007;11:442–450.

14. Tononi G, Cirelli C. Sleep function and synaptic homeostasis. *Sleep Med Rev.* 2006;10:49–62.

15. de Vivo L, Bellesi M, Marshall W, et al. Ultrastructural evidence for synaptic scaling across the wake/sleep cycle. *Science* 2017;355:507–510.

16. Yoo S-S, Hu PT, Gujar N, Jolesz FA, Walker MP. A deficit in the ability to form new human memories without sleep. *Nat Neurosci.* 2007;10:385–392.

17. Cousins JN, Sasmita K, Chee MWL. Memory encoding is impaired after multiple nights of partial sleep restriction. *J Sleep Res.* 2018;27:138–145.

18. Perrin F, García-Larrea L, Mauguière F, Bastuji H. A differential brain response to the subject's own name persists during sleep. *Clin Neurophysiol.* 1999;110:2153–2164.

19. Arzi A, Shedlesky L, Ben-Shaul M, et al. Humans can learn new information during sleep. *Nat Neurosci.* 2012;15:1460–1465.

20. Rudoy JD, Voss JL, Westerberg CE, Paller KA. Strengthening individual memories by reactivating them during sleep. *Science.* 2009;326:1079.

21. Rasch B, Buchel C, Gais S, Born J. Odor cues during slow-wave sleep prompt declarative memory consolidation. *Science.* 2007;315:1426–1429.

22. Bendor D, Wilson MA. Biasing the content of hippocampal replay during sleep. *Nat Neurosci.* 2012;15:1327–1329.

23. Ross J. Sleep on a problem . . . it works like a dream. *Psychologist.* 2006;19:738–740.

24. Wagner U, Gais S, Haider H, Verleger R, Born J. Sleep inspires insight. *Nature.* 2004;427:352–355.

25. Beijamini F, Pereira SIR, Cini FA, Louzada FM. After being challenged by a video game problem, sleep increases the chance to solve it. *PLOS ONE.* 2014;9:e84342.

26. Cai DJ, Mednick SA, Harrison EM, Kanady JC, Mednick SC. REM, not incubation, improves creativity by priming associative networks. *Proc Natl Acad Sci.* 2009;106:10130.

27. Stickgold R, Scott L, Rittenhouse C, Hobson JA. Sleep-induced changes in associative memory. *J Cogn Neurosci.* 1999;11:182–193.

28. Ritter SM, Strick M, Bos MW, VAN Baaren RB, Dijksterhuis A. Good morning creativity: Task reactivation during sleep enhances beneficial effect of sleep on creative performance. *J Sleep Res.* 2012;21:643–647.

PART II

Lifespan Development

8

Fetal and Infant Development

ROSEMARY S. C. HORNE ■

INTRODUCTION

The definitions of sleep states and ways they cycle across the sleep period (known as "sleep architecture") in infants are quite different from those in adults, due to the immaturity of the infant brain. Behavioral states of sleep and wakefulness in infants are defined by physiological and behavioral variables that are stable over time and occur repeatedly in an individual infant and also across infants [1]. This chapter provides an overview of the development of sleep in the fetus, preterm born infants, and infants born at term. Cardiorespiratory disturbances during infant sleep will also be described, including apnea of prematurity and its treatments, periodic breathing, and the different types of sleep apnea observed during infancy. The final section explains sudden infant death syndrome (SIDS) and factors that may make infants vulnerable to this tragedy.

DEVELOPMENT OF SLEEP

Sleep in the Fetus

Sleep-like activity evolves during fetal life as the brain matures and the neural network becomes more coherent [2]. Functional magnetic resonance imaging studies have demonstrated the existence of primitive neural networks in human fetuses as young as 21 to 24 weeks of gestational age (GA) [3]. Assessment by ultrasound demonstrates that preterm fetal behavior consists of random movements, and that by mid-gestation, defined rest and activity periods start to develop, with increasing prolongation of quiescence periods (i.e., reduced body movements) with advancing GA [4]. These patterns are also seen in infants born prematurely; thus, they are not a consequence of reduced intrauterine space, but rather reflect maturation of neuroinhibitory processes [4]. From at least 32 weeks GA, fetal behavior can be categorized into four states based on fetal heart rate and body and eye movements: *state 1F*, quiet sleep (QS; slow and regular heart rate, infrequent body movements, mostly startles, and no eye movements); *state 2F* active sleep (AS; regular heart rate, eye movements, frequently and periodic gross body movements, mostly stretches); *state 3F*, quiet awake (fast and regular heart rate, eye movements, no body movements); and *state 4F*, active awake (fast and irregular heart rate with prolonged periods of tachycardia, eye movements, continual body movements) [5, 6]. While the term *awake* is used in these definitions, there is limited evidence to support the presence of actual wakefulness during fetal life.

The emergence of sleep states depends on the central nervous system and is a good, reliable indicator of normal and abnormal development [7]. A gradual coordination between behaviors is seen from gestational weeks 25 to 30, with clear linkages seen after 32 to 34 weeks GA, and accelerated maturation at 34 to 36 weeks GA [6]. With maturation, the fetus spends most of its time (~90%) in stages 1F and 2F, with little time spent in 3F and 4F [6]. In late gestation, the fetus alternates between stages 1F and 2F following an ultradian cycle of 70 to 90 minutes [8] and the stability of concordant behaviors, along with organized short transition phases between states, can be used as indices of normal neurodevelopment [9].

In a long-term longitudinal study, more rapid, synchronized transitioning between these fetal states during late gestation was significantly associated with better self-regulation or effortful control (i.e., more effective emotional control and executive functioning) when these children were ages 8 to 9 and 14 to 15 years. This finding was independent of other socioeconomic factors [9]. These data emphasize that how sleep matters even before we are born and that how sleep develops before birth is important for later postnatal neurocognitive outcomes.

Sleep in Preterm Infants

Observations of infants born preterm, including with direct measurements of electroencephalographic (EEG), electromyographic, and electrooculographic activities, in addition to behavioral and heart rate measures, support findings from the previously described in utero studies.

Sleep states after birth are generally defined as QS (equivalent to 1F) and AS (equivalent to 2F); these states are the precursors to adult nonrapid eye movement (NREM) and rapid eye movement (REM), respectively, in adults. QS is characterized by high-voltage, low-amplitude EEG activity, the absence of eye movements, reduced muscle tone, and regular heart rate and respiration; AS is characterized by low-amplitude, high-frequency EEG activity, eye movements, reduced muscle tone, and irregular heart rate and respiration [10] as illustrated in Figure 8.1.

In addition, a third state, indeterminate sleep, is defined when the criteria for AS and QS are not met. Indeterminate sleep is usually considered a sign of immaturity and its incidence decreases with increasing postnatal age [10]. Distinctions between sleep states is very difficult to objectively assess before 30 weeks GA, due to difficulties identifying chin hypotonia, and because the majority of the sleep period is spent in AS. QS does not become clearly identifiable until about 36 weeks

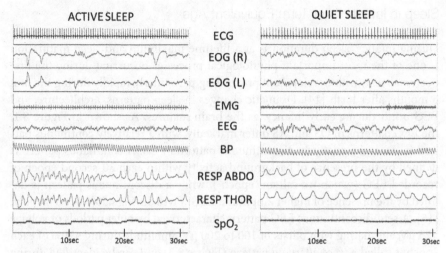

Figure 8.1 Cardio-respiratory parameters during infant active and quiet sleep. Note regular breathing and heart rate in quiet sleep compared to active sleep.
Abbreviations: ECG, electrocardiograph; EOG, electrooculograph; EMG, electromyograph; EEG, electroencephalograph; BP, blood pressure; RESP ABDO, abdominal respiratory effort; RESP THOR, thoracic respiratory effort; SpO2, oxygen saturation; HR, heart rate.

GA [11], consistent with maturation of the thalamocortical and intracortical pathways, and increased synaptogenesis [12]. This high proportion of time spent in AS by the preterm infant is important for brain growth and complexity of the neural network [13]. The percentage of time spent in QS increases, so that when the infant reaches its full-term age equivalence, they spend equal amounts of time in both AS and QS, alternating between these states throughout each sleep period (Figure 8.2).

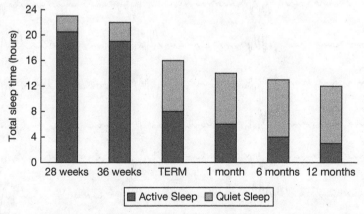

Figure 8.2 Total sleep time in active sleep and quiet sleep in preterm and term infants.
SOURCE: Redrawn from Sheldon SH, Spire JP, Levy H, eds. Pediatric Sleep Medicine. Philadelphia, PA: W. B. Saunders; 1992.

Sleep in Infants After Term Equivalent Age

During infancy, sleep duration is at a lifetime maximum and sleep maturation is one of the most important physiological processes occurring during the first postnatal year, with development proceeding particularly rapidly during the first 6 months after birth [14]. Dramatic changes in sleep patterns, architecture, and EEG occur during early infancy, as the brain matures. As shown in Figure 8.1, the EEG patterns of QS and AS differ markedly, with a relatively continuous pattern in AS and a relatively discontinuous pattern in QS. A continuous pattern is defined by the presence of background activity within each 30-second epoch of recorded EEG (which we call an "epoch"), while a discontinuous pattern is defined by the presence of higher amplitude EEG waves during <50% of each epoch [15]. A semidiscontinuous EEG pattern characterized by quiet periods of voltage >25 µV, alternating with bursts of 100 to 200 µV amplitude during ≤70% of each epoch is called a *tracé alternant* pattern (Figure 8.3) and can be identified during 32 to 34 weeks GA [15].

The *tracé alternant* pattern is not only prominent in preterm infants, but also occurs in infants born at term and disappears after 1 month after term-equivalent age. Sleep spindles appear coincidentally with the disappearance of *tracé alternant* [16]. True continuous delta frequency does not appear until 8 to 12 weeks postterm age, and it is not until this time when adult criteria for determining the stages of NREM sleep can be used [17].

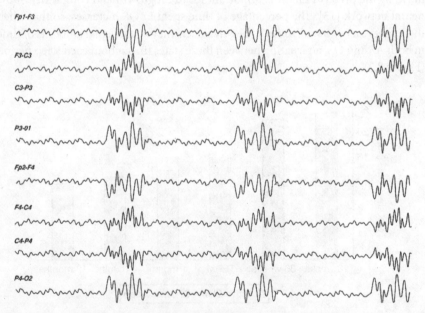

Figure 8.3 An example of trace alternant EEG pattern.
SOURCE: Sheldon SH, Spire JP, Levy H, eds. Pediatric Sleep Medicine. Philadelphia, PA: W. B. Saunders; 1992.

Table 8.1 THE EFFECTS OF SLEEP STATE ON CARDIORESPIRATORY
VARIABLES IN INFANTS

Cardio-respiratory variable	Active sleep	Quiet sleep
Heart rate	Increased	Decreased
Blood pressure	Increased	Decreased
Heart rate variability	Elevated	Decreased
Blood pressure variability	Elevated	Decreased
Baroreflex sensitivity	Similar	Similar
Respiratory rate	Increased	Decreased
Respiratory variability	Increased	Decreased
Hypoxic ventilatory response	Immature	Immature

At term, infants sleep about 16 to 17 hours out of every 24 [11]. There is a gradual decrease in total sleep time with infants sleeping 14 to 15 hours at 3 months of age and 13 to 14 hours by age 6 to 8 months (Figure 8.3). During the neonatal period, infants awaken every 2 to 6 hours for feeding, regardless of the time of day, and stay awake for 1 to 2 hours at a time [18]. The major change in sleep–wake pattern occurs between 6 weeks and 3 months postterm age [18]. During the first 6 months after term, consolidation and entrainment of sleep at night develops and sleep periods lengthen. At 3 weeks of age the mean length of the longest sleep period is about 3½ hours, increasing to 6 hours by 6 months of age [19]. The longest sleep period is randomly distributed between daytime and night-time at 3 months but moves to night-time by 6 months [19].

The proportion of AS decreases across the first 6 months to make up approximately 25% of total sleep time (similar to adults) [20]. In contrast, the proportion of QS increases with age to make up about 75% of total sleep time by 6 months [20].

CARDIORESPIRATORY DISTURBANCES DURING SLEEP

Sleep has a marked effect on cardiorespiratory control (Table 8.1). Cardiorespiratory disturbances occur predominantly in AS sleep, so the predominance of AS in early infancy may increase the risk of cardiorespiratory disturbances during this period of development.

Apnea of Prematurity

One of the major problems preterm infants face after birth is the immaturity of their cardiorespiratory system, which often leads to repeated apneic events. Apnea of prematurity is defined as either the cessation of breathing for >20 seconds or shorter breathing pauses which are associated with bradycardia, cyanosis, marked pallor, or hypotonia. Apnea of prematurity is extremely common, occurring in more than 85% of infants born prior to 34 weeks GA. The incidence of apnea of prematurity is inversely related to GA: 3% to 5% of term-born infants, 7% of infants born at 34 to 35 weeks, 15% of infants born at 32 to 33 weeks, 54% of infants born at 30 to 31 weeks, and nearly 100% of infants born at less than 29 weeks [21, 22]. There are also marked changes in apnea frequency with postnatal age, with few events in the first week after birth, and then a progressive increase during weeks 2 to 3, which plateau during weeks 4 to 6 and then decrease during weeks 6 to 8 [23].

Excessive or persistent apnea and bradycardia are associated with long-term neurodevelopmental problems [24]. It is well-known that obstructive sleep apnea in both children and adults is associated with neurocognitive deficits; the repetitive hypoxic events associated with this condition have been proposed as the primary mechanism for this effect. It is also possible that postnatal intermittent hypoxia affects cardiovascular control beyond the neonatal period, with studies in both rodent models [25] and human infants [26] demonstrating this.

Methylxanthines have been used since the 1970s to treat of apnea of prematurity and to facilitate extubation and weaning off mechanical ventilation [27, 28]. Methylxanthines cross the blood–brain barrier [29], and their primary action is to antagonize the A_1/A_{2a} adenosine receptors in the central nervous system. Methylxanthines improve apnea of prematurity by increasing minute ventilation and improving both hypercapnic and hypoxic ventilatory drive [30, 31].

Today, caffeine is the most commonly used methylxanthine in neonatal units worldwide. Caffeine's universal acceptance followed the 2006 randomized control trial Caffeine for Apnoea of Prematurity, which compared caffeine citrate (20 mg/kg loading dose followed by 5 mg/kg/day) to placebo in very low birth-weight preterm infants. The study demonstrated both significant short-term benefits (reduced incidence of bronchopulmonary dysplasia, medically and surgically treated ductus arteriosus) and long-term benefits (improved rates of survival without neurodevelopmental delay and significantly reduced incidences of cerebral palsy at 18 to 21 months) [32, 33]. Improved microstructural development of white matter has been also demonstrated in a subsample of these children who underwent brain magnetic resonance imaging at term equivalent age, a finding which may explain the improved neurodevelopmental outcomes [34]. However, when reassessed at age 5 years there was no longer any difference in rate of survival without disability between children who had been treated with caffeine and those who had not [35].

Periodic Breathing

Apneas during sleep can occur in isolation or in a repetitive pattern, termed "periodic breathing" (defined as three or more sequential central apneas each lasting ≥3 seconds). Periodic breathing is common in term infants during the first 2 weeks after birth and decreases significantly with age [36]. In term babies, the frequency of periodic breathing is low, making up <1% of total sleep time [36, 37]. Recent studies have shown that periodic breathing is associated with significant falls in cerebral oxygenation (Figure 8.4), is more common in ex-preterm infants and

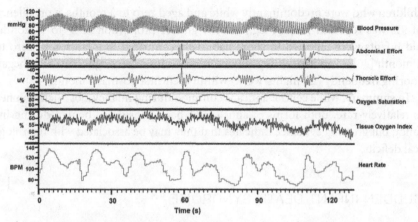

Figure 8.4 Example polysomnography epoch showing the effects of periodic breathing in an infant born at 27 weeks gestational age and studied at 2 to 4 weeks corrected age, after he had been discharged home. Periodic breathing is associated with repetitive oxygen desaturations, marked falls in cerebral tissue oxygenation index (measured with near infrared spectroscopy), and repetitive bradycardias, which may worsen over time. This infant spent 28% of his total sleep time in periodic breathing.

that the associated falls in cerebral oxygenation are greater in ex-preterm infants compared to term infants across the first 6 months of development [38], although any link to neurocognitive deficits has yet to be elucidated.

Sleep Apnea

Apneas are characterized as central, obstructive, or mixed. *Central* apneas are de-fined as a cessation of nasal and oral airflow in conjunction with an absence of respiratory effort. *Obstructive* apneas are defined as the cessation of nasal and oral airflow in the presence of continued respiratory effort, trying to move airflow against an obstruction in the airway. Central apneas are common in infancy and can occur spontaneously, although they occur more frequently after a movement [39, 40]. Traditionally, they are considered benign as they are not associated with significant desaturation and occur in healthy infants [40]. The frequency of central apneas declines with age. In a study by Brockmann et al., the median number of apneas per hour declined from 5.5 (minimum 0.9; maximum 44.3) at 1 month of age to 4.1 (minimum 1.2; maximum 27.3) at 2 months [37]. The authors suggested that these relatively high rates of central apnea may simply be due to the fact that the current definition of central apneas, while appropriate for older children, may not be appropriate for young infants.

Obstructive apneas are rare in infancy [37, 41]. However, snoring is common, with prevalence rates ranging from 5.6% to 26% [42–45]. This wide prevalence range may be due to confounders, with some studies including infants who had colds and others including infants of different ethnicities. In one study of healthy children who were predominantly white and aged zero to 3 months, a prevalence of 9% was reported [46]. A significantly greater proportion of 2- to 3-month-old infants were reported to snore habitually compared to infants aged zero to 1 month [46]. Cognitive ability at 6 months was lower among infants who began snoring frequently (≥3 nights/week) within their first postnatal month [47].

In summary, while central apnea is common during infancy, obstructive apnea is relatively rare. Both forms of apnea have been considered benign during infancy, but growing evidence indicates that they may be associated with neurological deficits.

SUDDEN INFANT DEATH SYNDROME

Sudden SIDS is defined as "the sudden unexpected death of an infant <1 year of age, with onset of the fatal episode apparently occurring during sleep, that remains unexplained after a thorough investigation, including performance of a complete autopsy and review of the circumstances of death and the clinical history" (p. 235) [48]. The incidence of SIDS reduced by more than half after public health campaigns publicized the known major risk factors: sleeping in the prone position, maternal smoking, prematurity, and overheating [49]. Despite this, SIDS remains the leading cause of unexpected death in infants in Western countries, contributing to almost 50% of all post-neonatal deaths.

As SIDS is a diagnosis of exclusion, there has been considerable research into the underlying mechanisms that may underpin known risk factors. SIDS is multifactorial in origin. The triple risk hypothesis [50] (Figure 8.5) proposes that when a vulnerable infant, such as one born preterm or exposed to maternal smoking, is at a critical but unstable developmental period in homeostatic control, and is exposed to an exogenous stressor, such as being placed prone to sleep, then SIDS may occur.

The model proposes that infants will die of SIDS only if all three factors are present and that the vulnerability lies dormant until they enter the critical developmental period and are exposed to an exogenous stressor. SIDS usually occurs during sleep, and the peak incidence is between 2 to 4 months of age, when sleep patterns are rapidly maturing. The final pathway to SIDS is widely believed to involve immature cardiorespiratory control, in conjunction with a failure to arouse from sleep [49]. Support for this hypothesis comes from numerous physiological studies showing that the major risk factors for SIDS (prone sleeping, maternal smoking, prematurity, head covering) have significant effects on blood pressure and heart rate and their control [51], and impaired arousal from sleep [52].

Vulnerable Infants

Neuropathologic findings from SIDS victims show significant deficits in brainstem and cerebellar structures involved in the regulation of respiratory drive,

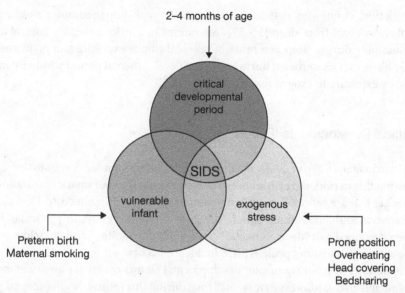

Figure 8.5 Triple risk model for SIDS, illustrating the three overlapping factors: (a) a vulnerable infant; (b) a critical developmental period; and (3) an exogenous stress. This model proposes that when a vulnerable infant, such as one born preterm or exposed to maternal smoking, is at a critical but unstable developmental period in homeostatic control, and is exposed to an exogenous stressor (e.g., being placed prone to sleep, overheated, having their head covered, are co-sleeping or have recently had an infection) then SIDS may occur.
SOURCE: Filiano JJ, Kinney H. A perspective on neuropathologic findings in victims of the sudden infant death syndrome: the triple risk model. *Biol Neonate*. 1994;65:194–197.

cardiovascular control, sleep–wake transition, and arousal from sleep [53]. Furthermore, genetic polymorphisms have been identified in SIDS victims, which affect the genes involved in autonomic function, neurotransmission, energy metabolism, and response to infection [54].

Prenatal and/or postnatal exposure to cigarette smoke is one factor that increases infant vulnerability to SIDS, with over 40 studies showing a positive association. This increased SIDS risk is likely due to the effects of nicotine exposure on autonomic control and arousal [53]. Few mothers change their smoking behavior postpartum; therefore, it is difficult to ascertain whether these physiological effects are caused by prenatal or postnatal smoke exposure. Studies of preterm infants have shown that before discharge home from the hospital—and thus prior to any postnatal smoke exposure—those whose mothers smoked already exhibit sleep pattern disruptions [55]. There is also considerable evidence from both animal and human studies suggesting that prenatal exposure to cigarette smoke has deleterious effects on the developing brain and cardiorespiratory system. It is suggested that these effects increase infant vulnerability to SIDS.

Maternal smoking may also be a confounding risk factor for SIDS due to its association with other risk factors, such as preterm birth and intrauterine growth restriction, conditions that are also associated with impaired autonomic control and arousal from sleep [56, 57]. Alterations in cardiorespiratory control and arousability during sleep as a result of prenatal smoke exposure and prematurity may be further exacerbated during a critical developmental period within infancy and by exposure to exogenous stressors.

Critical Developmental Period

Approximately 90% of SIDS deaths occur in infants under 6 months of age. During this period, the central nervous system undergoes dramatic maturational changes that are reflected in extensive alterations in sleep architecture, EEG characteristics, and autonomic control. The 2- to 4-month period, in particular, has been described as a "developmental window of vulnerability" and coincides with the age when a distinct peak in SIDS incidence occurs.

A number of other significant developmental factors may make an infant more vulnerable to a cardiorespiratory challenge during this critical developmental period. Studies of both preterm [58, 59] and term [60] infants have identified a nadir in basal blood pressure during sleep at 2 to 4 months of age, as compared to both earlier (2–4 weeks) and later (5–6 months) ages; a nadir in physiological anemia also occurs during this period. Blood pressure responses to a cardiovascular challenge (head-up tilting) are also impaired at 2 to 4 months compared to younger (2 to 4 weeks) and older (5 to 6 months) ages [61]. The maturational reduction in cerebral oxygenation is most marked between 2 to 4 weeks and 2 to 4 months of age, which may be due to limited or inadequate flow–metabolism coupling at this age [62]. Thus, the 2- to 4-month period could represent a critical period, when effects of low blood pressure may accentuate decrements in oxygen carrying capacity and delivery to critical organs [60]. These studies suggest that there is a postnatal age effect on cardiovascular control, with critical maturational changes occurring when the risk of SIDS is greatest.

Infants arouse from AS more readily compared to QS, a response also affected by postnatal age, although these maturational effects are sleep-state dependent. In response to respiratory (e.g., mild hypoxia), tactile (e.g., nasal air jet), and auditory stimulation, total arousability is reduced with increasing age during QS, while remaining unchanged in AS [52].

Exogenous Stressor(s)

An exogenous stressor constitutes the third aspect of the triple risk model for SIDS. Epidemiological studies have identified numerous factors common to SIDS victims, such as sleeping in the prone position, overheating, and recent infection, all of which may disrupt homeostasis [49].

The prone sleeping position has long been considered the major risk factor for SIDS, with some studies suggesting a causal relation. Several physiological changes ensue when infants sleep prone, including increased peripheral skin temperature, and increased baseline heart rate, together with decreased heart rate variability [53]. Furthermore, sympathetic effects on blood pressure and vasomotor tone are decreased in the prone sleeping position. Lower resting blood pressure and altered cardiovascular responses to head-up tilting have also been identified in term infants when sleeping in the prone position, compared with the supine position [60, 61]. Furthermore, cerebral oxygenation is reduced, and cerebrovascular control impaired in the prone position in both term [62, 63] and preterm infants [59, 64].

Studies of both term and preterm infants have consistently identified increases in sleep time, with significant reductions in spontaneous and induced arousability, to be associated with prone sleeping when compared with the supine position [53]. It has also been demonstrated that both spontaneous and induced arousal responses are similarly affected by sleep state and SIDS risk factors, suggesting that they are mediated through the same pathways [65]. The prone sleeping position also potentiates the risk of overheating, by reducing the exposed surface area available for radiant heat loss and reducing respiratory heat loss when the infant's face is covered.

Infant arousability is also affected by body and room temperature; decreased sleep continuity and increased body movements have been associated with exposure to cooler temperatures [66], while infants sleeping in warmer environments (28°C vs. 24°C) exhibited increased arousal thresholds to auditory stimuli [67].

Head covering has been identified as a major risk for SIDS with between 16% to 28% of SIDS infants found with their heads covered. Although a causal relationship with SIDS has not been established, it appears likely that rebreathing and impaired arousal are involved [68].

Bedsharing or co-sleeping significantly increases the risk of SIDS, particularly when the mother smokes; more than 50% of SIDS deaths occur in this situation [69]. Few studies have investigated the physiology behind this risk factor. In infants from nonsmoking families who were studied on successive bedsharing and solitary sleeping nights, bedsharing was associated with increased awakenings and transient arousals during slow wave sleep compared to solitary nights [70]. In contrast, another study found that bedsharing infants spent less time moving and were more likely to have their heads partially or fully covered by bedding than crib-sleeping infants [71]. More studies are required so that we can identify the exact physiological changes occurring during bedsharing.

Other external stressors, such as infection, fever and minor respiratory and gastrointestinal illnesses commonly occur in the days to weeks preceding the death of SIDS victims. Although not identified as an independent risk factor for SIDS, minor infections have been associated with an increased likelihood of SIDS when combined with head-covering or prone sleeping. In the prone sleeping position, minor infection, in combination with fever, could further exacerbate thermoregulatory effects on peripheral vasculature, which could increase susceptibility to a hypotensive episode. Thus, hypotension, in combination with a decreased ability to arouse from sleep, which has been documented in term infants immediately following an infection [72], could potentially further impair an infant's ability to appropriately respond to a life-threatening challenge such as circulatory failure or an asphyxial insult.

In summary, assessment of cardiovascular control and arousal processes during sleep is important toward understanding sleep-related pathologies such as SIDS. In otherwise healthy infants, studies have demonstrated impairment of these physiological mechanisms in association with all three aspects of the triple risk model, thus demonstrating the heterogeneous nature of SIDS. Altered cardiovascular and cerebrovascular control, in conjunction with a failure to arouse from sleep, may impair an infant's ability to appropriately compensate for life-threatening challenges, such as prolonged hypotension or asphyxia during sleep. The concept of a close relationship between SIDS and autonomic dysfunction has become more compelling with the demonstration of an apparent promotion of arousal from sleep by SIDS-protective factors, such as breastfeeding [52].

REFERENCES

1. Prechtl HF. The behavioural states of the newborn infant (a review). *Brain Res.* 1974;76:185–212.
2. Kostovic I, Judas M. The development of the subplate and thalamocortical connections in the human foetal brain. *Acta Paediatr.* 2010;99:1119–1127.
3. Jakab A, Schwartz E, Kasprian G, et al. Fetal functional imaging portrays heterogeneous development of emerging human brain networks. *Front Hum Neurosci.* 2014;8:852.
4. Ten Hof J, Nijhuis IJ, Mulder EJ, et al. Longitudinal study of fetal body movements: nomograms, intrafetal consistency, and relationship with episodes of heart rate patterns A and B. *Pediatr Res.* 2002;52:568–575.
5. Nijhuis JG, Prechtl HF, Martin CB, Jr., Bots RS. Are there behavioural states in the human fetus? *Early Hum Dev.* 1982;6:177–195.
6. Nijhuis IJ, ten Hof J, Nijhuis JG, et al. Temporal organization of fetal behavior from 24-weeks gestation onwards in normal and complicated pregnancies. *Dev Psychobiol.* 1999;34:257–268.
7. Curzi-Dascalova L, Challamel Marie-Josephe. Neurophysiological basis of sleep development. In: Loughlin GM, Carroll JL, Marcus CL, eds. *Sleep and Breathing in Children: A Developmental Approach.* New York, NY: Marcel Dekker; 2000:1–37.
8. Visser GH, Mulder EJ, Prechtl HF. Studies on developmental neurology in the human fetus. *Dev Pharmacol Ther.* 1992;18:175–183.
9. Van den Bergh BR, Mulder EJ. Fetal sleep organization: a biological precursor of self-regulation in childhood and adolescence? *Biol Psychol.* 2012;89:584–590.
10. Curzi-Dascalova L, Peirano P, Morel-Kahn F. Development of sleep states in normal premature and full-term newborns. *Dev Psychobiol.* 1988;21:431–444.
11. Parmelee AH, Stern E. Development of states in infants. In: Clemente CD, Purpura DP, Mayer FE, eds. *Sleep and the Maturing Nervous System.* New York, NY: Academic Press; 1972:199–228.

Fetal and Infant Development

12. Peirano P, Algarin C, Uauy R. Sleep-wake states and their regulatory mechanisms throughout early human development. *J Pediatr.* 2003;143:S70–S79.

13. Mirmiran M, Maas YG, Ariagno RL. Development of fetal and neonatal sleep and circadian rhythms. *Sleep Med Rev.* 2003;7:321–334.

14. Gaultier C. Cardiorespiratory adaptation during sleep in infants and children. *Pediatr Pulmonol.* 1995;19:105–117.

15. Curzi-Dascalova L, Mirmiran M. *Manual of Methods for Recording and Analysing Sleep–Wakefulness States in Preterm and Full Term Infants.* Paris, France: Les Edition INSERM; 1996.

16. Metcalf D. The ontogenesis of sleep–awake states from birth to 3 months. *Electroencephalogr Clin Neurophysiol.* 1970;28:421.

17. Grigg-Damberger M, Gozal D, Marcus CL, et al. The visual scoring of sleep and arousal in infants and children. *J Clin Sleep Med.* 2007;3:201–240.

18. Coons S, Guilleminault, SC. Development of sleep-wake patterns and non-rapid eye movement sleep stages during the first six months of life in normal infants. *Pediatrics.* 1982;69:793–798.

19. Coons S. *Development of Sleep and Wakefulness During the First 6 Months of Life.* New York, NY: Raven Press; 1987.

20. de Weerd AW, van den Bossche RA. The development of sleep during the first months of life. *Sleep Med Rev.* 2003;7:179–191.

21. Henderson-Smart D. The effect of gestational age on the incidence and duration of recurrent apnoea in newborn babies. *Aust Paediatr J.* 1981;17:273–276.

22. Picone S, Bedetta M, Paolillo P. Caffeine citrate: when and for how long: a literature review. *J Matern Fetal Neonatal Med.* 2012:11–14.

23. Martin RJ, Di Fiore JM, Macfarlane PM, Wilson CG. Physiologic basis for intermittent hypoxic episodes in preterm infants. *Adv Exp Med Biol.* 2012;758:351–358.

24. Pillekamp F, Hermann C, Keller T, von Gontard A, Kribs A, Roth B. Factors influencing apnea and bradycardia of prematurity - implications for neurodevelopment. *Neonatology.* 2007;91:155–161.

25. Soukhova-O'Hare GK, Cheng ZJ, Roberts AM, Gozal D. Postnatal intermittent hypoxia alters baroreflex function in adult rats. *Am J Physiol Heart Circ Physiol.* 2006;290:H1157–H1164.

26. Cohen G, Lagercrantz H, Katz-Salamon M. Abnormal circulatory stress responses of preterm graduates. *Pediatr Res.* 2007;61:329–334.

27. Al-Saif S, Alvaro R, Manfreda J, et al. A randomized controlled trial of theophylline versus CO_2 inhalation for treating apnea of prematurity. *J Pediatr.* 2008;153:513–518.

28. Henderson-Smart DJ, Steer P. Methylxanthine treatment for apnea in preterm infants. *Cochrane Db Syst Rev.* 2001:CD000140.

29. McCall AL, Millington WR, Wurtman RJ. Blood–brain barrier transport of caffeine: dose-related restriction of adenine transport. *Life Sci.* 1982;31:2709–2715.

30. Montandon G, Kinkead R, Bairam A. Adenosinergic modulation of respiratory activity: developmental plasticity induced by perinatal caffeine administration. *Respir Physiol Neurobiol.* 2008;164:87–95.

31. Chardon K, Bach V, Telliez F, et al. Effect of caffeine on peripheral chemoreceptor activity in premature neonates: interaction with sleep stages. *J Appl Physiol.* 2004;96:2161–2116.

32. Schmidt B, Roberts RS, Davis P, et al. Caffeine therapy for apnea of prematurity. *NEJM*. 2006;354:2112–2121.

33. Schmidt B, Roberts RS, Davis P, et al. Long-term effects of caffeine therapy for apnea of prematurity. *NEJM*. 2007;357:1893–1902.

34. Doyle LW, Cheong J, Hunt RW, et al. Caffeine and brain development in very pre-term infants. *Ann Neurol*. 2010;68(5):734–742.

35. Schmidt B, Anderson PJ, Doyle LW, et al. Survival without disability to age 5 years after neonatal caffeine therapy for apnea of prematurity. *JAMA*. 2012;307:275–282.

36. Kelly DH, Stellwagen LM, Kaitz E, Shannon DC. Apnea and periodic breathing in normal full-term infants during the first twelve months. *Pediatr Pulmonol*. 1985;1:215–249.

37. Brockmann PE, Poets A, Poets CF. Reference values for respiratory events in over-night polygraphy from infants aged 1 and 3 months. *Sleep Med*. 2013;14:1323–1327.

38. Horne RSC, Sun S, Yiallourou SR, Fyfe KL, Odoi A, Wong FY. Comparison of the longitudinal effects of persistent periodic breathing and apnoea on cerebral oxy-genation in term- and preterm-born infants. *J Physiol*. 2018;596:6021–6031.

39. Carskadon MA, Harvey K, Dement WC, Guilleminault C, Simmons FB, Anders TF. Respiration during sleep in children. *West J Med*. 1978;128:477–481.

40. Marcus CL, Omlin KJ, Basinki DJ, et al. Normal polysomnographic values for chil-dren and adolescents. *Am Rev Respir Dis*. 1992;146:1235–1239.

41. Kato I, Franco P, Groswasser J, Kelmanson I, Togari H, Kahn A. Frequency of ob-structive and mixed sleep apneas in 1,023 infants. *Sleep*. 2000;23:487–942.

42. Gislason T, Benediktsdottir B. Snoring, apneic episodes, and nocturnal hypoxemia among children 6 months to 6 years old: An epidemiologic study of lower limit of prevalence. *Chest*. 1995;107:963–966.

43. Kelmanson IA. Snoring, noisy breathing in sleep and daytime behaviour in 2–4-month-old infants. *Eur J Pediatr*. 2000;159:734–739.

44. Mitchell EA, Thompson JM. Snoring in the first year of life. *Acta Paediatr*. 2003;92:425–429.

45. Montgomery-Downs HE, Gozal D. Sleep habits and risk factors for sleep-disordered breathing in infants and young toddlers in Louisville, Kentucky. *Sleep Med*. 2006;7:211–219.

46. Piteo AM, Lushington K, Roberts RM, et al. Prevalence of snoring and associated factors in infancy. *Sleep Med*. 2011;12:787–792.

47. Piteo AM, Kennedy JD, Roberts RM, et al. Snoring and cognitive development in infancy. *Sleep Med*. 2011;12:981–987.

48. Krous HF, Beckwith JB, Byard RW, et al. Sudden infant death syndrome and un-classified sudden infant deaths: a definitional and diagnostic approach. *Pediatrics*. 2004;114:234–238.

49. Moon RY, Horne RS, Hauck FR. Sudden infant death syndrome. *Lancet*. 2007;370:1578–1587.

50. Filiano JJ, Kinney H. A perspective on neuropathologic findings in victims of the sudden infant death syndrome: the triple risk model. *Biol Neonate*. 1994;65:194–197.

51. Horne RS, Witcombe NB, Yiallourou SR, Scaillet S, Thiriez G, Franco P. Cardiovascular control during sleep in infants: implications for sudden infant death syndrome. *Sleep Med*. 2010;11:615–621.

52. Franco P, Kato I, Richardson HL, Yang JS, Montemitro E, Horne RS. Arousal from sleep mechanisms in infants. *Sleep Med.* 2010;11:603–614.

53. Horne RSC. Autonomic cardiorespiratory physiology and arousal of the fetus and infant. In: Duncan JR, Byard RW, eds. *SIDS sudden infant and early childhood death: the past, the present and the future.* Adelaide, Australia: University of Adelaide Press; 2018:449–490.

54. Brownstein CA, Poduri A, Goldstein RD, Holm IA. The genetics of sudden infant death syndrome. In: Duncan JR, Byard RW, eds. *SIDS sudden infant and early childhood death: the past, the present and the future.* Adelaide, Australia: University of Adelaide Press; 2018:711–730.

55. Stephan-Blanchard E, Telliez F, Leke A, et al. The influence of in utero exposure to smoking on sleep patterns in preterm neonates. *Sleep.* 2008;31:1683–1689.

56. Horne RSC. Cardiovascular autonomic dysfunction in sudden infant death syndrome. *Clin Auton Res.* 2018;28:535–543.

57. Cohen E, Wong FY, Horne RS, Yiallourou SR. Intrauterine growth restriction: impact on cardiovascular development and function throughout infancy. *Pediatr Res.* 2016;79:821–830.

58. Witcombe NB, Yiallourou SR, Walker AM, Horne RSC. Blood pressure and heart rate patterns during sleep are altered in preterm-born infants: implications for sudden infant death syndrome. *Pediatrics.* 2008;122:1242–1248.

59. Fyfe KL, Yiallourou SR, Wong FY, Odoi A, Walker AM, Horne RS. Cerebral oxygenation in preterm infants. *Pediatrics.* 2014;134:435–445.

60. Yiallourou SR, Walker AM, Horne RSC. Effects of sleeping position on development of infant cardiovascular control. *Arch Dis Child.* 2008;93:868–872.

61. Yiallourou SR, Walker AM, Horne RSC. Prone sleeping impairs circulatory control during sleep in healthy term infants; implications for sudden infant death syndrome. *Sleep.* 2008;31:1139–1146.

62. Wong FY, Witcombe NB, Yiallourou SR, et al. Cerebral oxygenation is depressed during sleep in healthy term infants when they sleep prone. *Pediatrics.* 2011;127:e558–e565.

63. Wong F, Yiallourou SR, Odoi A, Browne P, Walker AM, Horne RS. Cerebrovascular control is altered in healthy term infants when they sleep prone. *Sleep.* 2013;36:1911–1918.

64. Fyfe KL, Yiallourou SR, Wong FY, Horne RS. The development of cardiovascular and cerebral vascular control in preterm infants. *Sleep Med Rev.* 2014;18:299–310.

65. Richardson HL, Walker AM, Horne R. Stimulus type does not affect infant arousal response patterns. *J Sleep Res.* 2010;19:111–115.

66. Bach V, Bouferrache B, Kremp O, Maingourd Y, Libert JP. Regulation of sleep and body temperature in response to exposure to cool and warm environments in neonates. *Pediatrics.* 1994;93:789–796.

67. Franco P, Scaillet S, Valente F, Chabanski S, Groswasser J, Kahn A. Ambient temperature is associated with changes in infants' arousability from sleep. *Sleep.* 2001;24:325–329.

68. Franco P, Lipshutz W, Valente F, Adams S, Scaillet S, Kahn A. Decreased arousals in infants who sleep with the face covered by bedclothes. *Pediatrics.* 2002;109:1112–1117.

69. Carpenter R, McGarvey C, Mitchell EA, Tappin DM, Vennemann MM, Smuk M, et al. Bed sharing when parents do not smoke: is there a risk of SIDS? An individual level analysis of five major case-control studies. *BMJ Open.* 2013;3.

70. McKenna JJ, Mosko SS. Sleep and arousal synchrony and independence among mothers and infants sleeping apart and together (same bed): an experiment in evolutionary medicine. *Acta Paediatr Suppl.* 1994;397:94–102.

71. Baddock SA, Galland BC, Bolton DP, Williams SM, Taylor BJ. Differences in infant and parent behaviors during routine bed sharing compared with cot sleeping in the home setting. *Pediatrics.* 2006;117:1599–607.

72. Horne RS, Osborne A, Vitkovic J, Lacey B, Andrew S, Chau B, et al. Arousal from sleep in infants is impaired following an infection. *Early Human Dev.* 2002;66:89–100.

9

Child Development

YVONNE PAMULA, JOHN D. KENNEDY,
ALFRED J. MARTIN, AND KURT LUSHINGTON ∎

INTRODUCTION

Once considered a passive state of no particular importance or useful function, sleep is now known to be a highly dynamic and complex neurophysiological state that is vital to many aspects of human health and well-being. Numerous physiological, metabolic, and cellular processes are up- or downregulated during sleep, which, if disrupted due to insufficient or disturbed sleep, may lead to adverse *sequelae* across a range of physical, cognitive, and psychosocial domains [1–4]. This is particularly critical during childhood, which is characterized by rapid growth and development, and encompasses developmentally sensitive time periods. Inadequate or poor sleep during childhood is also associated with unfavorable health and behavioral outcomes in adolescence and adulthood; thus, sleep has not only immediate but also long-term effects on well-being [5–8].

The physiology, structure, and distribution of sleep changes markedly across the human lifespan, but the most profound changes occur during the period from birth to adolescence. That the highest proportion of sleep also occurs during childhood is unlikely to be happenstance. Indeed, increasing evidence suggests that sleep is crucial for normal central nervous system (CNS) development due to intrinsic neurophysiological processes that only occur during sleep, such as endogenous stimulation of neuronal networks and synaptic growth and remodeling [9–16]. While the evolution of sleep across childhood follows an organized progression reflecting underlying CNS development and maturation [17], genetic, biological, environmental, psychosocial, cultural, and health factors also influence and shape the development, structure and regulation of sleep. These intrinsic and extrinsic influences can act in isolation or interact in complex ways. Thus, sleep in children is most appropriately viewed within a biopsychological construct [18]. In this chapter, we will discuss normal sleep development and the consequence of inadequate sleep in children between the ages of 1 to 12 years.

NORMAL SLEEP AND SLEEP DEVELOPMENT

Electrophysiological Characteristics of Sleep

The human brain exhibits three major behavioral states: wake, nonrapid eye movement (NREM) sleep and rapid eye movement (REM) sleep (also known as paradoxical sleep). In normal healthy individuals each of these behavioral states are characterized by a recurring and relatively stable pattern of physiological and behavioral parameters that represent distinct modes of brain regulation and function [19–21]. The orchestration of wake, NREM and REM sleep is a complex neurophysiological process achieved by the modulation of neuronal activity in distinct brain regions facilitated by the release or inhibition of multiple neurotransmitters including acetylcholine, serotonin, norepinephrine, histamine, glutamate, and hypocretin [22]. However, sleep is not a uniform, homogenous process, as temporal and spatial variations in neuronal activity may result in local variations in sleep–wake states [23–25]. Sleep–wake states are conventionally defined by the features of three major electrophysiological signals acquired during polysomnography: the electroencephalograph (EEG), eye movements (electrooculogram) and chin muscle tone (submental electromyogram). As the anatomical origin and neurophysiology of NREM and REM sleep are fundamentally different these three parameters display a distinctive and concordant pattern of behavior enabling highly reproducible sleep state identification in normal healthy individuals.

The neurophysiology of sleep in children differs significantly from that of adults and the sleep EEG undergoes significant ontogenetic changes, particularly in the first few years of life. Features of the EEG which show developmental changes include the frequency (number of cycles per second or Hertz [Hz]), amplitude (or voltage) and morphology of waveforms observed. In addition to showing a greater variety of EEG waveforms, children often display different EEG frequencies and amplitudes [26]. In general, background EEG frequencies are a little slower, and EEG amplitudes are significantly higher than those seen in adults [17, 26]. Children also display EEG patterns of wakefulness and drowsiness, which are distinctly different to those observed in adults [17, 27].

Once past infancy, sleep begins with NREM sleep which, until recently, was divided into four stages approximating a continuum of sleep depth (as reflected by the EEG amplitude), stage 1 being the lightest and stage 4 being the deepest stage of sleep [28]. The classification of NREM sleep has since been reorganized with stages 3 and 4 combined into a single stage (N3) and the previous classification relabeled N1 to N3 [29]. N1 (stage 1 NREM) sleep is a transitional stage which does not represent a significant proportion of sleep in normal healthy children.

The majority of the sleep period is occupied by N2 (stage 2 NREM) sleep, which is characterized by two specific EEG oscillations: sleep spindles and K-complexes (Figure 9.1). In adults, sleep spindles appear as transient clusters of rhythmic activity, with a mean frequency range of 12 to 14 Hz, and a fusiform

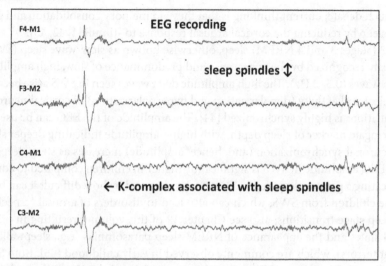

Figure 9.1 K-complex and sleep spindles seen in a child during NREM sleep (N2) throughout central (C4-M1/C3-M2) and frontal (F4-M1/F3-M2) electroencephalographic (EEG) derivations.

appearance. Rudimentary sleep spindles can first be seen in the sleep EEG of infants at around 4 weeks postterm and thereafter undergo numerous maturational changes with respect to morphology, frequency, amplitude, duration, density, and topographical scalp location [27, 30]. Sleep spindles are generated in the thalamus and are believed to play a key role in sleep maintenance via sensory gating [31]. In addition to ontogenetic changes, spindle behavior (e.g., frequency, amplitude, density) varies as a function of sleep pressure and circadian phase and can be altered by a range of factors including medical disorders and drugs [32–34]. Abnormalities in sleep spindle development or behavior are observed in children with neurodevelopmental and psychiatric disorders [35], and thus spindles have been touted as an indirect marker of neural development and a biomarker of emergent neuropsychiatric illness [36]. Sleep spindles have become the focus of much attention in recent years, as increasing evidence suggests they are mechanistically linked to both cognitive development and performance via memory consolidation during sleep [37–39].

N2 sleep is also characterized by the presence transient biphasic EEG waveform comprising a large sharp negative EEG wave (upward deflection on the EEG trace) followed immediately by a slower positive (downward) component, otherwise known as a K-complex. K-complexes may appear either spontaneously or in response to external stimuli and may have sleep spindles as part of the complex [40]. Clearly identifiable spontaneous K-complexes first appear in the infant EEG at around 6 months of age and undergo changes in morphology between the ages of 6 months and 2 years and again between 6 and 12 years of age [41]. Age-related changes are also seen in the frequency with which spontaneous K-complexes are generated [27]. The functional significance of K-complexes has been the subject of much debate; current thinking is that they aid memory consolidation and protect sleep by reducing the cortical arousal response to stimuli [1, 42, 43].

N3 (stages 3 and 4 NREM) sleep, otherwise known as slow-wave sleep (SWS), is easily recognized by the appearance and predominance of slow, high amplitude delta waves (0.5–2 Hz). The high amplitude delta waves seen in SWS arise because the electrical activity (depolarization and hyperpolarization) of cortical neuronal populations is highly synchronized [44]. The amplitude of the EEG can be used as a surrogate marker of sleep depth, with higher amplitude indicating deeper sleep as neuronal synchronization (and, hence, amplitude) increases as sleep deepens. The EEG amplitude in SWS is significantly higher in children compared to adults, indicating a greater sleep depth. This can be observed by how difficult it can be to rouse children from SWS, which can also lead to disorders of arousal (especially at sleep stage transitions; also see Chapter 19 of this volume) resulting in mixed EEG states and the appearance of NREM sleep parasomnias (e.g., sleepwalking, night terrors), which are commonly observed in early childhood [45]. Both SWS and slow-wave activity (EEG power between 0.75 and 4.5 Hz as derived from spectral analysis) show marked ontogenetic changes, which is believed to reflect cortical development and maturation [46]. Children exhibit significantly more SWS compared with adults, with a sharp decline during early adolescence (40% reduction between 11 and 14 years of age [47]), coinciding with a critical period of synaptic remodeling [46]. Growth hormone (GH) is secreted during SWS, with the timing and amount of GH secreted in early SWS temporally and quantitatively correlated with EEG delta wave activity [48] (although the putative relationship between SWS and GH has been debated [49]). In prepubertal children, GH is secreted exclusively during sleep, while in adolescence and adulthood it is also secreted during the day [50, 51].

More recently, the role of NREM sleep in memory formation and learning has received attention [52]. During NREM sleep, waking patterns of neuronal activity are reactivated, suggesting that information acquired during wakefulness is further processed during this sleep state [53]. Children are reported to show greater learning gains after sleep compared with adults, which has been attributed to their higher sleep slow-wave activity [54]. Also consistent with the hypotheses that NREM sleep is important for learning and memory, spectral analysis of slow wave activity (EEG power between 0.75 and 4.5 Hz) has revealed abnormalities in the topographical maturation of sleep wave activity in children with attention deficit/hyperactivity disorder [55], children at high risk of sociocultural handicap [56], and children with dyslexia [57].

The EEG of REM sleep is very different from that of NREM sleep and is characterized by low-voltage, mixed-frequency (mostly theta) activity, similar to that seen during wakefulness. Alpha activity is prominent in REM sleep but is typically 1 to 2 Hz slower than seen during wake [40] and trains of sawtooth waves in the theta frequency range (4–8 Hz), having a characteristic triangular/ serrated appearance, are commonly seen. Thus, during REM sleep the brain is significantly activated due to a high level of cortical activity. Neural firing is relatively desynchronized, resulting in a lower amplitude EEG signal. Two patterns of physiological behavior are seen in REM sleep: tonic and phasic. The tonic phase dominates REM sleep and is relatively quiescent, characterized by skeletal muscle atonia (a temporary paralysis) and the absence of eye movements. Phasic REM sleep is characterized by bursts of rapid, conjugate eye movements (REMS), transient muscle twitching and irregularities in respiration and heart rate [58]. In younger children and toddlers, blending of sleep states is not unusual, as various neuronal networks are still developing and maturing and thus features of NREM sleep such as spindles may be present in REM sleep [17]. One of the striking features of sleep in young children is the high amount of REM sleep they display, particularly in the first few years of life, leading to speculation that REM sleep plays a vital role in normal CNS development [11, 12]. The most compelling sources of evidence for this are that acetylcholine, an excitatory neurotransmitter released during REM sleep, is known to be important for neural development [59] and that REM sleep deprivation in animals corresponding to the human neonatal period results in abnormal structural and functional development of the CNS, especially the visual cortex [13, 60]. All terrestrial mammals studied to date demonstrate more REM sleep during early development compared with adulthood, with altricial species, such as humans and rats, showing comparatively higher proportions of REM to NREM sleep than precocial species, such as guinea pigs. Indeed, the proportion of REM to NREM sleep at birth in a species is used as a marker of brain maturity [61–63]. While newborns spend approximately 50% of the sleep period in active sleep (the developmental precursor to REM sleep; also see Chapter 8 of this volume), this has reduced to approximately 35% to 40% by 1 year of age, when the REM sleep EEG starts to display a more mature pattern. The proportion of REM sleep continues to decline during early childhood, reaching the adult level of 20% to 25% of total sleep time by approximately 5 years of age [17, 64].

In addition to the differences outlined above in the sleep EEG of children versus adults, a number of normal EEG patterns or variants can be seen during sleep in the pediatric age group that are not normally present in adults. These EEG patterns include anterior slow-wave activity, hypnagogic hypersynchrony, hypersynchronous theta, postarousal hypersynchrony, rhythmic anterior theta activity of drowsiness, and the frontal arousal rhythm [65]. While sleep development in normal children follows an organized and predictable pattern of change, beginning during fetal development and continuing into adolescence, there is significant interindividual variation in the trajectory of sleep maturation [17, 66]. Thus, variation is the rule rather than the exception.

Arousals

An important feature of sleep is arousals—discrete, generally transient events that may be associated with autonomic, motor/somatic, or EEG activation (e.g., an increase in heart rate, a change in body position and/or a reduction in sleep depth). Arousals are a normal feature of sleep that can be intrinsically generated (they often occur at sleep stage transitions), or they may be triggered by external events, particularly as a protective/defensive response (e.g., in response to hypoxia). Arousal generation is a graded process beginning with activation at the autonomic/brainstem level that progresses to the cortex (EEG) if the stimulus is sufficiently strong, resulting in a lightning of sleep or brief awakening. Arousal thresholds (i.e., the amount of stimulus required to activate an arousal) vary as a function of sleep stage and time of night: they are highest in SWS sleep and earlier in the night (a reflection of higher homeostatic sleep pressure at the start of the sleep period) and lower in REM sleep [67].

As with other aspects of sleep physiology, arousals demonstrate ontogenetic changes and differ from those of adults with respect to presentation, threshold, and frequency, particularly for protective arousals [68-74]. Children have been shown to have fewer cortical (EEG) arousals in the presence of pathological events such as episodes of abnormal breathing [75]; this may be due to sleep pressure being higher in children, meaning there are stronger protective mechanisms preventing EEG activation—possibly due to the importance of sleep-related CNS development during infancy and childhood [76, 77]. Arousal thresholds (and therefore frequency) are altered by a range of intrinsic and extrinsic factors including premature birth, sleeping position, thermal conditions, sleep deprivation, and drugs. Deficiencies in the arousal response are believed to play a role in the pathophysiology of sudden infant death syndrome (also see Chapter 8 of this volume) [78–81]. While arousals are a normal physiological feature of sleep and an important protective mechanism, excessive arousals result not only in fragmented and poor quality sleep but they also lead to wide-ranging adverse sequelae including metabolic/endocrine derangement, overactivation of the sympathetic nervous system, and disruption to numerous cellular processes that are crucial for normal physiological function and health [82] (Figure 9.2). Numerous intrinsic and extrinsic triggers can cause excessive arousals, including disorders of sleep (e.g., obstructive sleep apnea), behavioral factors (e.g., inability of a child to settle back to sleep), or external disturbances (e.g., noise, uncomfortable thermal environment).

While arousals are evident when viewing sleep EEG recordings in the conventional manner (i.e., visually in 30-second epochs) analysis of the microstructure of NREM sleep reveals that arousals are not just discrete, isolated events but rather are dynamically interwoven into the structure and behavior of NREM sleep—an endogenous arousal rhythm known as the cyclical alternating pattern (CAP) [83]. CAP is a periodic EEG pattern of arousal instability where transient EEG activation (phase A) alternates with the tonic background activity of NREM sleep (phase B). Three subtypes of phase A have been described based on the pattern of EEG activation [84]. Sleep periods that do not contain this biphasic EEG pattern (i.e., contain relatively few, randomly distributed episodes of EEG activation) are non-CAP and represent a period of stable sleep [85]. CAP is quantified using several parameters related to subtype frequency and rate, and normative data have been established across the human lifespan [84]. CAP parameters undergo maturational changes during infancy and childhood, when they show specific alterations

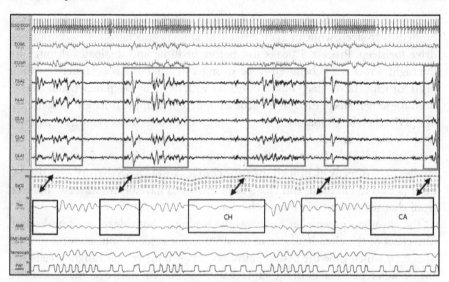

Figure 9.2 Two-minute recording derived from overnight polysomnography showing pathological cortical arousals during sleep in a child with sleep-disordered breathing. The 5 black lines in the upper panel are electroencephalography (EEG) recordings. The gray boxes show the appearance of cortical arousals in the EEG derivations while the flatter EEG periods in between the boxes show sleep. The arousals are occurring because the child is experiencing abnormal breathing events (central hypopneas and apneas), which can been seen in the bottom panel (black boxes) during sleep. Even though the hypopneas (CH—reduction in breathing effort) and apneas (CA—cessation of breathing effort) are not causing significant hypoxia (SaO2—pulse oximetry) the arousals are significantly fragmenting sleep. There is also significant activation of the sympathetic nervous system shown by the presence of tachycardia and bradycardia in the electrocardiographic (EKG) trace. Sleep fragmentation in the absence of significant hypoxia may contribute to the neurobehavioral deficits seen in some children with sleep disordered breathing.

in a variety of neurodevelopmental and sleep disorders commonly seen in the pediatric population [86–88]. Presently the clinical utilization of CAP is limited by our reliance on visual scoring of sleep, although advances in automated sleep detection will undoubtedly increase its applicability—not only in advancing our understanding of sleep neurophysiology but also in the diagnosis and management of sleep disorders.

Physiological Regulation of Sleep

Two major regulatory processes govern the timing and distribution of wake–sleep in healthy humans: a circadian process (Process C) and a sleep-wake homeostatic process (Process S; also see Chapter 4 of this volume). While there is no specific anatomical location for the homeostatic control of sleep, this system is regulated by an intrinsic neurophysiological process that is driven by the accumulation of prior sleep or wake time. As the duration of wakefulness increases, so does the propensity to sleep, while increased sleep duration is associated with a diminished drive for sleep. Process S peaks just before bedtime and dissipates throughout the night. Process S is believed to be stronger in children, as evidenced by their need for naps, faster sleep onset, difficulty with delaying sleep onset, and overall need for longer sleep. Process S becomes apparent at approximately 2 months of age [89]. As children mature, Process S diminishes with the cessation of napping, later bedtimes, consolidated sleep–wake pattern, and shorter sleep periods. N3 sleep and EEG SWS density are thought to be markers of Process S [90]. As yet, no studies have directly examined the time course of EEG SWS density over the 24-hour period in children, and changes in Process S have been indirectly inferred from changes observed in sleep behavior.

The circadian pacemaker regulates the timing of both sleep onset and offset. The effect of the circadian system on sleep is not evident until about 3 months of age, by which time the neural pathways between the retinal ganglion cells and the circadian pacemaker in the suprachiasmatic nucleus have become established thus permitting the entrainment of the circadian pacemaker by light exposure. The circadian system has a strong influence on timing of sleep over the developmental period from late infancy to preadolescence. In general, children struggle to delay sleep onset and typically fall asleep at the same time regardless of the day of the week, and, similarly, they spontaneously awaken at the same time regardless of whether it is a school versus nonschool night [91]. Despite this stability, there is nevertheless a trend with age toward later sleep onsets and offsets (i.e., a shift toward a more eveningness chronotype [92–94]). There is also a gradual increase in the phase angle between the circadian pacemaker and the timing of sleep onset [95] and a trend with age for larger differences in the timing of sleep onset/offset between school compared to nonschool nights [96].

In addition to the homeostatic and circadian regulation of sleep-wake, NREM and REM sleep display an ultradian rhythm (<24-hour cycle), alternating in a regular, predictable pattern throughout the sleep period. As with other aspects of sleep, the ultradian rhythm shows marked developmental changes across the human lifespan (Figure 9.3). By 1 year of age sleep has attained a more mature pattern; the proportion of NREM sleep is now greater than REM sleep, which is a reversal of the relationship seen at birth [64] with changes in sleep architecture occurring more slowly than seen in the first 12 months of life [17, 97]. During the preschool years, sleep shifts from a polyphasic to a monophasic modality and as childhood progresses sleep becomes more consolidated at night with fewer daytime naps. Sleep cycles become longer, sleep cycle length is approximately 60 minutes in duration at 2 to 3 years of age, which gradually increases to 90 minutes by age 5 years (Sheldon, 1996). As childhood progresses, SWS is reduced, with a preponderance of SWS early in the night and REM sleep later in the night [97] and sleep duration slowly decreases; the adult pattern of sleep is usually observed by the end of adolescence [98].

A marked change in sleep behavior over childhood is the consolidation of sleep with the reduction in the frequency and length of naps, diminution in the number

A. Newborn infant

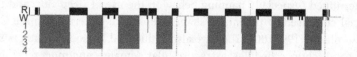

B. Two and a half years of age

C. Five years of age

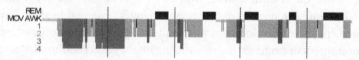

Figure 9.3 Normal ontogenetic changes in sleep architecture between birth to early childhood. Each of the three sleep hypnograms shows the progressive cycling of sleep throughout one night as recoded during overnight polysomnography in a sleep laboratory. *Hypnogram A*: The sleep EEG of infants is less differentiated compared to older children and adults with three main sleep states recognized: active sleep (black blocks), quiet sleep (dark gray blocks) and indeterminate sleep (light gray blocks). Sleep onset is usually via active sleep which occupies up to 50% of total sleep time in the neonatal period. Sleep cycles are relatively short with active sleep and quiet sleep being of similar duration. *Hypnogram B*: Differentiation of the sleep EEG occurs rapidly over the first twelve months of life and by two and a half years of age the sleep EEG has significantly matured. Quiet sleep has now become differentiated into nonrapid eye movement (NREM) sleep: N1 (medium gray blocks), N2 (light gray blocks), N3 or slow wave sleep (black periods). Black blocks represent rapid eye movement (REM) sleep. The proportion of REM sleep has declined markedly compared to birth with slow wave sleep occurring regularly during the night. Sleep cycles are now longer in duration and sleep onset begins with NREM sleep. *Hypnogram C*: By 5 years of age, the distribution of NREM and REM sleep has changed with a preponderance of slow-wave sleep in the first third of the night and REM sleep occurring more in the latter part of the sleep period (same color key as hypnogram B).

of nocturnal awakenings, reduced reliance on sleep aids (e.g., pacifiers), and establishment of a single nocturnal sleep period. These changes are partly culturally determined (especially napping behavior, the use of sleep aids, and the types of social cues used by parents to shape sleep–wake patterns; also see Chapter 5 of this volume) [99, 100]. They are also influenced by societal factors such as day care and school schedules, extracurricular demands and more recently the intrusion of digital technologies into the bedroom [101–104]. As previously discussed, they are also biologically driven as evinced by the developmental trajectories of Process S and Process C. During childhood, the capacity to self-regulate/self-soothe at night is learned [105], and approaching adolescence, the parental control of bedtime and especially wake-up times are increasingly devolved to the responsibility of the child [94, 106].

Pathological Sleep

Childhood sleep problems are very common and may present as insufficient sleep, disrupted sleep or abnormal timing of wake–sleep (also see Chapter 16 of this volume). The etiology of sleep disorders can be behavioral or physiological, or a combination of both factors, which can operate in a bidirectional or synergistic fashion. The normal maturational changes observed in sleep physiology may predispose the development of specific sleep disorders, some of which are more prominent or occur exclusively, during infancy and childhood. For example, rhythmic movement disorders often emerge in infancy and generally self-resolve by early childhood [107]; NREM sleep parasomnias are more common in early childhood when SWS and sleep depth are at their highest [108, 109]; sudden infant death syndrome occurs in infancy when relatively unstable cardiorespiratory control is coupled with high amounts of REM sleep (also see Chapter 8 of this volume). Various medical conditions increase the risk of developing sleep disorders and, while also seen in adulthood, often have different presentations and sequelae in children. These include structural or anatomical abnormalities of the upper airway which increase the risk of obstructive sleep apnea; neurological defects causing central sleep apnea; visual impairments which invariably result in circadian rhythm disorders; neurodevelopmental disorders such as epilepsy and cerebral palsy where CNS abnormalities can disrupt sleep regulation, particularly via irregularities in melatonin secretion [110, 111]. In addition to the previously described sleep problems, a higher incidence of sleep disorders are observed in children with chronic physical illness or impairment, especially if causing discomfort or pain (e.g., juvenile arthritis, eczema, asthma) where symptoms sometimes worsen at night [112–115]. Children with psychiatric and neurodevelopmental disabilities (e.g., attention-deficit/hyperactivity disorder, autism) demonstrate high rates of sleep disorders, which can be attributed to both psychosocial and physiological factors [110, 116].

In addition to any contemporaneous effects on daytime functioning, sleep problems early in life are reported to predict daytime deficits later in life. For example, longitudinal studies report that sleep problems in preschool children predict anxiety and depression in middle childhood [117] and socioemotional difficulties in adolescence [118].

Medications, especially psychotropic and antiepileptic drugs, can also have marked effects of sleep structure and behavior including causing significant sleepiness, increasing sleep fragmentation, suppressing REM sleep, altering arousal thresholds, and modifying the behavior of EEG oscillations such as sleep spindles [119, 120]. The long-term sequelae of these effects have not been well studied. Pharmaceuticals have also been shown to induce or worsen some sleep disorders in children such as insomnia, sleep walking, movement disorders, and sleep-disordered breathing [121–123].

CONSEQUENCES OF INADEQUATE SLEEP

The importance of sleep for health and optimal daytime functioning are now well recognized. Healthy sleep is characterized by optimal duration, consistent night-to-night timing and normally distributed sleep architecture. Notably, healthy sleep is sometimes assessed by the construct sleep quality which depending on the research study may encompass one or more of the elements making up healthy sleep or a conflation of the elements. In the literature there is an ongoing debate as to the relative importance of sleep quality versus duration for optimal daytime functioning. Sleep quality is difficult to define without the use of polysomnography to assess sleep architecture, sleep timing, and the presence or absence of an occult sleep disorder. In most child studies, sleep quality is assessed using parental report (also see Chapter 23 of this volume) with questions that typically assess whether sleep is restorative or disrupted (e.g. problems with sleep onset or awakenings at night) and, less frequently, by questions assessing the night-to-night consistency in the timing of sleep. Sleep quality may also be a surrogate measure of brain maturity and, therefore, some of the associations between measures of sleep quality and neurocognitive/behavioral functioning may reflect issues to do with brain maturity rather than sleep per se. This complicates the interpretation of findings, especially in very young children.

Findings from meta-analytical studies indicate that short sleep duration is associated with an increased risk of obesity, type 2 diabetes, difficult temperament, poor cognitive performance (although not memory or sustained attention), emotional dysregulation, behavioral problems, and poor academic performance [124–127]. Moreover, the effect of poor sleep on cognitive performance is reportedly more pronounced in younger compared with older children [128]. An emerging literature also indicates that short sleep duration is associated with decreased insulin sensitivity, elevated blood pressure, and potentially altered brain structure [9]. It is noteworthy that much of the literature has focused on short sleep as an explanation for daytime deficits in children. A less well-explored aspect is excessive sleep length. A U-shaped rather than linear relationship has been reported between child sleep length and externalized behavior, with both short and long sleep duration associated with higher level of behavioral problems and worse physical health [129].

Sleep architecture can be disrupted by both sociobehavioral and medical factors. Sociobehavioral factors include parental anxiety, insecure maternal–child attachment and maternal depression. Medical factors include arousals, parasomnias, pain, and atopy. The most thoroughly studied medical condition is sleep-disordered breathing, which is associated with impaired neuropsychological functioning and increased problematic behavior [130, 131]. Treatment of sleep-disordered breathing with adenotonsillectomy is reported to reverse behavioral but not neurocognitive deficits, suggesting that sleep fragmentation may have a stronger impact on cognitive function than hitherto thought [132, 133].

The importance of night-to-night sleep regularity for daytime functioning is less well studied and meta-analytical studies are lacking. Developmental changes in night-to-night variability in the timing of sleep are not especially evident in childhood. This can be attributed to the greater parental control over sleep behavior in this developmental period [94]. Nonetheless, there is compelling evidence that routine is important for sleep quality. Maintaining a constant bedtime routine, especially consistency over weekday and weekend nights, is reported to benefit sleep in young infants [134]. Conversely, greater night-to-night variability (especially large differences in sleep timing on school versus weekend nights) is associated with a higher frequency of behavioral problems [135]. Together with regularity, the timing of sleep may also be important. In children, irregular, together with late, bedtimes have been associated with poor sleep and a higher frequency of problematic behaviors [136–138]. Circadian-related sleep disorders such as delayed sleep phase syndrome are more commonly reported in adolescents (also see Chapter 15 of this volume). However, it is likely that a predisposition to an eveningness chronotype can occur much earlier in life with a consequential impact on sleep quality [95, 96]. The latter findings point to the often underappreciated contribution that "circadian hygiene" plays in maintaining healthy sleep and optimal daytime functioning.

A child's sleep can also affect family functioning. In young and otherwise healthy children, reduced family well-being has been associated with settling problems, ability to self-soothe after a nocturnal awakening and parasomnias (especially night terrors and sleepwalking) [139]. In later childhood, insomnia and parasomnias (such as nightmares) are more likely to impact family well-being [109]. Studies investigating the impact of child sleep on family functioning have mostly examined the impact on maternal well-being and typically report impaired mother–child attachment, reduced maternal well-being, and reduced marital satisfaction [140–143] (also see Chapter 13 of this volume). Only a few studies have examined the impact on fathers but generally report poorer well-being and health [143, 144]. The impact on siblings is poorly documented but disturbed sleep and increased stress are typically reported [145, 146].

It is noteworthy that the relationship between child sleep and daytime functioning is bidirectional [147]. For example, poor sleep is reported to have a persistent negative effect on emotional regulation, which itself can, in turn, contribute to ongoing sleep problems and poorer attentional regulation [148]. The same applies to the relationship between child sleep and family functioning. For example, weak maternal attachment and poor maternal health are associated with poor infant sleep [149, 150].

CONCLUSION AND FUTURE DIRECTIONS

Findings from many studies have shown that inadequate or disturbed sleep during childhood is associated with adverse outcomes across a range of physical, cognitive, and behavioral domains. While the pathophysiology underlying these observations is not yet fully understood due to the complex interplay of biological, environmental, and psychosocial factors influencing sleep, there is sufficient evidence to suggest that more research is needed to elucidate the causal pathways. Childhood sleep is increasingly viewed in a developmental context, with an emerging perspective that the early identification and management of inadequate or disturbed sleep has the potential to prevent the development of adverse functional outcomes/deficits later life and potentially ameliorate neurodevelopmental impairments in children with brain injury such as cerebral palsy [151, 152]. Childhood sleep represents a vulnerable time for normal growth and development, and the timely recognition and treatment of inadequate or disturbed sleep are therefore critical.

REFERENCES

1. Tononi G, Cirelli C. Sleep function and synaptic homeostasis. *Sleep Med Rev.* 2006;10:49–62.
2. Léger D, Debellemaniere E, Rabat A, Bayon V, Benchenane K, Chennaoui M. Slow-wave sleep: from the cell to the clinic. *Sleep Med Rev.* 2018;41:113–132.
3. Van Someren EJW, Cirelli C, Dijk D-J, Van Cauter E, Schwartz S, Chee MWL. Disrupted sleep: from molecules to cognition. *J Neurosci.* 2015;35:13889–13895.
4. Tononi G, Cirelli C. Modulation of brain gene expression during sleep and wakefulness: a review of recent findings. *Neuropsychopharmacology.* 2001;25:S28–S35.
5. Pfaff A, Schlarb AA. Does your childhood define how you sleep and love? *Somnologie.* 2018;22:175–182.
6. Thomas AG, Monahan KC, Lukowski AF, Cauffman E. Sleep problems across development: a pathway to adolescent risk taking through working memory. *J Youth Adolesc.* 2015;44:447–464.
7. Palagini L, Domschke K, Benedetti F, Foster RG, Wulff K, Riemann D. Developmental pathways towards mood disorders in adult life: is there a role for sleep disturbances? *J Affect Disord.* 2019;243:121–132.
8. Young J, Savoy C, Schmidt LA, Saigal S, Van Lieshout RJ. Child sleep problems and adult mental health in those born at term or extremely low birth weight. *Sleep Med.* 2019;53:28–34.

9. Dutil C, Walsh JJ, Featherstone RB, et al. Influence of sleep on developing brain functions and structures in children and adolescents: a systematic review. *Sleep Med Rev.* 2018;42:184–201.

10. Li W, Ma L, Yang G, Gan W-B. REM sleep selectively prunes and maintains new synapses in development and learning. *Nat Neurosci.* 2017;20:427.

11. Roffwarg HP, Muzio JN, Dement WC. Ontogenetic development of the human sleep-dream cycle. *Science.* 1966;152:604–619.

12. Marks GA, Shaffery JP, Oksenberg A, Speciale SG, Roffwarg HP. A functional role for REM sleep in brain maturation. *Behav Brain Res.* 1995;69:1–11.

13. Frank MG, Issa NP, Stryker MP. Sleep Enhances plasticity in the developing visual cortex. *Neuron.* 2001;30:275–287.

14. Blumberg M. Beyond Dreams: Do sleep-related movements contribute to brain development? *Front Neurol.* 2010;1:1–10.

15. Kilb W, Kirischuk S, Luhmann HJ. Electrical activity patterns and the functional maturation of the neocortex. *Eur J Neurosci.* 2011;34:1677–1686.

16. Campbell IG, Feinberg I. Maturational patterns of sigma frequency power across childhood and adolescence: a longitudinal study. *Sleep.* 2016;39:193–201.

17. Sheldon SH. Development of sleep structure. In: Sheldon SH, ed. *Evaluating Sleep in Infants and Children.* Philadelphia, PA: Lippincott-Raven; 1996:11–20.

18. Jenni OG, Carskadon MA. Normal human sleep at different ages: infants to adolescents. In: *SRS Basics of Sleep Guide.* Westchester, IL: Sleep Research Society 2005:11–20.

19. Parmelee AH, Stern E. Development of states in infants. In: Clemente CD, Pupura DP, Mayer FE, eds. *Sleep and the Maturing Nervous System.* New York: Academic Press 1972:199–228.

20. Prechtl HFR. The behavioural states of the newborn infant (a review). *Brain Res.* 1974;76:185–212.

21. Curzi-Dascalova L. Developmental trend of sleep characteristics in premature and full-term newborns. In: Mathew OP, ed. *Respiratory Control and Disorders in the Newborn.* New York, NY: Marcel-Dekker; 2003:149–182.

22. Brown RE, Basheer R, McKenna JT, Strecker RE, McCarley RW. Control of sleep and wakefulness. *Physiol Rev.* 2012;92:1087–1187.

23. Rector DM, Schei JL, Van Dongen HPA, Belenky G, Krueger JM. Physiological markers of local sleep. *Eur J Neurosci.* 2009;29:1771–1778.

24. Nir Y, Staba RJ, Andrillon T, et al. Regional slow waves and spindles in human sleep. *Neuron.* 2011;70:153–169.

25. Krueger JM, Nguyen JT, Dykstra-Aiello CJ, Taishi P. Local sleep. *Sleep Med Rev.* 2019;43:14–21.

26. Scholle S, Schaefer T. Atlas of sleep and wakefulness in infants and children. *Somnologie.* 1999;3:163–165.

27. Grigg-Damberger MM, Gozal D, Marcus CL, et al. The visual scoring of sleep and arousal in infants and children. *J Clin Sleep Med.* 2007;3:201–240.

28. Carskadon MA, Dement W. Normal human sleep: an overview. In: Kryger M, Roth T, Dement W, eds. *Principles and Practice of Sleep Medicine.* 6th ed. Philadelphia, PA: Elsevier Inc; 2017:15–24.

29. Division of Sleep Medicine, Harvard Medical School. Glossary. http://healthysleep. med.harvard.edu/healthy/glossary/n-p. Published 2009 Retrieved August 26, 2019.

30. Shinomiya S, Nagata K, Takahashi K, Masumura T. Development of sleep spindles in young children and adolescents. *Clin Electroencephal.* 1999;30:39–43.

31. Hobson JA, Pace-Schott EF. The cognitive neuroscience of sleep: neuronal systems, consciousness and learning. *Nat Rev Neurosci.* 2002;3:679–693.

32. Weiner OM, Dang-Vu TT. Spindle oscillations in sleep disorders: a systematic review. *Neural Plast.* 2016;2016:7328725.

33. Hirshkowitz M, John IT, Karacan I. Sleep spindles: pharmacological effects in humans. *Sleep.* 1982;5:85–94.

34. Brienza M, Pulitano P, Mecarelli O. Effects on EEG of drugs and toxic substances. In: Mecarelli O, ed. *Clinical Electroencephalography.* Cham, Switzerland: Springer International; 2019:715–729.

35. Barone I, Hawks-Mayer H, Lipton JO. Mechanisms of sleep and circadian ontogeny through the lens of neurodevelopmental disorders. *Neurobiol Learn and Mem.* 2019;160:160–172.

36. Wulff K, Gatti S, Wettstein JG, Foster RG. Sleep and circadian rhythm disruption in psychiatric and neurodegenerative disease. *Nat Rev Neurosci.* 2010;11:589.

37. Fogel SM, Smith CT. The function of the sleep spindle: a physiological index of intelligence and a mechanism for sleep-dependent memory consolidation. *Neurosci Biobehav Rev.* 2011;35:1154–1165.

38. Kurdziel L, Duclos K, Spencer RMC. Sleep spindles in midday naps enhance learning in preschool children. *P Natl Acad Sci USA* 2013;110:17267–1772.

39. Vermeulen MCM, Van der Heijden KB, Swaab H, Van Someren EJW. Sleep spindle characteristics and sleep architecture are associated with learning of executive functions in school-age children. *J Sleep Res.* 2019;28:e12779.

40. Rechtschaffen A, Kales A. *A Manual of Standardized Terminology, Techniques, and Scoring Systems for Sleep Stages of Human Subjects.* Los Angeles, CA: Brain Information/Brain Research Institute UCLA; 1968.

41. Metcalf DR, Mondale J, Butler FK. Ontogenesis of spontaneous K-complexes. *Psychophysiology.* 1971;8:340–347.

42. Colrain IM. The K-complex: a 7-decade history. *Sleep.* 2005;28:255–273.

43. Halász P. K-complex, a reactive EEG graphoelement of NREM sleep: an old chap in a new garment. *Sleep Med Rev.* 2005;9:391–412.

44. Kurth S, Jenni OG, Riedner BA, Tononi G, Carskadon MA, Huber R. Characteristics of sleep slow waves in children and adolescents. *Sleep.* 2010;33:475–480.

45. Kotagal S. Parasomnias in childhood. *Sleep Med Rev.* 2009;13:157–68.

46. Buchmann A, Ringli M, Kurth S, et al. EEG sleep slow-wave activity as a mirror of cortical maturation. *Cereb Cortex.* 2010;21:607–615.

47. Jenni OG, Carskadon MA. Spectral analysis of the sleep electroencephalogram during adolescence. *Sleep.* 2004;27:774–783.

48. Gronfier C, Luthringer R, Follenius M, et al. A quantitative evaluation of the relationships between growth hormone secretion and delta wave electroencephalographic activity during normal sleep and after enrichment in delta waves. *Sleep.* 1996;19:817–824.

49. Brandenberger G, Weibel L. The 24-h growth hormone rhythm in men: sleep and circadian influences questioned. *J Sleep Res.* 2004;13:251–255.

50. Sheldon SH. Sleep in infants and children. In: Teofilo LC, ed. *Sleep: A Comprehensive Handbook.* Hoboken, NJ: Wiley-Liss; 2005:507–510.

51. Copinschi G, Challet E. Endocrine rhythms, the sleep-sake cycle, and biological clocks. In: Jameson JL, De Groot LJ, de Kretser DM, Giudice LC, Grossman AB, Melmed S, et al., eds. *Endocrinology: Adult and Pediatric.* 7th ed. Philadelphia, PA: Elsevier Saunders; 2016:199–229.

52. Cirelli C, Tononi G. Cortical development, electroencephalogram rhythms, and the sleep/wake cycle. *Biol Psychiatr.* 2015;77:1071–1078.

53. Stickgold R, Walker MP. Sleep-dependent memory triage: evolving generalization through selective processing. *Nat Neurosci.* 2013;16:139.

54. Wilhelm I, Rose M, Imhof KI, Rasch B, Büchel C, Born J. The sleeping child outplays the adult's capacity to convert implicit into explicit knowledge. *Nat Neurosci.* 2013;16:391.

55. Ringli M, Souissi S, Kurth S, Brandeis D, Jenni OG, Huber R. Topography of sleep slow wave activity in children with attention-deficit/hyperactivity disorder. *Cortex.* 2013;49:340–347.

56. Otero GA. EEG spectral analysis in children with sociocultural handicaps. *Int J Neurosci.* 1994;79:213–220.

57. Bruni O, Ferri R, Novelli L, et al. Slow EEG amplitude oscillations during NREM sleep and reading disabilities in children with dyslexia. *Dev Neuropsychol.* 2009;34:539–551.

58. Rama AN, Cho SC, Kushida CA. NREM–REM sleep. *Handb Clin Neurophysiol.* 2005;6:21–29.

59. Jones BE. Arousal and sleep circuits. *Neuropsychopharmacology.* 2020;45(1):6–20.

60. Dang-Vu TT, Desseilles M, Peigneux P, Maquet P. A role for sleep in brain plasticity. *Pediatr Rehab.* 2006;9:98–118.

61. Jouvet-Mounier D, Astic L, Lacote D. Ontogenesis of the states of sleep in rat, cat, and guinea pig during the first postnatal month. *Dev Psychobiol.* 1969;2:216–239.

62. Kurth S, Dean DC, Achermann P, et al. Increased sleep depth in developing neural networks: new insights from sleep restriction in children. *Front Human Neurosci.* 2016;10:456.

63. Kurth S, Olini N, Huber R, LeBourgeois M. Sleep and early cortical development. *Curr Sleep Med Rep.* 2015;1:64–73.

64. Anders TF, Keener MA. Developmental course of nighttime sleep-wake patterns in full-term and premature infants during the first year of life: I. *Sleep.* 1985;8:173–192.

65. Grigg-Damberger MM. Ontogeny of sleep and its functions in infancy, childhood, and adolescence. In: Nevšímalová S, Bruni O, eds. *Sleep Disorders in Children.* Cham, Switzerland: Springer International; 2017:3–29.

66. Hoppenbrouwers T, Hodgman J, Arakawa K, Geidel SA, Sterman MB. Sleep and waking states in infancy: normative studies. *Sleep.* 1988;11:387–401.

67. Busby KA, Mercier L, Pivik RT. Ontogenetic variations in auditory arousal threshold during sleep. *Psychophysiology.* 1994;31:182–188.

68. Mograss MA, Ducharme FM, Brouillette RT. Movement/arousals: description, classification, and relationship to sleep apnea in children. *Am J Respir Crit Care Med.* 1994;150:1690–1696.

69. Boselli M, Parrino L, Smerieri A, Terzano MG. Effect of age on EEG arousals in normal sleep. *Sleep.* 1998;21:361–367.

70. Scholle S, Zwacka G. Arousals and obstructive sleep apnea syndrome in children. *Clin Neurophysiol.* 2001;112:984–991.

71. Guilleminault C, Poyares D. Arousal and upper airway resistance (UAR). *Sleep Med.* 2002;3:S15–S20.

72. Gilmartin GS, Thomas RJ. Mechanisms of arousal from sleep and their consequences. *Curr Opin Pulm Med.* 2004;10:468–474.

73. Montemitro E, Franco P, Scaillet S, et al. Maturation of spontaneous arousals in healthy infants. *Sleep.* 2008;31:47–54.

74. Wulbrand H, McNamara F, Thach BT. The role of arousal related brainstem reflexes in causing recovery from upper airway occlusion in infants. *Sleep.* 2008;31: 833–840.

75. Marcus CL, Lutz J, Carroll JL, Bamford O. Arousal and ventilatory responses during sleep in children with obstructive sleep apnea. *J Appl Physiol.* 1998;84:1926–1936.

76. McNamara F, Issa FG, Sullivan CE. Arousal pattern following central and obstructive breathing abnormalities in infants and children. *J Appl Physiol.* 1996;81: 2651–2657.

77. Ward SLD, Bautista DB, Keens TC. Hypoxic arousal responses in normal infants. *Pediatrics.* 1992;89:860–864.

78. Horne RSC, Ferens D, Watts A-M, et al. The prone sleeping position impairs arousability in term infants. *J Pediatr.* 2001;138:811–816.

79. Machaalani R, Waters KA. Neurochemical abnormalities in the brainstem of the sudden infant death syndrome (SIDS). *Paediatr Resp Rev.* 2014;15:293–300.

80. Vivekanandarajah A, Waters KA, Machaalani R. Cigarette smoke exposure effects on the brainstem expression of nicotinic acetylcholine receptors (nAChRs), and on cardiac, respiratory and sleep physiologies. *Resp Physiol Neurobiol.* 2019;259:1–15.

81. Franco P, Montemitro E, Scaillet S, et al. Fewer spontaneous arousals in infants with apparent life-threatening event. *Sleep.* 2011;34:733–743.

82. Kheirandish L, Gozal D. Neurocognitive dysfunction in children with sleep disorders. *Dev Sci.* 2006;9:388–399.

83. Terzano MG, Mancia D, Salati MR, Costani G, Decembrino A, Parrino L. The cyclic alternating pattern as a physiologic component of normal NREM sleep. *Sleep.* 1985;8:137–145.

84. Parrino L, Terzano MG. Central nervous system arousals and cyclic alternating patterns. In: Kryger M, Roth T, Dement WC, eds. *Principles and Practice of Sleep Medicine.* 6th ed. Philadelphia, PA Elsevier; 2017:1576–1587.

85. Ferri R, Parrino L, Smerieri A, et al. Cyclic alternating pattern and spectral analysis of heart rate variability during normal sleep. *J Sleep Res.* 2000;9:13–18.

86. Bruni O, Novelli L, Miano S, Parrino L, Terzano MG, Ferri R. Cyclic alternating pattern: A window into pediatric sleep. *Sleep Med.* 2010;11:628–636.

87. Parrino L, Ferri R, Bruni O, Terzano MG. Cyclic alternating pattern (CAP): the marker of sleep instability. *Sleep Med Rev.* 2012;16:27e45.

88. Ferri R, Novelli L, Bruni O. EEG and sleep during development. In: Gozal LK, Gozal D, eds. *Sleep Disordered Breathing in Children: A Comprehensive Guide to Evaluation and Treatment.* Totowa, NJ: Humana Press 2012;73–84.

89. Jenni OG, LeBourgeois MK. Understanding sleep–wake behavior and sleep disorders in children: the value of a model. *Curr Opin Psychiatr.* 2006;19:282.

90. Dijk DJ, Beersma DGM, Daan S. EEG power density during nap sleep: reflection of an hourglass measuring the duration of prior wakefulness. *J Biol Rhyth.* 1987;2:207–219.

91. Werner H, LeBourgeois MK, Geiger A, Jenni OG. Assessment of chronotype in four-to eleven-year-old children: reliability and validity of the Children's Chronotype Questionnaire (CCTQ). *Chronobiol Int.* 2009;26:992–1014.

92. Park YM, Seo YJ, Matsumoto K, Shinkoda H. Sleep and chronotype for children in Japan. *Percept Motor Skills.* 1999;88:1315–1329.

93. Simpkin CT, Jenni OG, Carskadon MA, et al. Chronotype is associated with the timing of the circadian clock and sleep in toddlers. *J Sleep Res.* 2014;23:397–405.

94. Russo PM, Bruni O, Lucidi F, Ferri R, Violani C. Sleep habits and circadian preference in Italian children and adolescents. *J Sleep Res.* 2007;16:163–169.

95. LeBourgeois MK, Carskadon MA, Akacem LD, et al. Circadian phase and its relationship to nighttime sleep in toddlers. *J Biol Rhyth.* 2013;28:322–331.

96. Kuula L, Pesonen A-K, Merikanto I, et al. Development of late circadian preference: sleep timing from childhood to late adolescence. *J Pediatr.* 2018;194:182–189.

97. Kahn A, Dan B, Groswasser J, Franco P, Sottiaux M. Normal sleep architecture in infants and children. *J Clin Neurophysiol.* 1996;13:184–197.

98. Scholle S, Beyer U, Bernhard M, et al. Normative values of polysomnographic parameters in childhood and adolescence: quantitative sleep parameters. *Sleep Med.* 2011;12:542–549.

99. Jenni OG, O'Connor BB. Children's sleep: an interplay between culture and biology. *Pediatrics.* 2005;115:204–216.

100. Sadeh A, Mindell J, Rivera L. "My child has a sleep problem": a cross-cultural comparison of parental definitions. *Sleep Med.* 2011;12:478–482.

101. Taras H, Potts-Datema W. Sleep and student performance at school. *J School Health.* 2005;75:248–254.

102. LeBourgeois MK, Hale L, Chang A-M, Akacem LD, Montgomery-Downs HE, Buxton OM. Digital media and sleep in childhood and adolescence. *Pediatrics.* 2017;140:S92–S96.

103. Carissimi A, Dresch F, Martins AC, et al. The influence of school time on sleep patterns of children and adolescents. *Sleep Med.* 2016;19:33–39.

104. Lushington K, Wilson A, Biggs S, Dollman J, Martin J, Kennedy D. Culture, extracurricular activity, sleep habits, and mental health: a comparison of senior high school Asian-Australian and Caucasian-Australian adolescents. *Int J Ment Health.* 2015;44:139–157.

105. Sadeh A, Tikotzky L, Scher A. Parenting and infant sleep. *Sleep Med Rev.* 2010;14:89–96.

106. Short MA, Gradisar M, Wright H, Lack LC, Dohnt H, Carskadon MA. Time for bed: parent-set bedtimes associated with improved sleep and daytime functioning in adolescents. *Sleep.* 2011;34:797–800.

107. Gwyther AR, Walters AS, Hill CM. Rhythmic movement disorder in childhood: an integrative review. *Sleep Med Rev.* 2017;35:62–75.

108. Markov D, Jaffe F, Doghramji K. Update on parasomnias: a review for psychiatric practice. *Psychiatry.* 2006;3:69–76.

109. Petit D, Touchette É, Tremblay RE, Boivin M, Montplaisir J. Dyssomnias and parasomnias in early childhood. *Pediatrics.* 2007;119:e1016–e1025.

110. Lélis ALPA, Cardoso MVLM, Hall WA. Sleep disorders in children with cerebral palsy: an integrative review. *Sleep Med Rev.* 2016;30:63–71.

111. van Golde EGA, Gutter T, de Weerd AW. Sleep disturbances in people with epilepsy; prevalence, impact and treatment. *Sleep Med Rev.* 2011;15:357–368.

112. Stores G, Ellis AJ, Wiggs L, Crawford C, Thomson A. Sleep and psychological disturbance in nocturnal asthma. *Arch Dis Child.* 1998;78:413–419.

113. Comas M, Gordon CJ, Oliver BG, et al. A circadian based inflammatory response: implications for respiratory disease and treatment. *Sleep Sci Pract.* 2017;1:18.

114. Camfferman D, Kennedy JD, Gold M, Martin AJ, Lushington K. Eczema and sleep and its relationship to daytime functioning in children. *Sleep Med Rev.* 2010;14:359–369.

115. van der Giessen L, Bakker M, Joosten K, Hop W, Tiddens H. Nocturnal oxygen saturation in children with stable cystic fibrosis. *Pediatr Pulmonol.* 2012;47:1123–1130.

116. Richdale AL, Schreck KA. Sleep problems in autism spectrum disorders: prevalence, nature, & possible biopsychosocial aetiologies. *Sleep Med Rev.* 2009;13:403–411.

117. Foley JE, Weinraub M. Sleep, affect, and social competence from preschool to preadolescence: distinct pathways to emotional and social adjustment for boys and for girls. *Front Psychol.* 2017;8:711.

118. Jung E, Jin B. Associations between sleep problems, cognitive, and socioemotional functioning from preschool to adolescence. *Child Youth Care Forum.* 2019;48(6):829–848.

119. Brown LW. Medications. In: Accardo JA, ed. *Sleep in Children with Neurodevelopmental Disabilities: An Evidence-Based Guide.* Cham, Swizterland: Springer International; 2019:319–329.

120. Nita DA, Weiss SK. Sleep and epilepsy. In: Accardo JA, ed. *Sleep in Children With Neurodevelopmental Disabilities: An Evidence-Based Guide.* Cham, Switzerland: Springer International; 2019:227–240.

121. Stallman HM, Kohler M, White J. Medication induced sleepwalking: a systematic review. *Sleep Med Rev.* 2018;37:105–113.

122. Owens JA, Rosen CL, Mindell JA, Kirchner HL. Use of pharmacotherapy for insomnia in child psychiatry practice: a national survey. *Sleep Med.* 2010;11:692–700.

123. Zutler M, C. Holty J-E. Opioids, sleep, and sleep-disordered breathing. *Current Pharma Design.* 2011;17:1443–1449.

124. El-Sheikh M, Philbrook LE, Kelly RJ, Hinnant JB, Buckhalt JA. What does a good night's sleep mean? Nonlinear relations between sleep and children's cognitive functioning and mental health. *Sleep.* 2019;42(6):zsz078.

125. Quist JS, Sjödin A, Chaput J-P, Hjorth MF. Sleep and cardiometabolic risk in children and adolescents. *Sleep Med Rev.* 2016;29:76–100.

126. Astill RG, Van der Heijden KB, Van Ijzendoorn MH, Van Someren EJW. Sleep, cognition, and behavioral problems in school-age children: a century of research meta-analyzed. *Psychol Bull.* 2012;138:1109–1138.

127. Geiger A, Achermann P, Jenni OG. Sleep, intelligence and cognition in a developmental context: differentiation between traits and state-dependent aspects. In: Kerkhof GA, van Dongen HPA, eds. *Progress in Brain Research.* Philadelphia, PA: Elsevier; 2010:167–179.

128. Dewald JF, Meijer AM, Oort FJ, Kerkhof GA, Bögels SM. The influence of sleep quality, sleep duration and sleepiness on school performance in children and adolescents: a meta-analytic review. *Sleep Med Rev.* 2010;14:179–189.

157

129. James S, Hale L. Sleep duration and child well-being: a nonlinear association. *J Clin Child Adolesc Psychol*. 2017;46:258–268.
130. Blunden S, Lushington K, Kennedy D, Martin J, Dawson D. Behavior and neurocognitive performance in children aged 5–10 years who snore compared to controls. *J Clin Child Adolesc Psychol*. 2000;22:554–568.
131. O'Brien LM, Gozal D. Behavioural and neurocognitive implications of snoring and obstructive sleep apnoea in children: facts and theory. *Paediatr Respir Rev*. 2002;3:3–9.
132. Kohler M, Kennedy D, Martin J, et al. The influence of body mass on long-term cognitive performance of children treated for sleep-disordered breathing. *Sleep Med*. 2018;51:1–6.
133. Kohler M, Lushington K, Kennedy JD. Neurocognitive performance and behavior before and after treatment for sleep-disordered breathing in children. *Nat Sci Sleep*. 2010;2:159–185.
134. Prokasky A, Fritz M, Molfese VJ, Bates JE. Night-to-night variability in the bedtime routine predicts sleep in toddlers. *Early Child Res Q*. 2019;49:18–27.
135. Biggs SN, Lushington K, van den Heuvel CJ, Martin AJ, Kennedy JD. Inconsistent sleep schedules and daytime behavioral difficulties in school-aged children. *Sleep Med*. 2011;12:780–786.
136. Owens JA, Jones C, Nash R. Caregivers' knowledge, behavior, and attitudes regarding healthy sleep in young children. *J Clin Sleep Med*. 2011;7:345–350.
137. Yokomaku A, Misao K, Omoto F, et al. A study of the association between sleep habits and problematic behaviors in preschool children. *Chronobiol Int*. 2008;25:549–564.
138. Hoyniak CP, Bates JE, Staples AD, Rudasill KM, Molfese DL, Molfese VJ. Child sleep and socioeconomic context in the development of cognitive abilities in early childhood. *Child Dev*. 2019;90(5):1718–1737.
139. Sadeh A, Anders TF. Infant sleep problems: origins, assessment, interventions. *Infant Ment Health J*. 1993;14:17–34.
140. Meltzer LJ, Mindell JA. Relationship between child sleep disturbances and maternal sleep, mood, and parenting stress: a pilot study. *J Fam Psychol*. 2007;21:67–73.
141. Kelly RJ, El-Sheikh M. Marital conflict and children's sleep: reciprocal relations and socioeconomic effects. *J Fam Psychol*. 2011;25:412–422.
142. El-Sheikh M, Buckhalt JA, Mark Cummings E, Keller P. Sleep disruptions and emotional insecurity are pathways of risk for children. *J Child Psychol Psychiatr*. 2007;48:88–96.
143. Martin J, Hiscock H, Hardy P, Davey B, Wake M. Adverse associations of infant and child sleep problems and parent health: An Australian population study. *Pediatrics*. 2007;119:947–955.
144. Bernier A, Bélanger M-È, Bordeleau S, Carrier J. Mothers, fathers, and toddlers: parental psychosocial functioning as a context for young children's sleep. *Dev Psychol*. 2013;49:1375–1384.
145. Drake CL, Scofield H, Roth T. Vulnerability to insomnia: the role of familial aggregation. *Sleep Med*. 2008;9:297–302.
146. Owens JA, Spirito A, McGuinn M, Nobile C. Sleep habits and sleep disturbance in elementary school-aged children. *J Dev Behav Pediatr*. 2000;21:27–36.

147. Zee PC, Turek FW. Sleep and health: everywhere and in both directions. *JAMA Intern Med.* 2006;166:1686–1688.
148. Williams KE, Berthelsen D, Walker S, Nicholson JM. A developmental cascade model of behavioral sleep problems and emotional and attentional self-regulation across early childhood. *Behav Sleep Med.* 2017;15:1–21.
149. Benoit D, Zeanah CH, Boucher C, Minde KK. Sleep disorders in early childhood: association with insecure maternal attachment. *J Am Acad Child Adolesc Psychiatr.* 1992;31:86–93.
150. Armstrong KL, O'Donnell H, McCallum R, Dadds M. Childhood sleep problems: association with prenatal factors and maternal distress/depression. *J Paediatr Child Health.* 1998;34:263–266.
151. Beebe DW. Cognitive, behavioral, and functional consequences of inadequate sleep in children and adolescents. *Pediatr Clin.* 2011;58:649–665.
152. Verschuren O, Gorter JW, Pritchard-Wiart L. Sleep: an underemphasized aspect of health and development in neurorehabilitation. *Early Human Dev.* 2017;113:120–128.

10

Adolescence and Emerging Adulthood

AMY R. WOLFSON AND TERRA ZIPORYN ■

INTRODUCTION

Insufficient and erratic adolescent sleep has been identified as a major public health concern by the American Psychological Association, Centers for Disease Control and Prevention (CDC), American Academy of Pediatrics (AAP), American Medical United States and worldwide. Sleep challenges in this age group stem partly from too-early and/or irregular class schedules and other social and cultural factors and partly from a developmental delay in the timing of sleep. Together these forces make it difficult for most adolescents to get the sleep they need at the times they most need it, particularly on school nights.

Our chapter will give you the opportunity to reflect on your middle and high school years and examine how your sleep–wake patterns have changed and how they compare with those of your peers. As you read, think about the following questions:

1. On average, what time did you fall asleep and wake up, and how much sleep did you get (school vs. nonschool nights) during high school? In college?
2. Were your school versus nonschool night sleep schedules different during high school?
3. Did your preference for morningness versus eveningness change over your adolescent years?
4. What time did your middle and/or high school start, and how did the start time align with your sleep schedule? What about your class times now?

5. How did you and your family, friends, and community value sleep relative to nutrition and exercise?

6. How can you as an individual improve your sleep health, and how can we as a society improve it for all adolescents and emerging adults?

In this chapter, we define adolescence and emerging adulthood; explain why sleep deprivation and its consequences are serious public health problems for adolescents; examine the sleep behavior and circadian timing changes occurring throughout this remarkable developmental period; and discuss interventions and countermeasures to improve the sleep health and overall lives of adolescents and emerging adults. Because we focus on the relationship between sleep science and social forces and institutions, particularly schools, we frame the discussion around the US education system. However, most of the content, including the science of adolescent sleep and many of the psychosocial forces affecting it, are relevant worldwide.

ADOLESCENCE AND EMERGING ADULTHOOD: DEFINITIONS

Adolescence, a critical developmental period, is conventionally understood as the period between the onset of puberty and the establishment of social independence [1]. Pioneering American psychologist G. Stanley Hall's original conception of adolescence in 1904 included ages of 14 to 24 years [2]. Today, the most commonly used chronologic definition of adolescence includes ages 10 to 18, although the term sometimes includes ages 9 to 26.[1]

For the purposes of our discussion, we define adolescence as the stage of life from 11 to 25 years of age, a definition that Alexa Curtis of the University of San Francisco helped create for use in research, education, and intervention [7] This definition considers early adolescence and emerging adulthood as substages that occur at the beginning and end, respectively, of this transitional period of life. While this is a useful definition grounded in developmental science, it is important to understand that there is not necessarily one correct definition and that any of the proposed definitions are subject to cultural and historical context. As developmental science evolves, so too will our understanding of adolescent development. Regardless of precise definition, moreover, adolescent developmental

---

1. More recent definitions of adolescence and what Jeffrey Arnett has defined as Emerging Adulthood vary depending on the source and often without theoretical bases [3]. As recently as 2015, several medical and healthcare organizations published papers defining adolescence. For example, the Society for Adolescent Medicine's position paper on adolescent health research defined adolescence as the ages 10 to 25 [4], whereas the AAP identified adolescence as the ages of 11 to 21 years [5].The World Health Organization defined "adolescents" as individuals between 10 and 19 years, "youth" between 15 and 24 years, and "young people" between 10 and 24 years [6].

science has bearing on your sleep experiences in middle and high school and on your sleep today.

DEVELOPMENTAL CHANGES IN SLEEP AND CIRCADIAN RHYTHMS

Adolescents need just as much sleep as younger children, a finding first demonstrated by our colleague (see Box 10.1) Mary A. Carskadon as part of her doctoral dissertation. Carskadon and colleagues' 6-year longitudinal summer sleep laboratory study gave children aged 10 to 17 a constant 10-hour sleep opportunity during a 3-night in-lab assessment [8]. The research hypothesis was that older youngsters would sleep less, reaching a normal adult sleep length of 7.5 or 8 hour by late adolescence. In fact, sleep quantity remained consistent at approximately 9.2 hours across all pubertal stages [8]. In a subsequent series of studies, Carskadon's team also found that slow-wave sleep time decreased by about 40% across this age span and level of daytime sleep tendency increased at mid-puberty, exemplified by faster sleep onset via the Multiple Sleep Latency Test in the afternoon [9, 10]. A field study of over 300 13- to 19-year-olds using daily self-reported measures has since confirmed these findings, showing that the overall "optimum" sleep for next-day mood ratings was about 9 hours [11].

In 1993, Carskadon's team also published a landmark study that documented an association between more mature pubertal development and delayed (i.e., later) circadian preference [12]. We now know that this association is rooted in two biological systems that change during adolescence. First, the sleep–wake homeostatic process (known as Process S; also see Chapter 3 of this volume), which creates sleep pressure (homeostatic sleep drive), builds more slowly in more mature (i.e., postpubertal) adolescents. This developmental change in intrinsic sleep–wake regulation allows older adolescents to stay awake longer, even though their sleep need remains constant.

A study [13] examining the speed of falling asleep following prolonged wakefulness in which pre-/early pubertal adolescents (mean 11 years old) fell asleep faster than postpubertal adolescents (mean 14 years old) supports this concept, as do longitudinal and cross-sectional studies modeling the decay of sleep pressure using sleep EEG slow wave activity [14–17] (also see Chapter 1 of this volume). This decrease in sleep pressure may feel familiar if you remember what it was like to sleep over at a friend's home on a Saturday night, staying up until about 2 AM and obtaining little sleep. A sleepover in sixth or seventh grade probably left you feeling cranky, distracted, and possibly falling asleep at lunch when you returned home Sunday. Under the same circumstances in high school, though, you more likely came home feeling relatively alert—even though you still needed 8.5 to 9.5 hours of sleep and certainly slept too little the night before.

Box 10.1

MARY A. Carskadon: Founder of The Study of Adolescent Sleep

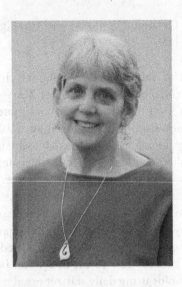

Mary A. Carskadon is considered the global founder of adolescent sleep research. In this chapter, we describe much of her pioneering work on sleep and circadian rhythms during childhood, adolescence, and young adulthood. Her timely and historic research, across several decades, have given us a clear and substantial understanding of the developmental changes in sleep and circadian rhythms over the course of adolescence. Dr. Carskadon's work has also led to important global conversations, policy decisions, and further research addressing healthy school start times and other ways in which sleep impacts adolescents' health, academic performance, and emotional well-being. Her research and leadership have influenced education policy, prompting the AAP, CDC, and other groups to call for later school timing for middle and high school students.

Dr. Carskadon studied psychology at Gettysburg College, graduating with honors in 1969. She then earned her PhD in neuro- and biobehavioral sciences in 1979 from Stanford University. With her mentor, William C. Dement, she developed the Multiple Sleep Latency Test (MSLT), which has since served as the primary objective measurement of sleepiness (also see Chapter 22 of this volume). Since 1985, she has been a Professor of Psychiatry and Human Behavior at the Warren Alpert Medical School at Brown University, and Director of the Sleep and Chronobiology Research Lab at E. P. Bradley Hospital.

The many awards Dr. Carskadon has received for her research also emphasize the variety of impacts that can be made during a career in sleep research: the American Sleep Disorders Association's Nathaniel Kleitman Distinguished Service Award (1991); the National Sleep Foundation's Lifetime Achievement Award (2003); the American Academy of Sleep Medicine's Mark O. Hatfield Public Policy Award 2003); and the Sleep Research Society's Distinguished

Scientist Award (2007) and Outstanding Educator Award (2005; which was later renamed the Mary A. Carskadon Outstanding Educator Award). In 2007, she was elected a Fellow of the Association of Psychological Sciences and the American Association for the Advancement of Science "for probing the nature of circadian rhythms in human adolescence."

In addition to teaching hundreds of undergraduates annually in her popular course, Introduction to Sleep, Dr. Carskadon offers a prestigious summer internship for undergraduate and early graduate students who are interested in sleep research. These students, named "Dement Fellows" after Dr. Carskadon's mentor, spend a summer training and working in her sleep lab—assisting with research studies on adolescents who live in the lab for up to 2 weeks and participate in summer camp-like activities while their sleep and waking performance and mood are monitored. At the end of this summer apprenticeship, Dr. Carskadon hosts a research retreat that brings together early career sleep and circadian rhythms investigators and the Dement Fellows for a weekend of conversation, mentoring, and the apprentices' research presentations (for details and opportunities, see the Sleep for Science Research Lab: http://www.sleepforscience.org/).

A second biologic change associated with puberty involves a phase delay in Process C or the circadian timing system, which regulates the timing of sleepiness and wakefulness (also see Chapter 4 of this chapter), shifting phase preference from "morningness" to "eveningness." Using self-reported pubertal development and phase preference scores from over 400 pre-/early pubertal sixth graders, Carskadon and Acebo showed that delayed phase preference correlated with maturation stage [12]. A subsequent laboratory study examining the circadian timing system more directly during early adolescents also associated a biological phase delay with puberty, measuring the timing of melatonin secretion in the absence of psychosocial factors [18]. This phase shift—seen in nonhuman mammals, too—explains why most teenagers are more alert later in the evening, have relatively later bedtimes, and, at least on vacations and nonschool days, later wake times [19]. These biological changes also largely explain why, after reaching puberty, adolescents are less likely to wake spontaneously, even after a full 9 hours of sleep.

Biologic changes continue to affect sleep timing into the early 20s. Two cross-sectional studies have reported a progressive sleep-phase delay from childhood through ages 18 to 21, the typical college years, with sleep phase beginning to advance only after age 19 or 20 [20, 21]. The first study to estimate the distribution and prevalence of individual chronotypes in the US population based on a large-scale, nationally representative sample recently estimated distribution of chronotypes by age and sex. Using 12 years (2003–2014) of pooled diary data from the American Time Use Survey, the research team confirmed that midpoint of sleep (i.e., halfway point between sleep onset time and sleep offset time; also see Chapter 4 of this volume) shifts later during adolescence, showing a peak in "lateness" at about 19 years and shifting earlier thereafter [22]. Variability in chronotype decreased with age, with males typically having later chronotypes than females before age 40, but earlier thereafter [22].

Together, these sleep behavior changes enable adolescents to stay up late socializing in person or virtually, refine skills, and handle high homework demands and pressures, extracurriculars, and evening jobs. They also keep many adolescents from getting sufficient sleep throughout the week, leading them to nap during the day and/or "sleep in" on weekends (and vacations) in a largely futile attempt to regain lost sleep. This pattern empowers adolescents by decreasing school-night sleep debt but may also create difficulties, particularly for middle and high school students who attend school that start before 8:30 AM.

ADOLESCENTS' ERRATIC AND INSUFFICIENT SLEEP: A PUBLIC HEALTH PROBLEM

Beginning in early adolescence, teenagers report obtaining less sleep than when they were younger, due largely to early school schedules that conflict with their biology [19, 23, 24]. Over the past four decades, numerous epidemiological studies have shown not only that adolescents get inadequate sleep but that sleep timing and quantity vary significantly between school nights and weekends [19, 23, 25–28]. Adolescent bed and rise times are also markedly delayed, especially on weekends, during summers, and over vacations [19, 28]. Insufficient sleep coupled with these erratic and misaligned school- versus nonschool-night sleep–wake schedules underlie many negative health, behavioral, and performance outcomes, including impaired school performance, physical and mental health challenges, substance misuse, risk-taking behaviors, and drowsy driving [19, 25, 28]. For these reasons, erratic and insufficient adolescent sleep is considered a public health problem.

Studies of adolescents around the world show that 53% of teenagers worldwide typically get under 8 hours of sleep on school nights [29]. Although adolescents generally need 8.5 to 9.5 hours of sleep nightly, two-thirds of US high school students recently surveyed reported getting 7 or fewer hours, and only about 10% reported getting 9 or more. When the CDC's Youth Risk Behavior Surveillance System asked students *how much sleep they usually got on school nights*, they defined sufficient sleep as 9 hours for ages 6 to 12 and 8 hours for ages 13 to 18. Even with these more lenient definitions, about 6 in 10 (57.8%) of middle schoolers (grades 6–8) and 7 in 10 (72.7%) of high schoolers reported insufficient sleep on school nights [30]. In many of these self-reports, older adolescents report obtaining less sleep than younger adolescents, and girls generally report the largest sleep deficits [31].

To find out whether adolescents today sleep fewer hours per night than adolescents in the past, psychologist Jean Twenge and colleagues examined data from two long-running, nationally representative, government-funded surveys of over 1 million teenagers: The Monitoring the Future Survey which asked US 8th, 10th, and 12th graders *how frequently they got at least 7 hours of sleep*, and the

Youth Risk Behavior Surveillance System, which asked 9th to 12th graders *how many hours of sleep they got on an average school night* [32, 33]. Results showed that 40% of adolescents in 2015 slept under 7 hours a night—58% more than in 1991 and 17% more than in 2009 [33].

SLEEP IN COLLEGE AND YOUNG ADULTHOOD

Most studies of emerging adults' sleep have focused on sleep quality, sleep deprivation, daytime sleepiness, sleep onset latency, sleep regularity, and the sleep environment [34–38]. Many of these studies involve college students, whose sleep, as with younger students, may be challenged by academic and social activities and expectations, as well as structural constraints of school and residential life. Approximately 69% of adolescents attend college in the United States [39]. Whether they live on campus or commute, they are rarely if ever required to attend extremely early morning classes every day like many younger adolescents. Nonetheless, the transition to college (or the work world) can also make sleep health challenging. These older adolescents, many of whom set their own sleep and wake times for the first time, need to navigate irregular class and work schedules, a late-night culture, widespread availability of caffeine and other stimulants, and dormitory living environments (e.g., noise and light) that can impact biological clocks and disrupt sleep [40–42].

At least 60% of college students have been characterized as poor-quality sleepers, reporting restricted sleep on weeknights versus weekends, frequent "all-nighters," and other unhealthy sleep practices [35, 36, 43, 44]. Researchers have portrayed college students as sleep-deprived, with 71% obtaining under 8 hours of sleep per night [36]. First-year college students sometimes report poorer sleep than second-year students [45, 46]. College students' total sleep has also declined from the 1960s into the 21st century [47].

Various longitudinal and/or cross-sectional designs comparing sleep patterns in high school and college students show significant differences, particularly in sleep timing. A 2010 assessment comparing sleep patterns of about 1,000 college students to high school data from the 2006 National Sleep Foundation's "Sleep in America" poll found similar total sleep times, but bedtimes and wake times shifted later by about 90 minutes on both weekdays and weekends [36]. Similarly, an actigraphic assessment of 24 students at the end of high school and again 5 years later while in college found a 45-minute delay in sleep onset, offset, and mid-sleep times without any change in total sleep time [48]. One of us (AW) analyzed data from an earlier study by Carskadon's lab, involving 515 students who had been accepted at an Ivy League university [49]. Students completed questionnaires about midpoint of time in bed (TIB), bedtime, and wake time on school and nonschool nights in May (i.e., before college) and again during the November of their first college term [49]. Over that time, midpoint TIB was delayed by approximately 2 hours on both school and nonschool nights, but absolute TIB changed minimally [49].

These and other studies show a clear delay in the timing, but not amount, of sleep needed from high school to college. They also highlight some unique challenges to sleep health during the college years, as well as opportunities to improve it. One study, for example, posed retrospective questions to college students in an introductory psychology class and found that those with evening chronotypes may have unusual advantages in a college setting [50]. These "owls" were more likely to utilize the increased flexibility in college to align their sleep–wake patterns with their circadian timing preference, shifting to later sleep–wake patterns on weekends.

CONSEQUENCES OF INSUFFICIENT, ERRATIC, AND MISALIGNED SLEEP

Adolescents' insufficient, ill-timed, and irregular sleep has potentially serious, and often unappreciated, implications—including academic and athletic performance deficits, poor judgment, risk-taking behaviors, lack of motivation, inattention, motor vehicle and other accidents, difficulties regulating emotions, substance misuse, and compromised immune systems, and increasing the odds of getting sick and staying sick longer [23, 25, 51, 52]. Complicating matters, the causes and consequences of chronic sleep loss are often closely intertwined. For example, consuming alcohol and other drugs can lead to insufficient and poor-quality sleep and subsequent daytime sleepiness, while sleep loss itself also increases the risk of using alcohol and other drugs [38].

Academic Performance and Cognitive Functioning

Because being in class presumably affects learning, many studies have examined the relationships among sleep behaviors, school start times, and attendance/tardiness. One study examined the sleep patterns and school performance of early adolescents attending two urban, public middle schools starting "early" (7:15 AM) versus "late" (8:37 AM). Based on transcript data and self-reports, students at the late-starting school had four times fewer tardies during both fall and spring, with 50 minutes more sleep each night and less daytime sleepiness [53]. Naturalistic surveys as well as experimental, laboratory-based approaches in various research settings around the world also demonstrate associations between decreased academic performance and poor sleep quality, daytime sleepiness, insufficient sleep, irregular sleep–wake patterns, and evening circadian preference and link sleep loss to impaired declarative and procedural learning and cognitive-behavioral performance (e.g., psychomotor reaction times, awareness of the extent of sleep loss, impulsivity, and sustained attention) [54–61]. These findings are hardly surprising, given that sufficient and quality sleep is required for acquiring, consolidating, stabilizing, filtering, and retrieving information (as discussed further in Chapter 7 of this volume).

In one survey-based study conducted over 20 years ago, we found that students who describe themselves as struggling or failing school (earning Cs or Ds/Fs, respectively) reported greater differences between their school- and nonschool-night schedules than students earning As and Bs [23]. Using a new approach to sleep regularity, Andrew Phillips and colleagues assessed 61 undergraduates for 30 days using sleep diaries, quantifying sleep regularity with a sleep regularity index (calculating the probability of being asleep or awake at any two time-points 24 hours apart). Not surprising, a higher sleep regularity index was associated with better academic performance [62].

Other survey-based studies link circadian preference and phase to cognitive functioning and academic performance. A review of studies examining school-aged versus university-aged participants, for example, associated eveningness with poorer academic performance (transcript, teacher or self-report grade point average [GPA], and/or standardized test scores) in both age groups [57]. Notably, school-aged students showed a stronger association between eveningness and low academic achievement, perhaps because, as the authors observe, university students or older adolescents often have more independence and flexibility in creating their daily schedules and can select classes that fit their sleep–wake preferences, avoiding "social jetlag" and obtaining more sleep [57]. Social jet lag refers to the discrepancy between school-night sleep and free or nonschool-night schedules or between social and biological time.

Supporting this hypothesis are findings that students who align their course schedule with their circadian schedule are more likely to do better academically. Researchers analyzed 2 years of data ($N = 14,894$) from an American university to assess how misalignment between circadian rhythms and older adolescents' course schedules affect their academic performance (i.e., GPA)—a misalignment amounting to social jetlag. After categorizing the students into "night owls," "day-time finches," and "morning larks," based on a learning management system activity during nonclass days, they compared class times to academic outcomes. Forty percent of the students' activity synced with their class times; 50% of students took classes before they were fully alert; and 10% had already peaked by the time their classes started. Moreover, 60% of students experienced over 30 minutes of social jet lag, with greater times associated with lower GPAs, especially for owls [63].

Recent laboratory-based studies have enhanced our understanding of the way sleep restriction, napping, and sleep timing affect adolescents' cognitive functioning. One study simulated nonschool-night "catch-up" sleep and afternoon naps, common to many adolescents, by examining neurobehavioral functioning during multiple-night periods of restricted and recovery sleep, respectively [64]. Fifty-seven male adolescents experienced two cycles of 5-hour TIB for 3 nights with a 9-hour TIB recovery for 2 nights per cycle; half the participants received the opportunity for a 1-hour afternoon nap following each sleep-restriction night. The nonnappers showed a progressive decline in sustained attention, working memory, and speed of processing, not returning to baseline even after 2 nights of recovery sleep. Napping improved but did not entirely eliminate dwindling performance [64]. In an earlier study, a sleep restriction group (TIB = 5 hours) demonstrated poorer sustained attention, working memory, and executive function, while the control group (TIB = 9 hours) maintained cognitive performance levels [65].

Another laboratory study examining the impact of cramming for exams instead of sleeping considered the interaction of study timing and TIB on vocabulary learning [66]. Fifty-six teenage boarding school students were randomly assigned to 1 week of either 5-hour (sleep restricted) or 9-hour TIB as part of a 14-day protocol. Participants studied college/graduate level vocabulary words on digital flashcards with word pairs spaced over 4 consecutive days or simultaneously during a single study session, with recall examined immediately, 24 hours, and 120 hours after studying. For all retention intervals, sleep-restricted adolescents had more impaired recall—although paced learning seemed to mitigate the effects of sleep restriction compared to studying over short intervals [66]. Together these lab-based studies demonstrate that for sleep-restricted adolescents, weekend catch-up sleep, even when combined with napping on school days, is inferior to sufficient and regular school-night sleep. They also suggest that sleep-deprived adolescents cramming for exams might have particular difficulties remembering new material, with learning deficits possibly minimized by studying over several days [64–66].

Athletic Performance

Whether you were one of the 8 million US high school students who participated in a sport, the approximately 7% who went on to play a varsity sport in college [67], or, like us, simply enjoy swimming, running, hiking, or lifting weights for physical and psychological health, you may have noticed that sleep is a tool you can use to your advantage. Accumulating evidence associates sufficient and quality sleep with both improved performance and competitive success, as well as a reduced risk of injury and illness. and faster recovery time in athletes [68, 69]. Perhaps that is why coaches (rather than teachers and professors) have been ahead of the curve in recommending sleep health, often reminding their athletes to keep regular sleep–wake schedules and to prioritize sleep a few nights before competitions since sleeping well the night before can be challenging.

Studies have taken different approaches to investigating how insufficient sleep and circadian disruption affect athletic performance. Some researchers have focused on physiological measures, while others assess athletic performance directly. Findings suggest that improved sleep duration improves reaction time, accuracy, and endurance, although sleep's effects on anaerobic power, strength, and sprint performance—required more for some sports than others—are less clear [68]. A recent review of the research on sleep patterns, circadian rhythms, and athletic performance concluded that athletic performance is best in the evening, close to the time when the core body temperature typically is at its peak [68] (also see Chapter 4 of this volume).

Despite this evidence, athletes often fail to obtain recommended amounts of sleep, threatening both performance and health. College athletes often face numerous challenges to maintaining sleep health, including training and competition schedules, travel, stress, academic demands, and overtraining. For example, the Patriot League student athletes whom we (AW) teach must travel often up and down the East Coast for games, making it difficult to keep a regular sleep–wake schedule.

Emotional Well-Being: Depression and Depressed Mood

You probably know first-hand that sleep affects your mood and behavior. After a night of insufficient sleep, you may be more irritable, easily annoyed, short-tempered, and vulnerable to stress and anxiety. Once you sleep well, your mood often returns to normal. While there are many components to emotional well-being, we focus here on depressed mood and depression because they are so common among adolescents. Poor quality and insufficient sleep have not only been associated with emotional well-being generally, but also with depressed mood specifically [70–73].

Numerous studies have independently associated depression with various features of adolescent sleep, including short sleep duration, delayed sleep timing, sleep disturbances, and insomnia [70–76]. Moreover, this relationship is bidirectional: not only do sleep disorders and sleep difficulties (e.g., insomnia, insufficient sleep, excessive daytime sleepiness, disrupted sleep, increased need for sleep) increase relative risk of developing depression, but insomnia and other sleep behavior difficulties can also predict relapse for those struggling with depression [71, 72, 76]. Although studies examining sleep architecture in depressed adolescents have not consistently replicated polysomnographic findings in depressed adults (i.e., increased rapid eye movement [REM] sleep, decreased REM onset latency), other polysomnographic variables, such as sleep spindle activity and cyclic alternating patterns, may be more relevant [77] (also see Chapter 20 of this volume).

Circadian factors may also play a role in mood regulation. Increased self-reported "eveningness," a marker of circadian phase delay, for example, has been associated with depression, less propensity to experience positive emotions, and lower responsiveness to behavioral therapy for depression [78]. Tamar Shochat at the University of Haifa, along with colleagues in the Carskadon lab, took a person-centered analytic approach to distinguish sleep symptom cluster groups and depressed mood in a sample of 1,451 adolescents [72]. Using a survey about sleep patterns completed near the end of high school that included questions about sleep patterns, with mood measured using the total score on the Center for Epidemiologic Studies Depression Scale, they found that groups with the fewest depressive symptoms had moderate sleep timing, shorter sleep-onset latencies, and fewer arousals [72].

Several recent studies have associated sleep problems with suicidal ideation [79, 80]. A recent systematic analysis of work on suicide risk and sleep among adolescents highlighted cross-sectional studies demonstrating that adolescents with sleep disturbances are at higher risk for suicidal ideation, plans, and attempts compared to peers without sleep disturbances [81]. These studies also associated sleeping fewer than 8 hours per night with an almost threefold increased risk of suicide attempts, even after controlling for confounding variables. Notably, prospective studies have also connected sleep disturbances and suicidal ideation, but not suicide attempts. Perhaps more important, while depression did not moderate associations between sleep problems and suicidal ideation or attempts, adolescents with a history of insomnia symptoms—regardless of mood—had a higher risk for suicidal ideation than those with other sleep disturbances [81].

Drowsy Driving

Driving is one of the most dangerous activities for adolescents and emerging adults, with motor vehicle crashes the leading cause of death among 12- to 19-year-olds in the United States [82]. Contributing factors include driving inexperience, age of licensing, high-risk driving situations, passengers, substance use, risk-taking behaviors, and—of greatest note here—drowsy driving and falling asleep at the wheel [83]. An estimated 1 in 25 adult drivers (aged 18 years or older) report having fallen asleep while driving in the previous month [84]. The National Highway Traffic Safety Administration estimates that drowsy driving was responsible for 72,000 crashes, 44,000 injuries, and 800 deaths in 2013; these are undoubtedly underestimates, it is more likely that up to 6,000 fatal crashes each year are caused by drowsy drivers [85]. A recent study examined survey data from 15- to 19-year-olds attending public schools in Fairfax County, Virginia, in which drowsy driving was defined as having ever *driven a car or motor vehicle while feeling drowsy* in the last year; the study revealed that 63% of these students drove at least several times a week and 48% reported drowsy driving. Drowsy driving rates were higher for students who slept fewer than 7 hours versus 8 or more hours on school nights, with drowsy driving rates highest in self-reported evening versus morning chronotypes [86].

Not surprisingly, adolescent drivers who start class earlier in the morning are involved in significantly more car accidents than their peers with a later class time [87]. One study found that school-day crash rates for adolescent drivers during the 2009–2010 school year were about 29% higher in Chesterfield County, Virginia, where classes began at 7:20 AM than in adjacent Henrico County, Virginia, with an 8:45 AM start time [87]. Results were similar the following academic year. In contrast, there was no difference in adult crash rates in the two counties during either year [87]. An earlier study demonstrated that delaying school start times in a Kentucky community decreased the average adolescent crash rate by nearly 17%, while the state as a whole increased by nearly 8% in the same period [88]. In 2014 a large, multistate prospective study found that moving bell times to 8:30 AM or later significantly reduced teen car crash rates, with the rate in Jackson Hole,

Wyoming, dropping by 70% in the first year after shifting from 7:35 to 8:55 AM starts [89].

SCHOOL START TIMES AND OTHER FACTORS AFFECTING ADOLESCENTS' LIVED SLEEP EXPERIENCE

The need to rise early in the morning for school is one of the best document factors in the "perfect storm" of bioregulatory mechanisms and psychosocial factors undermining healthy sleep for most adolescents today [10, 19, 28] (see Figure 10.1). Today most US middle and high schools are regularly required to wake at times when they would naturally still be sleeping. This chronic misalignment between natural sleep–wake schedules and externally imposed demands essentially guarantees short and ill-timed sleep, including social jetlag equivalent to traveling from New York to London and back every weekend, each week. As Troxel and Wolfson describe in their special issue of the journal *Sleep Health*, featuring research on school start time, Carskadon concluded that as far back as 1993, "[T]he starting time of school puts limits on the time available for sleep. This is a nonnegotiable limit established largely without concern for sleep" (p. 186) [90].

Increasing academic pressures, reduced parental control over bedtimes, and screen time and social media use may exacerbate these problems. With the popularity of binge TV series, computers, video game systems, and smartphone texting, adolescents (and adults for that matter) are almost always using digital technology [91, 92]. During a typical day, adolescents are exposed to nearly 12 hours of screen and audio media, with over a quarter of that time devoted to using

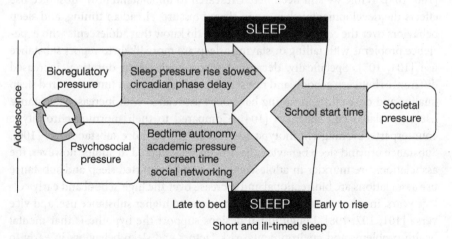

Figure 10.1 The perfect storm model.
SOURCE: First presented in Carskadon MA. Sleep in adolescents: the perfect storm. *Pediatr Clin.* 2011;58:637–647. Reprinted from Crowley SJ, Wolfson AR, Tarokh L, Carskadond MA. An update on adolescent sleep: new evidence informing the perfect storm model. *J Adolesc.* 2018;67:55–65.

more than one digital source simultaneously (i.e., media multitasking) [91, 92]. In the 21st century, adolescents' daily media exposure has increased by at least 2 hours. In a review of the compendium of research on digital technology use and sleep in adolescents and younger children around the world, over 90% of studies linked screen time to delayed bedtimes and reduced sleep [93–95]. Computer use was more consistently associated with poor sleep than was television, perhaps because television may be less interactive than computer-based activities. In a recent study of US 6- to 17-year-olds, technology (e.g., phones, computers) in a child or adolescent's bedroom overnight was a significant predictor of insufficient sleep [95, 96]. Twenge and colleagues also found that the more time young people reported spending online, the less sleep they got, with adolescents spending 5 hours online daily being 50% more likely to obtain insufficient sleep than those spending only an hour [33]. About 10 years into the 21st century, smartphone use skyrocketed, which Twenge argues might explain the 17% increase between 2009 and 2015 in the number of adolescents sleeping 7 hours or fewer [33].

While cause and effect remain unclear in these studies, there are a variety of ways digital technology might conceivably impair sleep. Digital technology time might interfere with time allotted for both sleep and exercise. The alerting aspects of some media content might fuel hyperarousal and decreased bedtime sleepiness [94, 97]. Lighting in smart phones and similar devices might alter circadian rhythms [98]. One study of emerging adults showed that reading on a light-emitting device before bedtime increased sleep onset latency, reduced REM sleep duration, and suppressed and delayed the release of melatonin, the sleep-promoting hormone that typically increases in the evening hours [99].

Contemporaneous with changes in sleep are increases in substance use during adolescence, most commonly alcohol, marijuana, tobacco, and caffeine [100–103]. While we still need better research to understand how substance use effects the developmental changes in sleep pressure, circadian timing, and sleep behaviors over the course of adolescence, we do know that adolescents who experience problems with falling or staying asleep are more likely to report substance use [104, 105]. Specifically, decreased school-night sleep duration, increased differences between school- and nonschool-night sleep onset times, lowered sleep quality, and delayed sleep timing have been associated with increased substance use and related consequences [104]. Compared to their morning-chronotype counterparts, evening-chronotype adolescents report more substance use [106]. Substance use and sleep behaviors have been well-studied in adults; however, the associations are murkier in adolescents. Certainly, reported sleep and substance use associations are bidirectional and increase over the high school and early college years; in other words, reduced sleep relates to higher substance use, and vice versa [101, 107, 108]. Longitudinal designs support the hypothesis that mental health problems and environmental risk factors and sleep behaviors in early to mid-adolescents who are substance-naïve prospectively predict level of substance involvement 5 or more years later [107, 109, 110].

While adolescents' caffeine consumption might seem innocuous or even helpful for attention, field and laboratory research on caffeine use in adolescents, specifically the impact on sleep, remains inadequate, and recommendations regarding caffeine intake for developing adolescents remain inconsistent. Regardless, caffeine consumption, including coffee, energy drinks, sodas, etc., in the United States is pervasive and difficult to avoid. A recent review of National Health and Nutrition Examination Survey data reported caffeine consumption prevalence as 75% for children and adolescents aged 6 to 17 [111]. Relative to body weight, adolescents, aged 12 to 17, consume 0.55 mg/kg, while average adult intake is 1.3 mg/kg [112]. The AAP discourages caffeine intake for children and adolescents, suggesting no more than 100 mg/day due to adverse impacts on sleep and blood pressure [113].

We have recently started investigating how caffeine might affect sleep and circadian timing development throughout adolescence. Not surprisingly, many studies link adolescent caffeine use to reduced sleep duration, and some associate moderate-to-high consumption, particularly in the evening, with disturbed and interrupted sleep and daytime sleepiness [103, 114, 115]. One of our studies surveyed nearly 200 high schoolers' regarding their caffeine use and, using cluster analysis, identified three groups differing on reasons and expectations for using caffeine [116]. Adolescents in the mixed-use and high soda-use groups consumed similar amounts of caffeine, both using significantly more caffeine than the low caffeine-use group. In contrast with high soda users, mixed users drank more coffee, expected more dependence symptoms and energy enhancement from caffeine, and were more likely to report early awakening, daytime sleepiness, and using caffeine to get through the day [116].

WHAT CAN YOU DO?

In general, two overarching types of countermeasures can improve sleep: individual approaches and societal/structural strategies. Individual approaches are aimed at changing behaviors or fixing personal issues, treating specific sleep disorders (see Part III of this volume), adopting healthy sleep habits, and educational or intervention programs aimed at promoting healthy sleep or preventing more serious sleep problems. Societal or structural countermeasures include more systemic, or population-level, changes, such as delaying school start times, developing sleep-healthy work or school environments (e.g., limited library and student center hours), and setting policies discouraging drowsy driving or regulating class times.

Individual/Group Approach: Preventive/Intervention Programs

Years ago, one of us (AW), as part of her doctoral work, evaluated the efficacy of a parenting program to help infants develop healthy sleep patterns [117]. As we write this chapter, several middle school sleep preventive/interventions programs are being developed and evaluated; some focus largely on sleep education, whereas others use motivational theory, social learning, or other behavioral change models to promote lasting "sleep smart" strategies and practices [118]. Two specific types of programs have emerged from recent reviews of these programs: those aiming to increase awareness, delivered to a general student population in a preventative fashion, and those targeting specific sleep behaviors and patterns [119, 120].

An example of the former is the Sleep Smart Program, developed by Wolfson and colleagues to improve sleep behaviors, academic performance, and behavioral well-being among early adolescents [118]. Using a social learning model, we randomly assigned a diverse group of seventh graders from two urban middle schools to an eight-session educational program or to a comparison group. Students assigned to the sleep-smart program group experienced significantly earlier bedtimes and greater sleep health, physiological and emotional sleep hygiene, and total sleep time than the comparison group [118]. The sleep-smart group also reported significantly fewer internalized behavior problems and sustained academic performance. While the comparison group's sleep health declined, program participants continued reporting improvements during the first three reporting periods, although not the fourth [118].

A review of sleep-education programs at the college level found insufficient evidence to determine their effects on sleep hygiene knowledge, sleep hygiene behavior, or sleep quality [121]. However, pilot data for Sleep 101, an interactive, online program co-designed by one of us (TZ) suggests that such programs can potentially reduce sleep problems among college students, with students reporting increased knowledge about caffeine use and reporting that they are less likely to pull all-nighters or drive drowsy after taking the course [122, 123]. This 45-minute, self-paced program explores the relationships with sleep among various areas critical to college life—including academics, athletics, mental and physical health, and social relationships—conveying the message that the college community values sleep and showing ways to use sleep to improve the college experience and overall well-being [122, 123].

Despite the significant resources devoted to studying and developing these kinds of programs; however, transfer of knowledge into largescale action remains slow and ineffective [120]. To date, no educational policy has been formulated regarding sleep, and very few sleep-health promotion programs have been integrated into school curricula. As Reut Gruber, a clinical psychologist at McGill University notes (and we concur), "until the necessary information is widely applied and disseminated, we will be missing an important opportunity to significantly improve health and well-being among our youth." (p. 26) Gruber advocates "Knowledge to Action," an evidence-based framework for knowledge transfer that has been successfully used with other health-related behaviors [120].

Structure Countermeasure: Delaying School Start Times

Although many psychosocial, cultural, and biological factors undermine the ability of middle school, high school, and college-aged students to obtain adequate and regular sleep, a large, broad, and consistent body of evidence strongly implicates early (i.e., before 8:30 AM) school start times as one of the key modifiable contributors [19, 23, 90, 124]. Not only does accumulating cross-sectional evidence show a linear relationship between school start time and sleep duration, but an extensive body of empirical research associates delaying school start times with increased sleep and more regular sleep–wake schedules, as well as improved physical and mental health school performance (test scores, graduation, and attendance), fewer car crashes, and less stimulant use [53, 125–128].

This research traces back to the 1990s. Just 1 year later after Carskadon's study documenting a delayed circadian preference at puberty, University of Minnesota neurologist Mark Mahowald and the Minnesota Medical Association urged Minnesota school districts to eliminate early-starting high school classes [90]. Based on this recommendation and under the leadership of superintendent Kenneth Dragseth, Edina, Minnesota, voted to delay its high school start time from 7:20 to 8:30 AM, beginning with the 1996–1997 academic year [129]. Seven Minneapolis high schools delayed their starts from 7:15 to 8:40 AM the following year. The districts asked Kyla Wahlstrom, director of the University of Minnesota's Center for Applied Research and Educational Improvement to study the impact of these changes in the different districts. Wahlstrom's study of over 18,000 high school students demonstrated increased attendance among 9th through 11th graders, improved enrollment, and slight improvement in grades [129, 130]. Moreover, the later-starting students had similar bedtimes to students from earlier starting schools, despite the start-time delay. In fact, on average, students at the later-starting schools got almost 1 hour more sleep each school night [129, 130]. These findings have been replicated in many other studies, to the point that numerous health, education, and civic organizations now recommend that middle and high schools begin classes at times that allow for healthy sleep.

Since Minnesota's lead, hundreds of additional school systems have worked on their own changes, often in collaboration with clinicians; researchers; private and public organizations, including the CDC and the National Sleep Foundation; and community advocates, to delay middle and high school start times. In addition to both grassroots and district-led efforts throughout the United States (see Box 10.2), interest in later start times is growing worldwide. In January 2019, one of us (AW) was invited to Tokyo to speak at a seminar for middle and high school teachers on adolescent sleep and school start times. In considering later bell times, Tokyo, similar to some other large metropolitan cities, must account for commute times since an overwhelming number of students use public transportation to get to and from schools, some spending up to 45 minutes to get to morning classes.

Although there is no systematic tracking of schools that have followed the evidence-based recommendations to ensure developmentally appropriate start times, an ever-growing number of school districts have already—or are actively considering—delaying their start times; these range from large and diverse districts (e.g., Seattle, Washington Public Schools, and Fairfax County, Virginia Public Schools) to smaller and rural or suburban districts. The increasing momentum in the movement for later start times has been spurred, in part, by

Box 10.2

THE START SCHOOL LATER MOVEMENT: TURNING SCIENCE INTO POLICY

Since the early 1990s, sleep researchers and health professionals have called for school start times that are compatible with the sleep needs and patterns of adolescents. Yet today, nearly 5 out of 6 American middle and high schools still start classes before 8:30 AM—the earliest bell time considered compatible with healthy sleep.[a] Over 10% of high schools start regular class before 7:30 AM, with nearly half starting before 8:30 AM Bus pickups begin as early as 5:00 AM in some districts.[b]

If the science is so clear, you might reasonably ask, *why do most schools still start so early*? The cumulative research showing that starting school before 8:30 AM is unhealthy and counterproductive is so extensive, broad, and consistent that major health organizations, including the AAP, the AMA, and the CDC now recommend that middle and high schools require attendance no earlier than 9:30 AM. However, even a compelling body of research and recommendations do not necessarily or immediately translate into policy changes. One reason for this is a *translation gap*—a lag between the time of an initial discovery by researchers and the time it takes for that discovery to reach clinicians, policymakers, and the general public. Even when new discoveries trickle down to the public, moreover, they are not always immediately or readily accepted. The history of public health is riddled with examples, such as the link between lung cancer and cigarette smoking, which was clear to scientists decades before any action was taken policy wise.[c]

When it comes to school start times, public ignorance about sleep, and adolescent sleep in particular, helps explain some of the resistance to change. In addition, there is a widespread ambivalence (and sometimes antipathy) toward sleep itself, and to some extent to teenagers as well. These feelings explain the public's reactions to proposals to start school later, such as "Are you kidding? We have to stop coddling these lazy kids and start being parents," "Get your kid to bed earlier and stop whining," and "Throw cold water on the kid, and I assure you he'll get up."

Even people who claim to value sleep are understandably concerned about how change in school schedules (later or earlier) will complicate their lives. Community life revolves around public school hours—even for those without children, leading to concerns over how a changed bell time will impact after-school jobs, childcare arrangements, sports practices, and even traffic. Some fear that change will be prohibitively expensive. These perceived obstacles almost all turn out to be unfounded or resolvable[d] but are politically powerful for preserving the status quo.

Even so, hundreds of schools have found feasible, affordable ways to delay bell times, while others never moved to such early hours in the first place. School leaders who have found solutions have done so by combining sleep education with change management tactics to prevent or allay community fears and concerns. If the history of other public health reforms is any guide, larger-scale changes also require an array of approaches to turn research into policy via a combination of public education about sleep, grassroots advocacy, position statements from key opinion leaders, legislation, and possibly even litigation. Through these approaches, a wide variety of stakeholders, including sleep researchers, health professionals, educators, policymakers, parents, and students, are already working together at local, state, and national levels to a create a climate in which communities prioritize sleep and sleep-friendly school hours. Many have joined forces through Start School Later, a US-based nonprofit organization, with nearly 130 local chapters, that aims to increase public awareness about the relationship between sleep and school hours, and to help ensure school start times that compatible with healthy sleep. Start School Later's website[e] includes a searchable research database; position statements on later start times from health, education, and civic organizations; a list of states introducing legislation to study, incentivize, or mandate later start times; and resources for community advocates and school leaders.[f]

[a]National Center for Education Statistics. Characteristics of public elementary and secondary schools in the united states: results from the 2015–16 National Teacher and Principal Survey. NCES 2017-071. Washington, DC: U.S. Department of Education; August 2017.

[b]Adolescent Sleep Working Group, Committee on Adolescence, Council on School Health. School start times for adolescents. *Pediatrics.* 2014;134:642–649.

[c]Berridge V. The policy response to the smoking and lung cancer connection in the 1950s and 1960s. *Hist J.* 2006;49:1185–1209.

[d]Start School Later. Why we must—and can—restore safe & healthy school hours. https://www.startschoollater.net/why-change.html. Accessed February 20, 2019.

[e]Start School Later. [Home page]. https://www.startschoollater.net/. Accessed May 14, 2019.

[f]Owens J, Drobnich D, Baylor A, Lewin D. School start time change: An in-depth examination of school districts in the United States. *Mind Brain Ed.* 2014;8:182–213.

---

increased messaging, integration, and resources provided by advocacy groups such as Start School Later and by recommendations issued by major medical organizations, including the AAP, AMA, and the American Academy of Sleep Medicine, all of whom recommend that middle and high schools start no earlier than 8:30 AM, to accommodate the known biological changes in adolescent sleep–wake cycles (e.g., [131]). Still, according to the CDC, the vast majority of middle and high schools still start before 8:30 AM, with 8:03 AM the average start time for middle and high schools combined and 7:59 AM the average for high schools [31].

There has also been enormous growth in regional, state, and national legislative efforts to ensure developmentally appropriate school start times in the United States, Europe, and Asia. Since 1998 California Congresswoman Zoe Lofgren has repeatedly introduced versions of a "ZZZs to As" bill and resolution to the US Congress, all proposing restrictions on hours at which high schools can begin required instruction. More recently, bills related to sleep and school start times have been introduced in state legislatures across the United States, including California, Connecticut, Florida, Hawaii, Indiana, Maryland, Massachusetts, New Jersey,

Maine, Minnesota, Nevada, Pennsylvania, Rhode Island, South Carolina, Texas, Utah, Virginia, and Washington. Some of these bills are studies, some incentive programs, and some mandates setting an earliest allowable opening hour [132].

CONCLUSIONS

The research reviewed in this chapter suggests the following conclusions, as well as steps individuals and institutions can take to improve adolescent sleep health.

1. Adolescents around the world are getting insufficient sleep, with markedly delayed bedtimes compared to younger children and significant variation between school nights and weekends.
2. Insufficient and erratic sleep in adolescents is a major public health concern associated with impaired physical and mental health, cognitive functioning, academic and athletic performance, and emotional regulation; risk-taking behaviors; drowsy driving; and unhealthy use of stimulants and other substances.
3. Many of these problems reflect a mismatch between biological changes in sleep needs and patterns at puberty and social and cultural factors including early school start times, irregular school and work hours, technology use, substance misuse, emotional challenges, light exposure, and social norms devaluing sleep.
4. Delaying school start times is the only public policy approach proven to improve adolescent sleep on a population level.
5. Although developmentally appropriate school start times cannot guarantee healthy sleep in all adolescents, they create the opportunity—one that many students use—for getting sufficient sleep and avoiding social jet lag.
6. To inform public policy and clinical practice, more research needs to explore the impact of light from increasing use of laptop computers, smartphones, and similar devices on the timing of sleep and wakefulness, as well as the impacts of caffeine and other substances.
7. Despite limited research on caffeine use and adolescent sleep, it makes sense to consider the timing of caffeine consumption carefully, especially limiting evening use, to reduce risk of impaired sleep duration or quality.
8. Pulling all-nighters, napping as your sole coping strategy, studying instead of sleeping before an exam or trying to write a paper on inadequate sleep will yield diminished returns, increasing sleep debt rather than grades.
9. When you think about getting up early to run or swim, or consider a late-night stint at the gym, make sure you are also prioritizing your sleep.
10. Sports medicine healthcare providers and coaches should prioritize scheduling, travel protocols, time and stress management, and healthy sleep practices to improve overall health and performance.

11. Having the freedom to select their class schedule can affect college students' sleep health.

12. Universities that want to improve student sleep health must take the initiative by creating sleep-healthy environments, from residence halls to class schedules to library hours.

ACKNOWLEDGMENT

Thank you to Abigail Cirelli, Loyola University Maryland, Class of 2020, for her work on the references and citations and final editing for this chapter.

REFERENCES

1. Steinberg L. *Age of Opportunity: Lessons from the New Science of Adolescence*. Boston, MA: Houghton Mifflin Harcourt; 2014.

2. Hall, G. S. *Adolescence: Its Psychology and Its Relations to Physiology, Anthropology, Sociology, Sex, CRIME, religion, And education* (Vols.1 & 2). New York, NY: D. Appleton; 1904.

3. Arnett, J. J. Emerging adulthood: A theory of development from the late teens through the twenties. *Am Psychol*. 2000;55:469–480.

4. Society of Adolescent Medicine. Guidelines for adolescent health research: A position paper of the society for adolescent medicine. *J Adolesc Health*. 2003;33:396–409.

5. American Academy of Pediatrics. Bright futures guidelines for health supervision of infants, children and adolescents. https://brightfutures.aap.org/Bright%20 Futures%20Documents/18-Adolescence.pdf. Published 2015. Accessed May 14, 2019.

6. World Health Organization. Adolescent health. http://www.who.int/topics/adolescent_health/en/. Published 2015. Accessed May 14, 2019.

7. Curtis C. Defining adolescence. *J Adolesc Fam Health*. 2015;7:2.

8. Carskadon MA, Harvey K, Duke P, Anders TF, Litt IF, Dement WC. Pubertal changes in daytime sleepiness. *Sleep*.1980;2:453–460.

9. Carskadon MA, Dement WC. The multiple sleep latency test: What does it measure? *Sleep*. 1982;5:S67–S72.

10. Carskadon MA, Acebo C. Regulation of sleepiness in adolescents: update, insights, and speculation. *Sleep*. 2002;25:606–614.

11. Fuligni AJ, Bai S, Kull JL, Gonzales NA. Individual differences in optimum sleep for daily mood during adolescence. *J Clin Child & Adolesc Psychol*. 2019;48(3):469–479.

12. Carskadon MA, Vieira C, Acebo C. Association between puberty and delayed phase preference. *Sleep*. 1993;16:258–262.

13. Jenni OG, Achermann P, Carskadon MA. Homeostatic sleep regulation in adolescents. *Sleep*. 2005;28:1446–1454.

14. Taylor DJ, Jenni OG, Acebo C, Carskadon MA. Sleep tendency during extended wakefulness: Insights into adolescent sleep regulation and behavior. *J Sleep Res*. 2005;14:239–244.

15. Campbell IG, Darchia N, Higgins LM, et al. Adolescent changes in homeostatic regulation of EEG activity in the delta and theta frequency bands during NREM sleep. *Sleep.* 2011;34:83–91.

16. Jenni OG, Carskadon MA. Spectral analysis of the sleep electroencephalogram during adolescence. *Sleep.* 2004;27:774–783.

17. Tarokh L, Carskadon MA, Achermann P. Dissipation of sleep pressure is stable across adolescence. *Neuroscience.* 2012;216:167–177.

18. Carskadon MA, Acebo C, Richardson GS, Tate BA, Seifer R. An approach to studying circadian rhythms of adolescent humans. *J Biol Rhythms.* 1997;12:278–289.

19. Crowley SJ, Wolfson AR, Tarokh L, Carskadon MA. An update on adolescent sleep: New evidence informing the perfect storm model. *J Adolesc.* 2018;67:55–65.

20. Roenneberg T, Kuehnle T, Pramstaller PP, et al. A marker for the end of adolescence. *Curr Biol.* 2004;14:R1038–R1039.

21. Tonetti L, Fabbri M, Natale V. Sex difference in sleep-time preference and sleep need: a cross-sectional survey among Italian pre-adolescents, adolescents, and adults. *Chronobiol Int.* 2008;25:745–759.

22. Fischer D, Lombardi DA, Marucci-Wellman H, Roenneberg T. Chronotypes in the US: influence of age and sex. *PLOS ONE* 2017;12:e0178782.

23. Wolfson AR, Carskadon MA. Sleep schedules and daytime functioning in adolescents. *Child Dev.* 1998;69:875–887.

24. Carskadon MA, Acebo C, Jenni OG. Regulation of adolescent sleep: implications for behavior. *Ann NY Acad Sci.* 2004;1021:276–291.

25. Owens J; Adolescent Sleep Working Group. Insufficient sleep in adolescents and young adults: an update on causes and consequences. *Pediatrics.* 2014;134:e921–e932.

26. Eaton DK, McKnight-Eily LR, Lowry R, Perry GS, Presley-Cantrell L, Croft JB. Prevalence of insufficient, borderline, and optimal hours of sleep among high school students: United States, 2007. *J Adoles Health.* 2010;46:399–401.

27. Short MA, Weber N, Reynolds C, Coussens S, Carskadon MA. Estimating adolescent sleep need using dose-response modeling. *Sleep.* 2018;41:zsy011.

28. Carskadon MA. Sleep in adolescents: the perfect storm. *Pediatr Clin.* 2011;58:637–647.

29. Gradisar M, Gardner G, Dohnt H. Recent worldwide sleep patterns and problems during adolescence: a review and meta-analysis of age, region, and sleep. *Sleep Med.* 2011;12:110–111.

30. Centers for Disease Control and Prevention. Youth risk behavior survey questionnaire. www.cdc.gov/yrbs Published 2015. Accessed May 14, 2019.

31. Wheaton AG, Chapman DP, Croft JB. School start times, sleep, behavioral, health, and academic outcomes: a review of the literature. *J School Health.* 2016;86:363–381.

32. The Monitoring the Future Survey. http://monitoringthefuture.org/. Accessed May 14, 2019.

33. Twenge JM, Martin GN, Campbell WK. Decreases in psychological well-being among American adolescents after 2012 and links to screen time during the rise of smartphone technology. *Emotion.* 2018;8:765–780.

34. Forquer LM, Camden AE, Gabriau KM, Johnson CM. Sleep patterns of college students at a public university. *J Am College Health.* 2008;56:563–565.

35. Hershner SD, Chervin RD. Causes and consequences of sleepiness among college students. *Nat Sci Sleep.* 2014;6:73–84.

36. Lund HG, Reider BD, Whiting AB, Prichard JR. Sleep patterns and predictors of disturbed sleep in a large population of college students. *J Adolesc Health.* 2010;46:124–132.

37. Philips AJ, Clerx WM, O'Brien CS, et al. Irregular sleep/wake patterns are associated with poorer academic performance and delayed circadian and sleep/wake timing. *Sci Rep.* 2017;7:3216.

38. Singleton RA, Wolfson AR. Alcohol consumption, sleep, and academic performance among college students. *J Stud Alcohol Drugs.* 2009;70:355–363.

39. Bureau of Labor Statistics. https://www.bls.gov/opub/ted/2017/69-point-7-percent-of-2016-high-school-graduates-enrolled-in-college-in-october-2016.htm. Published 2017. Accessed May 14, 2019.

40. Carney CE, Edinger JD, Meyer B, Lindman L, Istre T. Daily activities and sleep quality in college students. *Chronobiol Int.* 2006;23:623–637.

41. Sexton-Radek K, Hartley A. College residential sleep environment. *Psychol Rep.* 2013;113:903–907.

42. Brown C, Qin P, Esmail S. "Sleep? Maybe Later . . ." A cross-campus survey of university students and sleep practices. *Educ Sci.* 2017;7:66.

43. Pilcher JJ, Ginter DR, Sadowsky B. Sleep quality versus sleep quantity: relationships between sleep and measures of health, well-being and sleepiness in college students. *J Psychosom Res.* 1997;42:583–596.

44. Thacher PV. University students and the "all nighter": Correlates and patterns of students' engagement in a single night of total sleep deprivation. *Behav Sleep Med.* 2008;6:16–31.

45. Suen LK, Ellis Hon KL, Tam WW. Association between sleep behavior and sleep-related factors among university students in Hong Kong. *Chronobiol Int.* 2008;25:760–775.

46. Trockel MT, Barnes MD, Egget DL. Health-related variables and academic performance among first-year college students: Implications for sleep and other behaviors. *J Am College Health.* 2000;49:125–131.

47. Hicks RA, Fernandez C, Pellegrini RJ. Striking changes in sleep satisfaction of university students over the last two decades. *Percept Mot Skills.* 2001;93:660.

48. Urner M, Tornic J, Bloch, KE. Sleep patterns in high school and university students: a longitudinal study. *Chronobiol Int.* 2009;26:1222–1234.

49. Wolfson, AR, Futterman, A, Gredvig, C., Barker DH, Carskadon, MA. Large magnitude delay in sleep across the transition to college explained in part by high school sleep "struggles." *Sleep.* 2018;41:A101.

50. Zimmermann LK. Chronotype and the transition to college life. *Chronobiol Int.* 2011;28:904–910.

51. Beebe DW. Cognitive, behavioral, and functional consequences of inadequate sleep in children and adolescents. *Pediatr Clin.* 2011;58:649–665.

52. Orzech KM, Acebo C, Seifer R, Barker D, Carskadon MA. Sleep patterns are associated with common illness in adolescents. *J Sleep Res.* 2014;23:133–142.

53. Wolfson AR, Spaulding NL, Dandrow C, Baroni EM. Middle school start times: the importance of a good night's sleep for young adolescents. *Behav Sleep Med.* 2007;5:194–209.

54. Abraham J, Scaria J. Influence of sleep in academic performance–an integrated review of literature. *J Nurs Health Sci.* 2015;4:78–81.
55. Curcio G, Ferrara M, De Gennaro L. Sleep loss, learning capacity and academic performance. *Sleep Med Rev* 2006;10:323–337.
56. Dewald JF, Meijer AM, Oort FJ, Kerkhof GA, Bögels SM. The influence of sleep quality, sleep duration and sleepiness on school performance in children and adolescents: A meta-analytic review. *Sleep Med Rev.* 2010;14:179–189.
57. Tonetti L, Fabbri M, Filardi M, Martoni M, Natale V. Effects of sleep timing, sleep quality and sleep duration on school achievement in adolescents. *Sleep Med.* 2015;16:936–940.
58. Wolfson AR, Carskadon MA. Understanding adolescent's sleep patterns and school performance: a critical appraisal. *Sleep Med Rev.* 2003;7:491–506.
59. Fallone G, Acebo C, Arnedt JT, Seifer R, Carskadon MA. Effects of acute sleep restriction on behavior, sustained attention, and response inhibition in children. *Percept Mot Skills.* 2001;93:213–229.
60. Radazzo AC, Muehlbach MJ, Schweitzer PK, Waish, JK. Cognitive function following acute sleep restriction in children ages 10–14. *Sleep* 1998;21:861–868.
61. Sadeh A, Gruber R, Raviv A. The effects of sleep restriction and extension on school-age children: what a difference an hour makes. *Child Dev.* 2003;74:444–455.
62. Philips AJK, Clerx WM, O'Brien CS, et al. Irregular sleep/wake patterns associated with poorer academic performance and delayed circadian sleep/wake timing. *Sci Rep.* 2017;7:3216.
63. Smarr BL, Schirmer AE. 3.4 million real-world learning management system logins reveal the majority of students experience social jet lag correlated with decreased performance. *Sci Rep.* 2018;8:4793.
64. Lo JC, Lee SM, Teo LM, Lim J, Gooley JJ, Chee MW. Neurobehavioral impact of successive cycles of sleep restriction with and without naps in adolescents. *Sleep.* 2017;40:zsw042.
65. Lo JC, Ong JL, Leong RL, Gooley JJ, Chee MW. Cognitive performance, sleepiness, and mood in partially sleep deprived adolescents: the need for sleep study. *Sleep.* 2016;39:687–698.
66. Huang S, Deshpande A, Yeo SC, Lo JC, Chee MW, Gooley JJ. Sleep restriction impairs vocabulary learning when adolescents cram for exams: the need for sleep study. *Sleep.* 2016;39:1681–1690.
67. NCAA Research. Estimated probability of competing in college athletics http://www.ncaa.org/about/resouces/research/estimated-probility-competing-college-athletics. Accessed May 14, 2019.
68. Thun E, Bjorvatn B, Flo E, Harris A, Pallesen S. Sleep, circadian rhythms, and athletic performance. *Sleep Med Rev.* 2015;23:1–9.
69. Watson NF, Martin JL, Wise MS, et al. Delaying middle and high school start times promotes student health and performance: an American Academy of Sleep Medicine Position Statement. *J Clin Sleep Med.* 2017;13:623–625.
70. Fredriksen K, Rhodes J, Reddy R, Way N. Sleepless in Chicago: tracking the effects of adolescent sleep loss during the middle school years. *Child Dev.* 2004;75:84–95.
71. Roberts RE, Duong HT. The prospective association between sleep deprivation and depression among adolescents. *Sleep.* 37(2):239–244.

72. Shochat T, Barker DH, Sharkey KM, Van Reen E, Roane BM, Carskadon MA. An approach to understanding sleep and depressed mood in adolescents: person-centered sleep classification. *J Sleep Res* 2017;26:709–717.

73. Tzischinsky O, Shochat T. Eveningness, sleep patterns, daytime functioning, and quality of life in Israeli adolescents. *Chronobiol Int.* 2011;28:338–343.

74. Ojio Y, Nishida A, Shimodera S, Togo F, Sasaki T. Sleep duration associated with the lowest risk of depression/anxiety in adolescents. *Sleep.* 2016;39:1555–1562.

75. Díaz-Morales JF, Escribano C. Consequences of adolescent's evening preference on school achievement: A review. *Ann Psychol.* 2014;30:1096–1104.

76. Sivertsen B, Lallukka T, Salo P, et al. Insomnia as a risk factor for ill health: Results from the large population-based prospective HUNT Study in Norway. *J Sleep Res.* 2014;23:124–132.

77. Palagini, L, Baglioni C, Ciapparelli A, Gemignani A, Riemann D. REM sleep dysregulation in depression: state of the art. *Sleep Med Rev.* 2013;17:377–390.

78. Hasler BP, Allen JJ, Sbarra DA, Bootzin RR, Bernert RA. Morningness-eveningness and depression: preliminary evidence for the role of BAS and positive affect. *Psychiatry Res* 2010;176:166–173.

79. Owens JA, Weiss MR. Insufficient sleep in adolescents: causes and consequences. *Minerva Pediatrica.* 2017;69:326–336.

80. Park W-S, Yang KI, Hyeyun K. Insufficient sleep and suicidal ideation: A study of 12,046 female adolescents. *Sleep Med.* 2019;53:65–69.

81. Liu CH, Stevens C, Wong SHM, Yasui M, Chen JA. The prevalence and predictors of mental health diagnoses and suicide among U.S. college students: Implications for addressing disparities in service use. *Depress Anxiety.* 2018;36:8–17.

82. Centers for Disease Control and Prevention (CDC). Drowsy driving—19 states and the District of Columbia, 2009–2010. *Morb Mortal Wkly Rep.* 2013;61:1033–1037.

83. Herschner, S. Impact of sleep on the challenges of safe driving in young adults. In: Wolfson AR, Montgomery-Downs H, eds. *The Oxford Handbook of Infant, Child, and Adolescent Sleep and Behavior.* New York, NY: Oxford University Press; 2013:441–454.

84. Wheaton AG, Perry GS, Chapman DP, Croft JB. Self-reported sleep duration and weight-control strategies among US high school students. *Sleep.* 2013;36:1139–1145.

85. Tefft BC, AAA Foundation for Traffic Safety. *Prevalence of Motor Vehicle Crashes Involving Drowsy Drivers. United States, 2009–2013.* Washington, DC: AAA Foundation for Traffic Safety; 2014.

86. Owens JA, Dearth-Wesley T, Herman A, Whitaker RC. Drowsy driving, sleep duration, and chronotype in adolescents. *J Pediatr* 2019;205:224–229.

87. Vorona RD, Szklo-Coxe M, Lamichhane R, Ware JC, McNallen A, Leszczyszyn D. Adolescent crash rates and school start times in two central Virginia countries, 2009–2011: a follow-up study to a southeastern Virginia study, 2007–2008. *J Clin Sleep Med.* 2014;10:1169–1177.

88. Danner F, Philips B. Adolescent sleep, school start times, and teen-motor vehicle crashes. *J Clin Sleep Med.* 2008;4:533–535.

89. Wahlstrom K. Examining the impact of later high school start times on the health and academic performance of high school studies: a multi-site study. http://hdl.handle.net/11299/162769. Published 2014. Accessed May 14, 2019.

90. Troxel W, Wolfson A. Sleep science and policy: a focus on school start times. *Sleep Health*. 2016;2:186.

91. Martin S, Oppenheim K. Video gaming: general and pathological use. *Trends & Tudes*. 2007;6:1–7.

92. Rideout VJ, Foehr UG, Roberts DF. Generation M 2: Media in the Lives of 8-to 18-year-olds. Henry J. Kaiser Family Foundation. Available at https://kaiserfamilyfoundation.files.wordpress.com/2013/01/8010.pdf. Published 2010. Retrieved May 14, 2019.

93. Hale L. Guan S. Screen time and sleep among school-aged children and adolescents: A systematic literature review. *Sleep Med Rev*. 2015;21:50–58.

94. LeBourgeois MK, Hale L, Chang AM, Lameese DA, Montgomery-Downs HE, Buxton, OM. Digital media and sleep in childhood and adolescence. *Pediatrics*. 2017;140: S92–S96.

95. Li X, Buxton OM, Lee S, Chang AM, Berger LM, Hale L. Sleep mediates the association between adolescent screen time and depressive symptoms. *Sleep Med*. 2019;57:51–60.

96. Buxton OM, Chang AM, Spilsbury JC, Bos T, Emsellem H, Knutson KL. Sleep in the modern family: protective family routines for child and adolescent sleep. *Sleep Health*. 2015;1:15–27.

97. Weaver E, Gadisar M, Dohnt H, Lovato N, Doublas P. The effect of presleep video-game playing on adolescents sleep. *J Clin Sleep Med*. 2010;6:184–189.

98. Higuchi S, Motohashi Y, Liu Y, Maeda A. Effects of playing a computer game using a bright display on presleep physiological variables, sleep latency, slow wave sleep and REM sleep. *J Sleep Res*. 2005;14:267–273.

99. Chang AM, Aeschbach D, Duffy JF, Czeisler CA. Evening use of light-emitting eReaders negatively affects sleep, circadian timing, and next-morning alertness. *P Natl Acad Sci* 2015;112:1232–1237.

100. McKnight-Eily LR, Eaton DK, Lowry R, Croft JB, Presley-Cantrell L, Perry GS. Relationships between hours of sleep and health-risk behaviors in US adolescent students. *Prevent Med*. 2011;53:271–273.

101. Terry-McElrath YM, Maslowsky J, O'Malley PM, Schulenberg JE, Johnston LD. Sleep and substance use among US adolescents, 1991–2014. *Am J Health Behav*. 2016;40:77–91.

102. Johnston LD, Miech RA, O'Malley PM, Bachman JG, Schulenberg JE, Patrick ME. Monitoring the Future national survey results on drug use, 1975-2017: Overview, key findings on adolescent drug use. Available at: http://www.monitoringthefuture.org/pubs/monographs/mtf-overview2017.pdf. Published 2017. Accessed May 14, 2019.

103. Bonnar D, Gradisar M. Caffeine and sleep in adolescents: A systematic review. *J Caffeine Res* 2015;5:105–14.

104. O'Brien EM, Mindell JA. Sleep and risk-taking behavior in adolescents. *Behav Sleep Med*. 2005;3:113–133.

105. Roane BM, Taylor DJ. Adolescent insomnia as a risk factor for early adult depression and substance abuse. *Sleep*. 2008;31:1351–1356.

106. Pieters S, Van Der Vorst H, Burk WJ, Wiers RW, Engels RC. Puberty-dependent sleep regulation and alcohol use in early adolescents. *Alcohol Clin Exp Res*. 2010;34:1512–1518.

107. Nyguen-Louise TT, Brumback T, Worley MJ, et al. Effects of sleep on substance use in adolescents: a longitudinal perspective. *Addict Biol.* 2018;23:750–760.

108. Singleton RA, Wolfson AR. Alcohol consumption, sleep, and academic performance among college students. *J Stud Alcohol Drugs.* 2009;70:355–363.

109. Hasler BP, Kirisci L, Clark DB. Restless sleep and variable sleep timing during late childhood accelerate the onset of alcohol and other drug involvement. *J Stud Alcohol Drugs.* 2016;77:649–655.

110. Wong MM, Brower KJ, Fitzgerald HE, Zucker RA. Sleep problems in early childhood and early onset of alcohol and other drug use in adolescence. *Alcohol Clin Exp Res.* 2010;28:578–587.

111. Ahluwalia N, Herrick K. Caffeine intake from food and beverage sources and trends among children and adolescents in the United States: review of national quantitative studies from 1999 to 2011. *Adv Nutr.* 2015;6:102–111.

112. Frary CD, Johnson RK, Wang MQ. Food sources and intakes of caffeine in the diets of persons in the United States. *J Acad Nutr Diet.* 2005;105:110–113.

113. Adolescent Sleep Working Group, Committee on Adolescence, and Council on School Health. American Academy of Pediatrics Policy statement: school start times for adolescents. *Pediatrics.* 2014;134:642–648.

114. Malinauskas BM, Aeby VG, Overton RF, Carpenter-Aeby T, Barber Heidal K. A survey of energy drink consumption patterns among college students. *Nutr J.* 2007;6:35.

115. Sojar SH, Shrier LA, Ziemnik RE, Sherritt L, Spalding AL, Levy S. Symptoms attributed to consumption of caffeinated beverages in adolescents. *J Caffeine Res.* 2015;5:187–191.

116. Ludden A, Wolfson AR. Understanding adolescent caffeine use: connecting use patterns with expectancies, reasons, and sleep. *Health Ed Behav.* 2010;37:330–342.

117. Wolfson A, Lacks P, Futterman A. Effects of parent training on infant sleeping patterns, parents' stress, and perceived parental competence. *J Consult Clin Psychol.* 1992;60:41.

118. Wolfson AR, Harkins E, Johnson M, Marco C. Effects of the young adolescent sleep smart program on sleep hygiene practices, sleep health efficacy, and behavioral well-being. *Sleep Health* 2015;1:197–204.

119. Blunden S, Rigney G. Lessons learned from sleep education in schools: A review of dos and don'ts. *J Clin Sleep Med.* 2015;11:671–680.

120. Gruber R. School-based sleep education programs: a knowledge-to-action perspective regarding barriers, proposed solutions, and future directions. *Sleep Med Rev.* 2017;36:13–28.

121. Dietrich SK, Francis-Jimenez CM, Knibbs MD, Umali IL, Truglio-Londrigan M. Effectiveness of sleep education programs to improve sleep hygiene and/or sleep quality in college students: a systematic review. *JBI Db Sys Rev Implement Rep.* 2016;14:108–134.

122. Quan SF, Ziporyn PS. The impact of an online prematriculation sleep course (Sleep 101) on sleep knowledge and behaviors of college freshmen: a pilot study. *Southwest J Pulmon Sleep Med.* 2017;14:159–63.

123. Quan SF, Ziporyn PS, Czeisler CA. Sleep education for college students: the time is now. *J Clin Sleep Med.* 2018;14:1269.

124. Carskadon MA, Wolfson AR, Acebo C, Tzischinsky O, Seifer R. Adolescent sleep patterns, circadian timing, and sleepiness at a transition to early school days. *Sleep* 1998;21:871–881.

125. Nahmod NG, Lee S, Master L, Chang AM, Hale L, Buxton OM. Later high school start times associated with longer actigraphic sleep duration in adolescents. *Sleep.* 2018;42:zsy212.

126. Gariépy G. Janssen I, Sentenac M, Elgar FJ. School start time and sleep in Canadian adolescents. *J Sleep Res.* 2016;26:195–201.

127. Dunster GP, de la Iglesia L, Ben-Hamo M, Nave C, Fleischer JG, Panda S, Horacio O. Sleepmore in Seattle: Later school start times are associated with more sleep and better performance in high school students. *Sci Advance.* 2018;4:eeau6200.

128. KcKeever PM, Clark L. Delayed high school start times later than 8:30 AM and impact on graduation rates and attendance rates. *Sleep Health.* 2017;3:119–125.

129. Wahlstrom KL. *Adolescent Sleep Needs and School Starting Times.* Bloomington, IN: Phi Delta Kappa International; 1999.

130. Wahlstrom KL. Accommodating the sleep patterns of adolescents within current educational structures: An uncharted path. In Carskadon MA, ed. *Adolescent Sleep Patterns: Biological, Social, and Psychological Influences.* New York, NY: Cambridge University Press; 2002:172–197.

131. Start School Later. Key position statements. https://www.startschoollater.net/key-position-statements.html. Published 2019. Accessed May 21, 2019.

132. Start School Later. Legislation. Available at: https://www.startschoollater.net/legislation.html. Published 2019. Accessed May 14, 2019.

11

Adulthood

KEVIN R. PETERS ■

INTRODUCTION

The purpose of the chapter is twofold. The first goal is to provide a general overview of the changes in sleep that occur in adulthood (i.e., from 18 to 65 years of age). Sleep is broadly defined here and includes changes in sleep macroarchitecture (e.g., total sleep time [TST], percentage of time spent in sleep stages, etc.) and sleep microarchitecture (e.g., the density of sleep spindles, the amount of electroencephalogram [EEG] activity in certain frequency bands). The second goal is to provide a more selective review of the effect of caffeine on sleep in adults. Given that caffeine is the most commonly ingested psychoactive drug in the world, documenting its impact on sleep is important.

SLEEP MACROARCHITECTURE IN ADULTHOOD

In 1969 a well-known sleep researcher named Irwin Feinberg wrote: "The changes in sleep patterns with age far exceed in magnitude those produced by any pathological conditions compatible with life" [1, p. 39]. This is quite a statement, and it is as true today as it was back then. It also reflects just how much sleep changes over the lifespan. It should come as no surprise then that several chapters in this textbook are devoted to discussing how sleep develops over the lifespan.

Polysomnographic Measures of Sleep

This section focuses on changes in sleep macroarchitecture in adulthood. Perhaps the best place to start is with the very comprehensive meta-analysis on changes in sleep across the human lifespan that was published by Ohayon, Carskadon, Guilleminault, and Vitiello [2]. Meta-analyses are helpful because researchers combine the results of many studies to obtain an overall summary estimate of the population effect. Although meta-analyses have their own limitations, researchers place more confidence in the results of meta-analyses than they do in the results of individual studies. The Ohayon et al. [2] meta-analysis covered a rather large age range, including participants aged 5 years to 102 years, but we focus here on the 47 studies that examined participants that were 19 years or older ($N = 2,391$). In terms of patterns, the following sleep variables decrease significantly with age: TST, sleep efficiency (SE), the percentages of sleep time spent in slow-wave sleep (SWS) and rapid eye movement (REM) sleep, and REM latency. In contrast, the following sleep variables increase significantly with age: sleep latency, the amount of time spent awake after sleep onset, and the percentages of sleep time spent in stages N1 and N2. These results highlight that sleep becomes lighter and more fragmented as we get older.

Although statistical significance (i.e., p values less than some cut-off, usually 0.05) is the most commonly used benchmark in science for determining whether a given result is important, researchers also look at measures of *effect size* to help gauge the meaningfulness of a given result. In the Ohayon et al. [2] meta-analysis, Cohen's d values were computed as the summary effect size measures. To compute a d value, one takes the difference between two means and divides that difference by the pooled standard deviation (usually an average of the two standard deviations that takes into account the sample sizes of the groups), so that one is left with a standardized mean difference. For context, a d value of zero indicates that the two means are the same. Cohen [3] proposed the following guidelines to assist with interpretation: d values of 0.20, 0.50, and 0.80 are considered small, medium, and large effect sizes, respectively.

Using this framework, small effects in the Ohayon et al. [2] meta-analysis included the decreases in REM latency (–0.15) and percentage of REM sleep (–0.46), and the increases in sleep latency (0.27), percentage of stage N2 (0.28), and percentage of stage N1 (0.28). Medium effect sizes included the decreases in TST (–0.60) and SE (–0.71). Finally, the decrease in percentage of SWS (–0.85) and the increase in the amount of time spent awake after sleep onset (0.89) showed large effect sizes. The d values reported in this meta-analysis are shown graphically in Figure 11.1. In this figure, small effects are in white bars, medium effects are in grey bars, and large effects are in black bars. Bars to the left are decreases with age; bars to the right are increases with age. Here we can see the value added by the effect size indices: All of these age differences were statistically significant (i.e., for each variable, the probability of obtaining the age difference would be very low if the values were randomly drawn from two populations that had equal means), but the Cohen d values help us to see which effects are smaller and which are larger. Accordingly, we know from this meta-analysis that the decreases in SWS are of a much larger magnitude that the decreases in REM latency. Knowing this type of additional information is important in trying to understand how sleep changes as we age—not all changes are the same!

One important point to keep in mind is that most studies on sleep and aging focus on group differences in the mean or average, which is consistent with

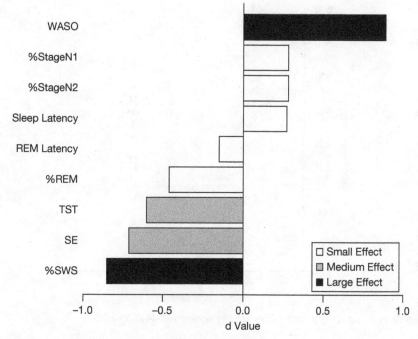

Figure 11.1 Cohen's *d* values reported in Ohayon et al. [2].
Abbreviation: WASO, time spent awake after sleep onset.

most other areas in science. There is a very good rationale for comparing group averages—after all, if we had to choose one number to represent the scores for a group, the average is a good place to start. When one looks at all data points, however, there is often considerable overlap between age groups even in the presence of significant differences in the group means. To illustrate this point, consider the following data from 24 younger adults and 24 older adults. Note that these data are from the study published by Peters, Ray, Fogel, Smith, and Smith [4]. The mean TST for the younger adults was 472.88 minutes, while the mean TST for older adults was 391.42 minutes. This is a large effect, as the Cohen's *d* value is 1.14 (it is also larger than the effect size report in the meta-analysis by Ohayon et al. [2] as previously described). The individual TST values for the two age groups are shown in Figure 11.2. As can be seen, despite the large difference between the group means, there is still considerable overlap between the two age groups.

Cohen's *d* is one of the most commonly used measure of effect size, but it is not the only measure of effect size. An alternative measure is the probability of superiority [5]. Basically, if we were to randomly select one younger adult from our sample and one older adult from our sample, the probability that the TST in the younger adult would be greater than the TST of the older adults would be 0.79. In other words, if we were to randomly select TST scores from each age group many times, the TST from the younger adult would be greater than the TST of the older adult 79% of the time, which also means that the TST for the younger adult would be less than the older adult 21% of the time. The probability

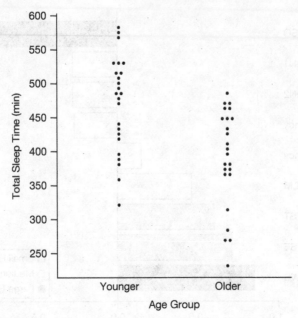

Figure 11.2 Total sleep time values for 24 younger and 24 older adults.

of superiority is consistent with Cohen's *d*, but it provides a different perspective on how the groups compare to one another. The presence of overlap is interesting and suggests that the TST does not drop very much for some older adults. In other words, the next question becomes, "Why does age seem to impact the sleep of some adults more than others?" A comprehensive theory of age differences or changes in sleep needs to consider this important question.

Subjective Reports of Sleep

The results of the Ohayon et al. [2] meta-analysis are largely consistent with studies that have examined subjective sleep quality in adults. To illustrate, consider the study by Lemola and Richter [6]. These researchers followed 14,179 participants, aged 18 to 85 years, over 4 years. In addition to a number of other questions, participants answered the question "How satisfied are you with your sleep?" using an 11-point scale at each time point. The researchers divided the sample into 17 age groups (e.g., 18–21 years, 22–25 years—up to 82–85 years). Across age groups, an interesting nonlinear pattern emerged: subjective sleep quality ratings declined from young adulthood until age 60, from which there was actually an increase in sleep quality until age 65, which was then followed by a decline. The researchers noted that the bump in sleep quality ratings coincided with the typical age of retirement, which makes sense as people would have less stress impacting their sleep just after they retire. Almost half of the age groups (7 of the 17) also showed a significant drop in sleep quality over the 4-year study period, with most of these age groups falling in the middle to older age groups. Thus, this study was able to look at both age differences (i.e., cross-sectional data) and age changes (i.e., longitudinal data) in subjective sleep quality.

In an attempt to examine why sleep quality declines with age, a number of variables have been correlated with subjective sleep quality in adults. We cannot review all such variables in this chapter, rather we focus on a few select examples. In a longitudinal study of 521 healthy women, Owens and Mathews [7] reported that women who transitioned from pre- to postmenopause during the study and who did not undergo hormone replacement therapy reported significantly more sleep disturbances than those who did not make this transition. These results suggest that hormonal changes may accompany declines in subjective sleep quality as women age.

In terms of psychological variables, Troxel, Buysse, Hall, and Matthews [8] reported that higher levels of reported marital happiness were associated with better subjective sleep quality in a sample of 2148 middle-aged women. Allen, Magee, and Vella [9] examined the associations between subjective sleep quality and a host of personality variables in a nationally representative sample of 14,065 adults in Australia. The strongest relationship was between high neuroticism scores and low sleep-quality scores, and this association was stronger in males than in females. Other personality variables such as higher extraversion scores and lower openness to experience scores were associated with better sleep quality. Positive and negative affect (i.e., hedonic balance) mediated the relationships between personality and sleep quality. One example of this mediation was that the strength of the relationship between neuroticism and sleep quality depended, in part, on the degree of negative affect the participants endorsed. In other words, the association was stronger in participants who reported higher levels of negative affect. We cannot draw causal conclusions from these studies, but we can say that subjective sleep quality in adults has a number of interesting biological and psychological correlates that are worth investigating further.

The previously reviewed studies focused on the associations between subjective sleep quality and other variables in adults either concurrently (i.e., at the same time in middle-aged adults) or prospectively (i.e., measuring sleep quality in middle-aged adults and then documenting subsequent changes). Some studies have taken a different perspective, examining the association between childhood/adolescent experiences with subsequent sleep quality in adulthood. These studies reveal some interesting patterns. Dregan and Armstrong [10] examined a sample of 7,781 UK participants at ages 16, 23, 33, and 42. Even after controlling for a wide range of variables, sleep disturbances at the first wave were a significant predictor of sleep problems later on, at each of the subsequent time points. Specifically, the odds ratios for having sleep problems at later time points based on the presence of such problems at age 16 were 1.77 (age 23), 1.35 (age 33), and 1.24 (age 44). In other words, having sleep problems at age 16 increases the odds of having similar problems at age 44 by 24%. The researchers reported that depression may be an important factor in the continuation of sleep problems into adulthood. There is also some evidence that childhood adversities (e.g., parents divorcing, having problems with alcohol or finances) or abuse (i.e., physical, emotional, or sexual) is associated with sleep problems in adulthood [11, 12] and that some of these adversities are associated with sleep disorders such as insomnia [13]. It is important to remember that correlation does not equal causation. These studies are not true experiments. It would be unethical to randomly assign half of the child participants to one condition and the other half to a control condition to see what impact that condition has on sleep in adulthood. Nonetheless, these studies underscore the importance of linking childhood experiences with subsequent sleep quality as we get older.

Where do the studies on subjective sleep quality leave us? Compared to studies that measure sleep objectively using polysomnography, studies that ask participants to subjectively rate their sleep quality have the advantage of being able to recruit much larger samples that can often be more representative of the population (i.e., have greater external validity). However, these studies have a major disadvantage in that participants may not be as accurate in rating their own sleep quality (i.e., have lower internal validity). For example, in a well-controlled study of 33 participants over several nights, Akerstedt, Kecklund, and Axelsson [14] examined the ability of 13 polysomnographic sleep variables to predict each participant's subjective sleep rating for each corresponding night. Interestingly, they found that the percentage of time spent awake was the best predictor of subjective sleep quality each night, with SE being the next-best predictor. Although the correlation coefficients between percent of time spent awake and subjective sleep quality were medium to large range (i.e., ranged from –0.39 to –0.57), they are still smaller than one would hope for given how often we examine subjective sleep quality in research studies. None of the other polysomnographic variables were significant predictors of subjective sleep quality. Clearly, more work is needed to understand the relationships between subjective and objective sleep quality.

Before moving on, one additional question to consider relates to the changes in sleep that accompany aging and sleep need. We have known for a long time that we tend to sleep less as we get older, and this is verified in studies that have examined sleep with polysomnography and subjectively. The traditional, and perhaps common sense, reason for this finding is that we simply need less sleep as we get older. There are some problems with this explanation, however. Equating one's sleep need with how long they sleep for is not that straightforward. Really, think about it. Can you honestly say that you get enough sleep to satisfy your sleep need? I would be surprised if this was the case for many readers. While our brains (and bodies) require a certain amount of sleep, there will usually be environmental restrictions or constraints that interfere with us meeting this need (e.g., the stress of school and/or work-related deadlines, family matters, etc.). How does one actually determine a person's "true" sleep need? Even if I let you sleep for as long as you like for several days, then took an average TST for you, I would likely still not know your true sleep need as you are probably a bit sleep deprived, so you might be oversleeping to "catch-up" on missed sleep. I would probably have to let you live somewhere with minimal external demands for a month and let you sleep as long as you wish to try to figure out how much sleep you actually need. This kind of experiment is simply not practical for most people, although some sleep researchers do this kind of study.

Returning to our question about why we tend to sleep less as we get older, one alternative view is that we sleep less as we age because our brains simply are unable to generate sleep as efficiently as it did when we were younger. Studies have shown that daytime napping increases with age. For example, Ohayon and Zulley [15] examined self-report measures in 4,115 adults between ages 15 to 99 years and reported that the prevalence of daytime napping increases across adulthood, with the increases becoming statistically significant in the mid-50s and older. They also reported that daytime napping was positively correlated with daytime sleepiness. These results are not consistent with the view that older adults need less sleep; rather, they suggest that older adults are not able to meet their sleep need in one nocturnal sleep period. Also, remember that sleep is an active process that is generated at multiple levels within the brain, so it stands to reason that some of the decline if TST is explained by brain aging. We do not hesitate to try to explain some of our in age-related declines in memory and other cognitive abilities as being the result of age-related changes to our brains, so why should sleep be any different. Something to think about!

SLEEP MICROARCHITECTURE IN ADULTHOOD

In addition to examining age differences in sleep macroarchitecture (e.g., SE, percentage of time spent in each stage), researchers have documented age differences in sleep microarchitecture. These studies focus on very specific events or waveforms within the EEG. We will not cover all of these age differences, but rather focus on several interesting examples.

One very well-established finding on sleep microarchitecture .is that the number and/or density of sleep spindles decreases with age. Studies that have compared extreme age groups (e.g., a group of younger adults vs. a group of older adults) have found that the number and density of sleep spindles is reduced in older adults [4, 16–18]. Spindle density in these studies is typically defined as the number of spindles per minute of stage N2, which takes into account age differences in the amount of stage N2. To help fill in the gaps between young and older adults, Nicolas, Petit, Rompre, and Montplaisir [19] examined participants who ranged from 10 to 69 years of age, categorized into the groups: 10 to 19 years, 20 to 29 years, 30 to 39 years, 40 to 49 years, 50 to 59 years, and 60 to 69 years. Consistent with the previously cited studies, the mean density of spindles of spindles showed a progressive and significant decrease across the age groups. In addition, the mean duration of spindles decreased significantly across the age groups. So, older adults tend to have fewer spindles than younger adults and the spindles that they do have tend to be shorter in duration.

While the average score for many variables changes with age, it is also known that the variability increases with age for many variables. In the study by Nicolas et al. [19], for example, the mean spindle density was quite a bit lower in the older adults than in the younger adults (1.62 vs. 4.44), but the standard deviation was also considerably larger in the older group than in the younger group (1.42 vs. 0.57). In other words, age does not affect all adults equally when it comes to spindle density. As previously mentioned, and shown in Figure 11.1, it is important to consider more than the average when comparing two or more groups.

The cause(s) of the age-related decreases in the density and duration of sleep spindles remain unknown. There has been speculation that these decreases are the result of compromises in the functioning of two key brain regions, the thalamus and the cortex, that are involved in generating sleep spindles, which may also be related to problems maintaining sleep [16, 17, 19]. Others have posited that spindles changes are possibly due to lower levels of melatonin that also accompany aging [20, 21]. Still others have tried to link age-related changes in sleep spindles with changes in cognitive abilities as we get older [18]. More research is clearly needed in this area.

Focusing on more global age-related EEG changes, Carrier, Land, Buysse, and Kupfer [22] examined quantitative EEG measures in 100 adults between ages 20 and 60 years. Quantitative EEG involves looking at the power (or area under the curve) for each individual frequency to see how much activity is present at that frequency. In general, higher power values indicate greater EEG activity. The analysis typically starts at around 1 Hz and then goes up to around 30 Hz, in 1 Hz bins. These researchers reported a number of interesting findings, but here we focus on three main results. First, there were deceases in EEG power with age for a wide range of lower to middle EEG frequencies in the delta, theta, and higher spindle frequency range. These results are consistent with age-related decreases in SWS and spindle density measures. Second, age was related to an increase in higher frequencies (e.g., beta activity), which is associated with cortical activation. This result is consistent with the "lightening" of sleep in older adults (e.g., more awakenings, more time spent in stages 1 and 2). Third, although females had higher power values than males for most of the EEG frequencies, there were no age by gender interactions, suggesting that age does not affect males and females differently. The results of this study on quantitative EEG are quite consistent with the results of the Ohayon et al. [2] meta-analysis that focused on sleep microarchitecture.

In the previous macroarchitecture section, it was noted that the percentage of time spent in SWS (stages N3 and N4 combined) decreases with age. An interesting study by Dube and colleagues [23] suggests that part of this decrease in SWS may be due to changes in brain structure. In this study, 30 young and 33 older adults completed both sleep polysomnography as well as structural magnetic resonance imaging for brain imaging. One of the main findings was that participants with greater slow-wave EEG activity (less than 4 Hz) in their sleep EEG also tended to have thicker cortical areas that are involved in producing SWS. In addition, age-related changes in slow-wave activity were mediated by cortical thickness. These results suggest that part of the age-related decrease in SWS may in fact be due to age-related decreases in gray matter in the brain areas that produce SWS.

CAFFEINE AND SLEEP

Perhaps the first study of the effects of caffeine on sleep was published by Hollingworth in 1912 [24]. When the Coca-Cola company was considering adding caffeine to its now famous beverage, there were serious concerns raised by the US federal government—caffeine was thought to be a dangerous and toxic chemical back then. Harry Hollingworth and his wife, Leta, were asked by the Coca-Cola company to study the effect of caffeine on a number of psychological variables, including sleep quality. The studies they carried out are now famous and included a number of methodologically sound principles that we take for granted today: counterbalancing, placebo controls, and the double-blind procedure [25]. The study involved 16 participants (6 women) over 40 days. Subjective measures of sleep duration (self-reported number of hours of sleep) and sleep quality ("better than usual," "normal," or "worse than usual") were recorded each morning. So, what did they find? First, the amount of caffeine mattered: small doses had little effect on sleep duration or quality, but larger doses did. Second, even with only 16 participants, they observed individual variability in the effect of caffeine: the sleep of a few participants was negatively affected even at lower doses, while larger doses appeared to have little effect on a few of the participants. This individual variability effect has been reported in research since this landmark study. Third, the effect of caffeine on sleep was more pronounced when the caffeine was ingested on an empty stomach. Fourth, the effect became more prominent over several days of ingestions (i.e., the effect was cumulative). Fifth, the effect of caffeine on sleep varied with body weight: the heavier the participant, the less pronounced the impact of caffeine on sleep.

Since the Hollingworth study in 1912, the effect of caffeine on subjective measures of sleep duration and/or quality have been replicated many times. Clark and Landolt [26] performed a systematic review of 58 studies on the association/effect of caffeine on sleep quality.

Like meta-analyses, systematic reviews attempt to rigorously review studies on a given topic; unlike meta-analyses, they do not report summary statistics from the combined studies (in other words, they provide a qualitative review of studies on a given topic, not a quantitative review). In large-scale survey studies, caffeine consumption in adolescents was associated sleep disturbances such as increased time to fall asleep, greater number of awakenings, shorter sleep duration, and poor sleep quality overall. In similar studies on adults, the negative effects of caffeine on sleep are more prominent in those individuals who consumed larger amounts of caffeine (e.g., 500 mg/day in one study and greater than 8 cups a day in another study). These results are consistent with those reported in the Hollingworth [24] study: for most people, small doses of caffeine have little impact on sleep, but negative effects are more common with larger doses of caffeine.

The Clark and Landolt [26] systematic review also examined studies that used more objective measures of sleep (EEG or actigraphy). The vast majority of these studies also reveal that caffeine does have negative impacts on sleep. In terms of sleep macroarchitecture, the effects of caffeine are similar to the effects of aging that were reviewed above: sleep becomes lighter and more fragmented following caffeine ingestion (i.e., increases in sleep latency, wakefulness, arousals, and stage N1 sleep, along with decreases in the SWS and TST). The effect of caffeine on REM is less clear.

The lightening effects of caffeine are consistent with studies that have examined EEG activity (microarchitecture) during sleep: in the studies reviewed by Clark and Landolt [26], caffeine ingestion reduces delta wave or slow wave activity (frequencies <5 Hz) and increases sigma/beta activity (13–30 Hz). In their interesting study, Landolt Weth, Borbely, and Dijk [27] showed that 200 mg of caffeine (a little more that the equivalent of a cup of coffee) ingested in the morning was sufficient to have an impact on sleep later that night. Compared to placebo, the caffeine group showed significant reductions in SE and sleep time. The effect on caffeine on the EEG during non-REM sleep was a significant reduction in slow wave activity (<1 Hz) along with a significant increase in EEG activity in the spindle range (11.25–14 Hz). The EEG during REM sleep was also impacted: Significant reductions in slow wave (<5 Hz) and theta activity (5–6 Hz) were observed.

In keeping with the developmental theme of this chapter, there is some evidence that the effects of caffeine on sleep are more pronounced in middle-aged adults than in young adults. Robillard, Bouchard, Cartier, Nicolau, and Carrier [28] examined the effect of low (200 mg) and high (400 mg) doses of caffeine on sleep polysomnography in 22 young adults (mean age = 24 years) and 24 middle-aged adults (mean age = 52 years). In general, the negative impacts of caffeine on sleep were consistent with those reported above, but this study also revealed that the effects of the higher dose of caffeine were larger in the middle-aged adults than in the younger adults, suggesting that these middle-aged adults were more sensitive to the effects of higher levels of caffeine. Thus, aging seems to have a lightening effect on sleep, which may be exacerbated by consuming caffeine (i.e., aging and caffeine seem to have a "double whammy" effect on sleep).

The effects of caffeine on sleep are consistent with how caffeine affects the brain. Without going into too much detail, caffeine binds to, and blocks, the activity of adenosine receptors, which are widely distributed throughout the brain and parts of the body. Adenosine normally has an inhibitory effect (i.e., it reduces the rate of neuronal activity). It is believed that adenosine has a role in sleep homeostasis in that it inhibits brain areas that keep us awake and alert. Thus, while adenosine helps to promote sleep, caffeine blocks this activity, which helps to keep us alert and reduce sleepiness [29]. Of course, the antagonistic effect of caffeine on adenosine reverses after the effects of caffeine have worn off. In other words, the effects of caffeine are temporary. Over the past decade, there has been some fascinating research examining how individual sensitivities to caffeine and the effect of caffeine on sleep may be mediated by different types of adenosine receptors [26].

CONCLUSION

In conclusion, age has well-documented effects on sleep. As we get older, sleep becomes lighter: we have more arousals, spend more time awake during the night, and spend more time in stages N1 and N2, less time in SWS and our TST decreases. Consistent with these microarchitecture changes, the EEG shows similar changes: power in the slow-wave frequency bands decreases and power in the higher frequency bands increases with age. Caffeine appears to have similar effects on sleep. Caffeine ingestion, especially at higher doses, increases sleep onset latency, decreases TST, increase time spent in stage N1 and decreases in SWS. At the EEG level, caffeine also reduces slow-wave activity and increases higher frequency activity. Subjectively, both older age and caffeine ingestion are associated with poorer reports of sleep quality. Finally, there is some limited evidence that age and caffeine seem to interact with one another. Higher doses of caffeine seem to be more disruptive to our sleep as we get older. These results highlight the complexity of sleep. Although advancing age and caffeine ingestion have similar effects on sleep, the precise mechanisms behind these effects are likely quite different. In other words, there is more than one way to negatively impact sleep.

ACKNOWLEDGMENTS

I would like to dedicate this chapter to Dr. Robert Ogilvie, Professor Emeritus in the Psychology Department at Brock University. Bob was the person who first introduced me to the scientific study of sleep—I took his third-year undergraduate course on sleep and he was my honors thesis supervisor. He showed me just how interesting sleep research could be, and I will always be grateful to him for that.

REFERENCES

1. Feinberg I. Effects of age on human sleep patterns. In Kales A, ed. *Sleep: Physiology and Pathology*. Philadelphia PA: Lippincourt; 1969:39–52.
2. Ohayon MM, Carskadon MA, Guilleminault C, Vitiello MV. Meta-analysis of quantitative sleep parameters from childhood to old age in healthy individuals: developing normative sleep values across the human lifespan. *Sleep*. 2004;27:1255–1273.
3. Cohen J. *Statistical Power Analysis for the Behavioral Sciences*. 2nd ed. Mahwah NJ: Erlbaum; 1988.
4. Peters KR, Ray L, Fogel S, Smith V, Smith CT. Age differences in the variability and distribution of sleep spindle and rapid eye movement densities. *PLOS ONE*. 2014;9:e91047.
5. Grissom RJ. Probability of superiority. *J Appl Psychol*. 1994;79:314–316.
6. Lemola S, Richter D. The course of subjective sleep quality in middle and old adulthood and it's relation to physical health. *J Gerontol B-Psychol*. 2013;68:721–729.
7. Owens JF, Matthews KA. Sleep disturbance in healthy middle-aged women. *Maturitas*. 1998;30:41–50.
8. Troxel WM, Buysse DJ, Hall M, Matthews KA. Marital happiness and sleep disturbance in a multi-ethnic sample of middle-aged women. *Behav Sleep Med*. 2009;7:2–19.

9. Allen MS, Magee CA, Vella SA. Personality, hedonic balance and the quality and quantity of sleep in adulthood. *Psychol Health.* 2016;31:1091–1107.

10. Dregan A, Armstrong D. Adolescence sleep disturbances as predictors of adulthood sleep disturbances: A cohort study. *J Adolesc Health.* 2010;46:482–487.

11. Greenfield EA, Lee C, Friedman EL, Springer KW. Childhood abuse as a risk factor for sleep problems in adulthood: evidence from a U.S. national study. *Ann Behav Med.* 2011;42:245–256.

12. Koskenvuo K, Hublin C, Partinen M, Paunio T, Koskenvuo, M. Childhood adversities and quality of sleep in adulthood: A population-based study of 26,000 Finns. *Sleep Med.* 2010;11:17–22.

13. Bader K, Schafer V, Schenkel M, Nissen L, Schwander J. Adverse childhood experiences associated with sleep in primary insomnia. *J Sleep Res.* 2007;16:285–296.

14. Akerstedt T, Kecklund G, Axelsson J. Subjective and objective quality of sleep. *Somnologie.* 2008;12:104–109.

15. Ohayon MM, Zulley J. Prevalence of naps in the general population. *Sleep Hypnosis.* 1999;1:88–97.

16. Crowley K, Trinder J, Kim Y, Carrington M, Colrain IM. The effects of normal aging on sleep spindle and K-complex production. *Clin Neurophysiol.* 2002;113:1615–1622.

17. Guazzelli M, Feinberg I, Aminoff M, Fein G, Floyd TC, Maggini C. Sleep spindles in normal elderly: comparison with young adult patterns and relation to nocturnal awakening, cognitive function and brain atrophy. *Electroencephal Clin Neurophysiol.* 1986;63:526–539.

18. Peters KR, Ray L, Smith V, Smith C. Changes in the density of stage 2 spindles following motor learning in young and older adults. *J Sleep Res.* 2008;17:23–33.

19. Nicolas A, Petit D, Rompre S, Montplaisir J. Sleep spindle characteristics in healthy subjects of different age groups. *Clin Neurophysiol.* 2001;112:521–527.

20. Dijk D-J, Roth C, Landolt HP, Werth E, Aeppli M, Achermann P, Borbely AA. Melatonin effect on daytime sleep in men: suppression of EEG low frequency activity and enhancement of spindle frequency activity. *Neurosci Lett.* 1995;201:13–16.

21. Landolt HP, Dijk D-J, Achermann P, Borbely AA. Effect of age on the sleep EEG: slow-wave activity and spindle frequency activity in young and middle-aged men. *Brain Res.* 1996;73:205–212.

22. Carrier J, Land S, Buysse DJ, Kupfer DJ. The effects of age and gender on sleep EEG power spectral density in the middle years of life (ages 20 to 60 years old). *Psychophysiology,* 2001;38:232–242.

23. Dube J, Lafortune M, Bedetti C, et al. Cortical thinning explains changes in sleep slow waves during adulthood. *J Neurosci.* 2015;35:7795–7807.

24. Hollingworth HL. The influence of caffeine alkaloid on the quality and amount of sleep. *Am J Psychol.* 1912;23:89–100.

25. Goodwin CJ, Goodwin KA. *Research in Psychology: Methods and Design.* 7th ed. Hoboken NJ: Wiley; 2013.

26. Clark I, Landolt HP. Coffee, caffeine, and sleep: a systematic review of epidemiological studies and randomized controlled trials. *Sleep Med Rev.* 2017;21:70–78.

27. Landolt HP, Werth E, Borbely AA, Dijk D-J. Caffeine intake (200 mg) in the morning affects human sleep and EEG power spectra at night. *Brain Res.* 1995;67:67–74.

28. Robillard R, Bouchard M, Cartier A, Nicolau L, Carrier J. Sleep is more sensitive to high doses of caffeine in the middle years of life. *J Psychopharmacol.* 2015;29:688–697.

29. Roehrs T, Roth T. Caffeine: sleep and daytime sleepiness. *Sleep Med Rev.* 2008;12:153–162.

12

Aging

MICHAEL K. SCULLIN AND ALEXANDRIA M. REYNOLDS ■

INTRODUCTION

No human being ever cared as much about sleep as Nathaniel Kleitman, the father of modern sleep research. He lived to be 104 years old. By contrast, his graduate student Eugene Aserinsky lamented that sleep was "the least desirable of the scientific areas [he] wished to pursue" [1]. Perhaps Aserinsky's low prioritization of sleep as a research area also manifested as a low prioritization of personal sleep hygiene: after all, he is suspected to have died because he fell asleep while driving his car.

These "case studies" illustrate a sobering finding that is now supported by hundreds of empirical studies: how you sleep in your 20s, 30s, 40s, and so forth impacts how long and how well you live. In this chapter, we will cover how sleep typically changes across the adult lifespan, the causes and consequences of age-related sleep changes, and solutions for improving sleep even in older age.

CHARACTERISTICS OF SLEEP IN NORMAL AGING

If you ask older adults what they most want to change about their sleep, they will almost certainly express frustration with waking in the middle of the night. Nocturia, or the need to use the bathroom during the night, is the primary sleep complaint among older adults, with half of older adults reporting nocturia every, or almost every, night [2]. As can be expected, frequent disruptions lead to shallower sleep, increased daytime sleepiness, and lower overall satisfaction with sleep. But do older adults sleep worse because of a full bladder, or do they wake up due to other causes and then attribute the awakening to needing to use the bathroom?

Laboratory polysomnography studies affirm older adults' reports that their sleep is highly fragmented (i.e., lower sleep efficiency, higher wake after sleep

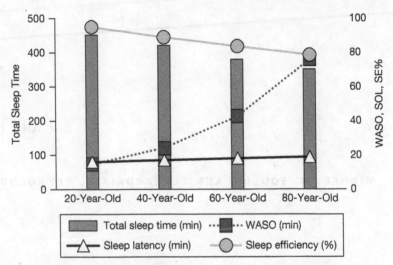

Figure 12.1 Aging does not affect difficulty falling asleep, but it does affect difficulty maintaining sleep (sleep fragmentation).

Abbreviations: WASO, wake after sleep onset; SE%, sleep efficiency percentage; SOL, sleep onset latency.

SOURCE: Modified from Gao C, Scullin MK, Bliwise DL. Mild cognitive impairment and dementia. In Savard J, Ouellet MC. Handbook of Sleep Disorders in Medical Conditions. London, UK: Elsevier; 2019. Used with permission from Elsevier.

onset, many night-time awakenings; Figure 12.1) [3–4]. But laboratory studies also help pinpoint the mechanisms for these nighttime awakenings. One such mechanism is that older adults have a lower arousal threshold. For example, some 20-year-olds sleep through sounds played at 80 decibels (equivalent to a garbage disposal), whereas many 80-year-olds awaken to sounds played at 55 decibels (equivalent to a quiet conversation) [5]. This partially explains why your roommate sleeps through everything when you return to the dorm at 2 AM, but your grandpa will awaken from his nap when the golf show switches to a commercial. The arousal threshold issue is exacerbated by age-related alterations in sleep architecture. Figure 12.2 illustrates that older adults spend longer in N1 and N2 than young adults, which is important because it is easier to awaken someone from shallower stages of sleep (N1, N2) than from deeper stages of sleep (slow-wave sleep [SWS] or rapid eye movement [REM] sleep; hence the name "deep") [5–6].

Is shallow sleep overactive or is deep sleep underactive in older adults? If shallow sleep is overactive, then one is faced with the dilemma of identifying a means to suppress shallow sleep without affecting deep sleep. However, if deep sleep is underactive, then one might increase SWS/REM sleep in older adults by pharmacological or behavioral interventions. The literature points to deeper stages of sleep being underactive in older adults. For example, with increasing age, slow waves decrease in amplitude and density to the extent that adults experience cortical thinning in the frontal and lateral fissure brain regions that are known to promote SWS [7–8]. Similarly, the neurotransmitter systems needed to generate

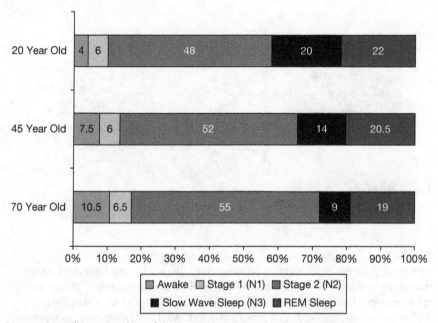

Figure 12.2 Changes in sleep architecture percentages with increasing age.
SOURCE: Scullin MK, Bliwise DL. Sleep, cognition, and normal aging: integrating a half-century of multidisciplinary research. *Persp Psychol Sci.* 2015;10:97–137. Reprinted with permission from SAGE.

REM sleep—particularly acetylcholine—decline with increasing age and in age-related diseases such as Alzheimer's disease [4]. Therefore, the density of REM sleep progressively declines as well.

In the midst of these general changes, it is important to recognize the extent of inter- and intraindividual variability in sleep changes over time. Not everyone gets the same quantity or quality of SWS and/or REM sleep every night, and the extent to which sleep architecture declines over time differs among individuals. Due to the expensive nature of polysomnography and the difficulties studying sleep longitudinally, almost all aging studies using polysomnography have been cross-sectional in nature (e.g., comparing a group of 20-year-olds to a group of 80-year-olds). The Sleep Heart Health Study represents an important exception [9]. From 1995 to 2003, more than 2,500 adult participants underwent polysomnography measurement at two time points, separated by approximately 5 years. The general patterns identified in this longitudinal study confirmed general cross-sectional findings: aging leads to greater sleep fragmentation, less total sleep time at night, and altered sleep architecture [10]. Figure 12.3 illustrates an arguably more important theme: Individual trajectories across time are remarkably variable. Furthermore, not all aspects of sleep change at the same rate or even in the same direction. For example, though there was an overall 9% decrease in SWS, about half of the adults who showed decreased SWS showed an increase in REM sleep over the same time period. One possible explanation is that REM

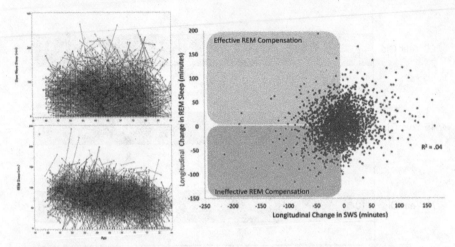

Figure 12.3 Longitudinal data from the Sleep Heart Health Study, with each line representing a single participant's 5-year trajectory. The top left and bottom left panels show inter- and intra-individual variability in levels of slow-wave sleep (SWS) and rapid eye movement (REM) sleep. The right panel shows that SWS and REM sleep do not decline uniformly, suggesting that preserved or enhanced REM sleep might compensate for some loss of SWS.
SOURCE: Scullin MK, Gao C. Dynamic contributions of slow wave sleep and REM sleep to cognitive longevity. *Curr Sleep Med Rep*. 2018;4:284–293. Figure reprinted with permission from Springer Nature.

sleep helps to support processes normally subserved primarily by SWS but can no longer do so because of cortical thinning (as well as alterations in older adult's neurochemistry and neural connectivity during SWS). For example, many studies show that SWS is vital to cognitive functioning in young adults, yet when similar studies are conducted in older adults, REM sleep is often a stronger predictor of cognitive functioning [6].

CLINICAL SLEEP DISORDERS IN OLDER ADULTS

Up to this point, we have considered sleep changes with "normal" aging, that is, how the healthiest older adults sleep. A reality of aging, however, is the accumulation of medical conditions such as hypertension, diabetes, cancer, stroke, and others. Consistent with this general theme, most sleep disorders also increase in prevalence as we age. Insomnia is more common in older adults—not because they have difficulty initially falling asleep—but because they wake up more during the night and are unable to return to sleep.

Although there are numerous predisposing and precipitating factors for insomnia (described in the next section), a core challenge for addressing insomnia in older adults is that they show advanced circadian rhythms [11]. Many older adults feel tired early in the evening (e.g., 8 PM) and are ready to awaken early in the morning (e.g., 4 AM). This circadian phase advance in subjective sleepiness/ alertness is partially caused by age-related changes in the suprachiasmatic nucleus (the "master clock" in your brain), which have downstream effects that cause an earlier secretion of the sleepiness-inducing hormone melatonin. Moreover, there are age-related changes in expression of circadian genes (e.g., CLOCK gene) and older adults may not be exposed to as much natural light throughout the day as are young adults (natural light helps to synchronize the suprachiasmatic nucleus). Any shifts in circadian timing have the potential to disrupt sleep, as you might have experienced with the spring and fall daylight saving time shifts. Figure 12.4 shows how the circadian advance coincides with changes in waking activity, suprachiasmatic nucleus firing rates, and release of melatonin.

Perhaps the most significant sleep-related medical concern for older adults is the increased prevalence of sleep disordered breathing, such as obstructive sleep apnea (OSA). With OSA, breathing reduces (hypopnea) or completely ceases (apnea) for 10 seconds, 20 seconds, 30 seconds, or even longer. Eventually, the person's brain detects a significant shift in cerebral oxygen and carbon dioxide

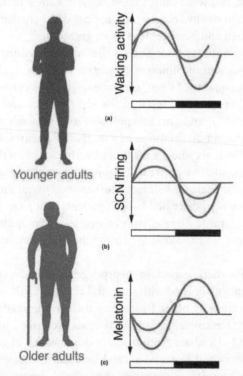

Younger adults

Older adults

Figure 12.4 Age-related changes in the brain advances the circadian rhythm, which impacts waking activity (a), suprachiasmatic nucleus (SCN) firing rate and amplitude (b), and melatonin level and timing of release (c) over the course of 24 hours (dark side of the bars signify nighttime.

SOURCE: Figure modified from Hood S, Amir S. The aging clock: circadian rhythms and later life. *J Clin Invest*. 2017;127:437–446.

levels, causing them to awaken, often with a gasp for air. Yet, such individuals typically return to sleep within seconds and the next day may not remember waking at all. Adults with moderate OSA show approximately 100 apneas or hypopneas across a single night; adults with extreme OSA show 100 or more events every hour (<1% of cases). Each apnea fragments sleep, stresses the cardiovascular system, and causes cerebral hypoxia. Although population-based estimates of the prevalence of OSA vary substantially, the National Health and Aging Trends Study (NHATS) recently estimated that more than 50% of older adults are at high risk for OSA [12]. Alarmingly, perhaps more than 75% of adults with severe sleep apnea are undiagnosed, meaning that they can have tens of thousands of apneas prior to ever being treated.

DISEASE-RELATED PHYSIOLOGICAL CAUSES OF POOR SLEEP IN OLDER ADULTS

Lower arousal thresholds, cortical thinning, and altered circadian rhythms all cause poorer sleep, but what causes these causes? Rather than being one single factor, a combination of physiological, situational, and behavioral factors dynamically influence when and how we sleep as we grow older.

One major contributor to poor sleep is that, with increasing age, many adults develop one or more chronic illnesses. Nearly every disease and disorder can disrupt the timing and quality of sleep, as do the medications prescribed to treat the disease/disorder. For example, think of the last time you were in pain at night (headache, injury, etc.), and you will probably also remember having difficulty sleeping. Pain is a common symptom of a myriad of diseases, and it consistently disrupts sleep. Individuals who are diagnosed with conditions that typically cause high levels of pain, such as arthritis, fibromyalgia, multiple sclerosis, and neuropathy, often report increased sleep disturbances. Opioid and benzodiazepine medications commonly prescribed to such patients alter sleep architecture. Even in the absence of chronic disease, pain caused by acute or chronic injury (e.g., falls) can cause increased awakenings during the night, resulting in shallow and unrestful sleep.

Neurological disorders, especially neurodegenerative disorders, can damage the areas in the brain associated with sleep and circadian rhythms; severe damage can render medication or other treatments useless for treating the underlying sleep condition. For example, melatonin is often prescribed to patients who experience sleep and circadian rhythm disruptions, which is commonly seen in diseases like Alzheimer's disease. As neurodegenerative diseases progress, areas of the brain atrophy, or waste away (hence, the term "degenerative"). If areas of the brain that are involved with producing, processing, regulating, or receiving melatonin (i.e., pineal gland or suprachiasmatic nucleus) are damaged or atrophied, then exogenous melatonin (taken outside of the body) will have little to no effect on those brain regions.

One controversial argument is that Alzheimer's disease is caused by OSA through years of fragmented sleep and intermittent hypoxia. There is growing evidence that sleep fragmentation, reduction in REM and SWS, and circadian disturbances (e.g. day–night reversal) are evident in the preclinical stage of Alzheimer's disease. For example, in rat model of Alzheimer's disease, the animals developed sleep architecture disruptions similar to those experienced by humans who have Alzheimer's disease: non-REM (especially SWS), decreased REM sleep, and greater time awake compared to the control group [13]. The results of this study support the idea that sleep disruptions that are comorbid with Alzheimer's disease are not a consequence of the progression of the disease. Instead, sleep architecture changes and circadian rhythm issues likely occur earlier and contribute to the progression and development of the disease.

Sleep disturbances are also commonly reported in related dementias [4]. Neurodegenerative disease patients, such as adults with frontotemporal dementia, vascular dementia, dementia with Lewy bodies, and Parkinson's disease, often experience an increased frequency of insomnia and daytime sleepiness. Patients with Parkinson's disease also commonly report nightmares, periodic limb movement disorder, restless leg syndrome, and even a condition in which they act out their dreams (known as REM sleep behavior disorder). The association between the aforementioned neurodegenerative diseases and REM sleep behavior disorder is so high—approximately 73% convert over 12 years—that this sleep disorder is often considered the prodromal stage of neurodegenerative diseases [14]. While researchers are still working to identify the mechanisms by which sleep disturbances and disease progression interact, it is important to note that there are also many modifiable factors that contribute to poor sleep across the adult lifespan.

PSYCHOLOGICAL, SOCIAL, AND BEHAVIORAL CAUSES OF POOR SLEEP IN AGING

Acute and chronic illnesses, along with the medications used to treat them, often cause poor sleep; however, as Figure 12.3 illustrated, worsening sleep is not a simple consequence of getting older.

Certainly, our behaviors surrounding sleep also can impact the timing and quality of sleep. Yet, up until recently, the public has not been well educated on the importance of sleep or how to engage in proper sleep practices referred to as "sleep hygiene." Good sleep hygiene practices include making enough time for sleep, keeping bedtimes and wake times consistent over the course of the week, avoiding bright light in the evening, and avoiding alcohol, stimulants, and heavy meals before bedtime.

One of the most important aspects of healthy sleep is simply making room for adequate sleep time. Western society values making the most of every minute, including sacrificing sleep to engage in many other aspects of life (i.e., social events, completing work deadlines, studying for upcoming final exams, etc.). For example, at least 60% of college students have pulled an "all-nighter" (i.e., exceeding 24 hours without sleep) to cram for exams, complete papers, and submit assignments before hard-pressed deadlines [15]. This type of behavior is not only common but expected. Although all-nighters may be unique to high school and college, poor sleep practices are not limited to students. Decades of poor practices add up to a lifetime of bad habits and many nights of accrued sleep debt.

When we accrue sleep debt, we usually engage compensatory behaviors that are beneficial in the short term but perpetuate poor sleep in the long term (e.g., excessive caffeine). As adults enter middle age and older adulthood, many nap to compensate for their poor nighttime sleep and daytime sleepiness. While napping attenuates daytime sleepiness and reduces sleep debt, excessive napping (i.e., greater than 90 minutes) increases sleep latency at night, especially when the napping occurs in the late afternoon or evening. Older adults may experience anxiety from this increased difficulty falling asleep, leading to even less sleep at night and increased need for even longer naps during the day; this process disrupts circadian rhythms and can become a never-ending cycle. Interestingly, the literature has identified that greater frequency of napping during middle, and older age is associated with increased risk for Alzheimer's disease and mortality, although the causal direction of these effects is a matter of scientific debate (e.g., subtle neuropathological processes may cause sleepiness, leading the person to take more naps).

Psychological states, like depressed mood and stress, can also alter sleep timing, duration, and quality. Most people can relate to how stressful life events, such as the week of final exams, can precipitate sleepless nights. Although middle-aged adults do not have to cram for exams, the stress of their careers, finances, marital separation/divorce, and other life events can profoundly influence their sleep. Furthermore, approximately 43.5 million adults in the United States serve as a caregiver for a child, aging family member, spouse, or friend [16]. Caregiving adds significant stress, worsens sleep, and strains the caregiver's health. Consider the "night life" of a caregiver to someone with dementia: the caregiver will experience severely fragmented sleep if he or she must wake several times during the night to administer medication, assist with bathroom breaks, and tend to various other needs of the care recipient. Caregivers' significant sleep fragmentation during the night can lead to disrupted circadian rhythms, which may put them at higher risk for major depression and other health consequences.

Depression negatively impacts sleep, whether it is caused by situational factors (i.e., grief) or other biological factors. Individuals who are depressed may sleep too much or too little. They often have difficulties falling asleep or staying asleep, and they typically experience excessive daytime sleepiness. Several sleep disorders are associated with depression, including OSA, restless leg syndrome, and insomnia. Moreover, depression is associated with cognitive impairment and dementia in older adults. Middle-aged and older adults are more vulnerable to experiencing depression as a result of the death of someone close to them.

Adjustment to the loss of a partner or spouse, friends, and/or family members (bereavement) adds to the aging adult's physical and psychological stress.

Additional stress occurs when bereaved individuals are forced to learn new skills (e.g., cooking, laundry, money management etc.) and have to adjust to new schedules, as many spouses synchronize their lives with each other (including sleep patterns). Grief often manifests into physical symptoms, including sleep disturbances, depression, and problems with memory and attention. Bereaved individuals are more likely to report sleep disturbances, depression, and pain, particularly in the more acute stages of grief. Seiler and colleagues [17] even found that fatigued bereaved individuals had higher levels of systemic inflammation. Elevated systemic inflammation (e.g., C-reactive protein), which can be triggered by poor sleep quality, is linked to increased risk of diabetes, cardiovascular events, fatigue, and other health outcomes. If the physiological and psychological effects of bereavement cause difficulty falling asleep and staying asleep, then poor sleep quality would also subsequently exacerbate those symptoms (e.g., emotional regulation, inflammation, cognitive functioning, cardiovascular health).

Physicians often prescribe medications to treat depression. Antidepressant medications may be prescribed to treat the symptoms of depression (i.e., social withdrawal, low mood, decreased motivation, changes in appetite) and/or the sleep issues that are often reported with the depressive symptomology (i.e., trouble falling asleep and/or sleeping too much or too little). However, antidepressants, such as selective serotonin reuptake inhibitors, have been shown to suppress REM sleep; in some cases, they even cause dream enactment by decreasing muscle atonia.

Even nonprescription drugs often have detrimental effects on sleep quality. Many middle-aged and older adults "self-medicate" for daytime sleepiness by using stimulants like caffeine and nicotine. Caffeine enhances wakefulness by blocking the receptors for the sleep-promoting neurotransmitter adenosine. Caffeine and tobacco use can impact sleep by making it more difficult to fall asleep, reducing total sleep time, and making sleep lighter. There is also evidence that tobacco use can lead to insomnia and that heavy addiction to nicotine may lead to increased awakenings during the night to smoke. Use of such stimulants might mask sleep problems, as they are quick, albeit transient, remedies for daytime sleepiness. Furthermore, middle-aged and older adults may use alcohol to help them fall asleep (often referred to as a "nightcap"). Although alcohol initially decreases sleep latency, it leads to increased awakenings during the night due to the speed at which the body metabolizes it. Thus, as with napping, using these nonprescription drugs may feel like a short-term solution, but they often perpetuate poor sleep in the long term.

CONSEQUENCES OF POOR SLEEP IN AGING

Although we might not know the principal reason for why humans sleep, we do know that restful sleep serves many restorative functions. Disrupting sleep, therefore, can have cumulative effects across the lifespan that impact quality of life, development/progression of disorders and/or diseases, and overall mental and physical health.

One important function that occurs during sleep is the activation of the glymphatic system, which clears metabolic waste from the brain to achieve metabolic homeostasis. Proteins, such as β-amyloid and tau (associated with Alzheimer's disease) and α-synuclein (associated with Parkinson's disease), accumulate in the interstitial spaces between cells throughout the day. During sleep, fluids in the brain (specifically, cerebrospinal and interstitial fluids) exchange to clear out these proteins. Fragmented sleep disrupts this waste clearing process, which can lead to an accumulation of protein waste that becomes toxic to the brain cells. This accumulation of proteins can further interrupt other neurological processes, causing cognitive decline, memory impairment, and poor decision-making, all of which are seen in several neurodegenerative conditions (e.g., Alzheimer's disease). As a result, sleep quality declines even further, thus continuing to exacerbate the metabolite-clearance process.

There is increasing evidence of a relationship between cortical thickness in the brain and sleep factors, such as increased sleepiness and sleep disturbances. Some studies have shown relationships between sleepiness and sleep quality with atrophy in the prefrontal cortex (Figure 12.5). In the Baltimore Longitudinal Study of Aging, adults who reported short sleep duration (5–6 hours per night) and long sleep duration (8–9 hours per night) showed thinner cortices in the frontal and temporal regions of the brain, as compared to those who reported sleeping 7 hours per night [18]. It is still unclear whether this cortical thinning is a consequence or cause of short sleep duration; it is more likely that the relationship is bidirectional.

You may find it surprising that long sleep duration is associated with greater cortical thinning. It turns out that most epidemiological studies on sleep and co-morbidities report a U-shaped curve (Figure 12.6), indicating that long sleep duration (>9 hours per night) is just as foreboding of declining health as short sleep duration (≤6 hours per night). Long sleep durations have been associated with an increased risk for developing cardiovascular disease, cancer, diabetes, stroke, depression, and cognitive impairment, as well as all-cause mortality. Yet too much sleep per se is probably not the root cause (as opposed to eating too much). Some of the mechanisms proposed to explain why long sleep might be harmful include sedentary behavior, light exposure, sleep fragmentation, and underlying pathologies. Long sleepers tend to spend more time in bed compared to individuals who sleep 7 hours per night, which could lead to systemic inflammation (related to heart disease, stroke, depression, anxiety, etc.). Individuals who sleep longer are exposed to a shorter photoperiod (day-length), and decreased exposure to light could interfere with circadian synchronization, perpetuating longer sleep durations. Furthermore, when an older adult experiences fragmented sleep, he or she may try to compensate for this by spending more time in bed to make up for the daytime sleepiness. In this case, the costs of the poor sleep quality offset any potential benefits of a longer sleep duration. Finally, sleeping longer can be indicative of an underlying health issue; just as you feel the increased need to sleep when you have a bad cold, sleeping longer is important for the acute healing process. The mechanisms of how sleep duration is related to disorders, diseases,

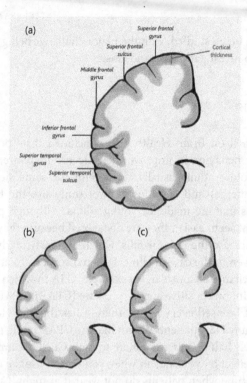

Figure 12.5 Coronal slice of the left hemisphere cortex demonstrating normal cortical thickness (gray matter) (a). Cortical thinning in older individuals who reported sleeping less than 7 hours per night is visible in superior temporal, inferior frontal, and middle frontal regions (b). Cortical thinning in older adults who reported sleeping more than 7 hours per night was most pronounced in superior frontal and middle frontal regions (c). SOURCE: Data were derived from Spira AP, Gonzelez CE, Venkatraman VK, et al. Sleep duration and subsequent cortical thinning in cognitively normal older adults. *Sleep*. 2016;39:1121–1128, and the figure was drawn by A. Reynolds.

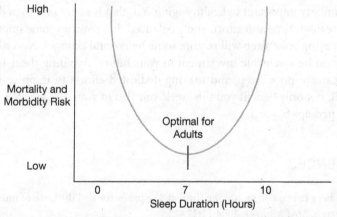

Figure 12.6 U-shaped curve demonstrating that mortality and morbidity risks are increased in short and long sleepers. Epidemiological studies of older adults indicate that 7 hours/night is an optimal sleep duration (in contrast with adolescents who need 8 to 10 hours/night).
SOURCE: Figure by A. Reynolds.

and death are still being studied, with the major challenge being designing experimental studies to investigate cause and effect.

CONCLUSIONS

The Global Council on Brain Health [19] concluded that "people, at any age, can change their behavior to improve their sleep." Therefore, correcting poor sleep quality in older adults usually starts with the same sleep hygiene (e.g., avoid evening caffeine) and stimulus control (only use the bed for sleeping) recommendations that are made for young adults. Although prescription sleep medications might seem easier, they are disfavored because they change sleep architecture and increase the risk for falls, which are particularly dangerous with advancing age. Even in the case of clinical sleep disorders, treatments usually require behavioral changes. Consider, for example, OSA in which most patients are treated with continuous positive airway pressure (CPAP). CPAP effectively treats OSA, but it must be used every night. Therein lies the behavioral-change challenge: because many OSA patients do not like the CPAP mask, pressure, or noise, only approximately half of patients adhere to their CPAP treatment. Just as going to a gym has no effect on your health when you do not use the equipment, CPAP works 0% of the time when patients do not wear it at night. Currently, the best-known means for increasing adherence is through motivational interviewing, a technique by which the clinician provides empathetic counseling to spur internal motivation and commitment to use CPAP (beyond simple education about the harms of OSA) [20].

For decades, the public has been told that aging gracefully requires one to maintain a balanced diet, exercise regularly, and stay engaged mentally and socially. Looking at the life of the sleep research pioneer Nathaniel Kleitman, and the extensive body of research that followed his career, we should conclude that sleeping well is similarly important to healthy aging. Yet, that is easier said than done. Just as exercise takes time and effort, and a balanced diet requires some impulse control, improving your sleep will require some behavioral changes. Nevertheless, to do so would be a valuable investment in your future. Avoiding short-term fixes that perpetuate poor sleep, and making dedicated efforts to improve sleep hygiene, will not only benefit you this week, but also in your 30s, 40s, 50s, 60s, 70s, 80s, and perhaps beyond.

REFERENCES

1. Lamberg L, Hagelberg, M. The student, the professor and the birth of modern sleep research. *Med Midway.* 2004;11:17–25.
2. Bliwise DL, Foley DJ, Vitiello MV, Ansari FP, Ancoli-Israel S, Walsh JK. Nocturia and disturbed sleep in the elderly. *Sleep Med.* 2009;10:540–548.

3. Ohayon MM, Carskadon MA, Guilleminault C, Vitiello MV. Meta-analysis of quantitative sleep parameters from childhood to old age in healthy individuals: developing normative sleep values across the human lifespan. *Sleep.* 2004;27:1255–1274.
4. Gao C, Scullin MK, Bliwise DL. Mild cognitive impairment and dementia. In Savard J, Ouellet MC. *Handbook of Sleep Disorders in Medical Conditions.* London, UK: Elsevier; 2019:253–276.
5. Zepelin H, McDonald CS, Zammit GK. Effects of age on auditory awakening thresholds. *J Gerontol.* 1984;39:294–300.
6. Scullin MK, Bliwise DL. Sleep, cognition, and normal aging: integrating a half-century of multidisciplinary research. *Persp Psychol Sci.* 2015;10:97–137.
7. Dubé J, Lafortune M, Bedetti C, et al. Cortical thinning explains changes in sleep slow waves during adulthood. *J Neurosci* 2015,35:7795–7807.
8. Mander BA, Winer JR, Walker MP. Sleep and human aging. *Neuron.* 2017;94:19–36.
9. Quan SF, Howard BV, Iber C, et al. The Sleep Heart Health Study: design, rationale, and methods. *Sleep* 1997;20:1077–1085.
10. Scullin MK, Gao C. Dynamic contributions of slow wave sleep and REM sleep to cognitive longevity. *Curr Sleep Med Rep.* 2018;4:284–293.
11. Hood S, Amir S. The aging clock: circadian rhythms and later life. *J Clin Invest.* 2017;127:437–446.
12. Braley TJ, Dunietz GL, Chervin RD, Lisabeth LD, Skolarus LE, Burke JF. Recognition and diagnosis of obstructive sleep apnea in older Americans. *J Am Geriatr Soc.*2018;66:1296–302.
13. Cui SY, Song JZ, Cui XY, et al. Intracerebroventricular streptozotocin-induced Alzheimer's disease-like sleep disorders in rats: role of the GABAergic system in the parabrachial complex. *CNS Neurosci Therapeut.* 2018; 24:1241–1252.
14. Postuma RB, Iranzo A, Hu M, et al. Risk and predictors of dementia and parkinsonism in idiopathic REM sleep behaviour disorder: a multicentre study. *Brain.* 2019;142:744–759.
15. Thacher PV. University students and the "All Nighter": Correlates and patterns of students' engagement in a single night of total sleep deprivation. *Behav Sleep Med.* 2008;6:16–31.
16. The National Alliance for Caregiving (NAC): Caregiving in the U.S. https://www.aarp.org/content/dam/aarp/ppi/2015/caregiving-in-the-united-states-2015-report-revised.pdf. Published 2015.
17. Seiler A, Murdock KW, Fagundes CP. Impaired mental health and low-grade inflammation among fatigued bereaved individuals. *J Psychosom Res.* 2018;11:40–46.
18. Spira AP, Gonzelez CE, Venkatraman VK, et al. Sleep duration and subsequent cortical thinning in cognitively normal older adults. *Sleep.* 2016;39:1121–1128.
19. Global Council on Brain Health. The brain–sleep connection: GCBH recommendations on sleep and brain health. www.GlobalCouncilOnBrainHealth.org. Published 2016.
20. Bakker JP, Wang R, Weng J, et al. Motivational enhancement for increasing adherence to CPAP: a randomized controlled trial. *Chest.* 2016;150:337–345.

13

Women's Health

BEI BEI AND FIONA C. BAKER ■

INTRODUCTION

Women and men share common features in sleep, but the female sex is also linked to unique sleep characteristics and changes in sleep depending on reproductive stage. Compared to men, women are more likely to be morning chronotype [1], report needing more sleep [2], sleeping longer [3, 4], and more likely to experience sleep difficulties [5]. Women have a higher risk of insomnia (ratio women to men is 1.41:1), which emerges after menarche [6] and persists across a woman's lifespan, even after taking into account underlying psychiatric disorders [7]. Several factors may contribute to these differences, including sex hormones acting on the brain, sex-linked genetic mechanisms, and sex differences in psychosocial factors [8]. In this chapter, we will focus on sleep characteristics in women during the menstrual cycle, pregnancy and postpartum, and during the approach to menopause, because each of these phases are accompanied by major changes in hormones and psychosocial environment.

MENSTRUAL CYCLE

Menstrual cycles are regulated by the hypothalamic–pituitary–ovarian axis to co-ordinate ovarian follicular development, ovulation, luteinization, and luteolysis [9]. Each menstrual cycle lasts about 28 days and includes the follicular or pro-liferative phase (first day of menses until ovulation), and the luteal or secretory phase (ovulation until the onset of menstruation) [9]. Distinctive hormone profiles during these phases are shown in Figure 13.1. Receptors for estrogen and progesterone exist in many sleep–wake regulatory nuclei in the central nervous system, and studies in rodents have shown that administration of estradiol and progesterone impacts sleep [8]. Estradiol, for example, induces increased arousal

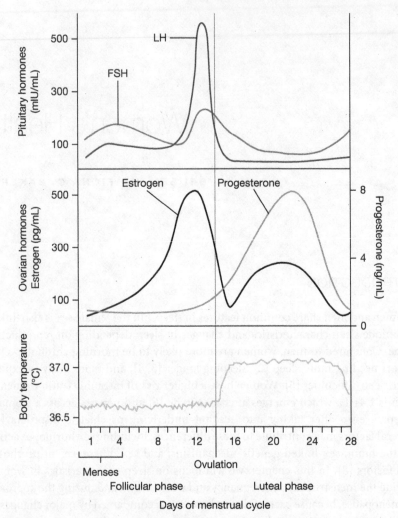

Figure 13.1 Mean daily plasma concentrations of estradiol, progesterone, follicle-stimulating hormone (FSH), and luteinizing hormone (LH) and basal body temperature throughout a "typical" 28-day ovulatory menstrual cycle.
SOURCE: Modified from Pocock G, Richards CD. *Human Physiology: The Basis of Medicine*. New York, NY: Oxford University Press; 1999:450.

in rodents [10]. The changes in reproductive hormones during the menstrual cycle, therefore, have the potential to influence sleep.

Sleep During the Menstrual Cycle

A seminal study in healthy young women showed that polysomnography (PSG) measures of slow-wave sleep (SWS), sleep onset latency (SOL), total sleep time (TST), and sleep efficiency (SE) were all stable across the menstrual cycle [11].

Rapid eye movement (REM) sleep showed a tendency to decrease in the luteal phase when body temperature was raised [11]. A more detailed analysis of the data showed that the decrease in REM sleep was related to a significant shortening of REM sleep episodes in the luteal phase, while non-REM episode duration was unchanged [12]. Other studies later confirmed the reduction in REM sleep in the luteal phase [13–15]. The amount of REM sleep correlates negatively with levels of both estradiol and progesterone in the luteal phase [14] and may be mediated by the changing sex hormone profile or increase in body temperature [11].

In addition to changes in REM sleep, electroencephalogram (EEG) activity within the upper spindle frequency range (14.25–15 Hz) increases during the luteal phase, often associated with increased stage 2 sleep [11]. Increased spindle activity may reflect an interaction between endogenous progesterone metabolites and GABAA membrane receptors [11], with the latter being critical in spindle generation [16]. In support of this hypothesis, synthetic progestin (medroxyprogesterone) use is associated with greater upper spindle frequency activity [17], and combined progestin–estradiol contraceptive pills are linked to more stage 2 sleep in women [18]. However, progesterone levels and spindle frequency activity are not correlated, at least in the late luteal phase of women with ovulatory menstrual cycles [14]. Alternatively, higher body temperature in the luteal phase may explain the increased spindle frequency activity [12]. Regardless of cause, more spindles may help maintain sleep quality in the presence of substantial physiological and hormonal changes during this period [19].

While most studies have been done in young women, findings from one PSG study in midlife women approaching menopause suggest that sleep may be more vulnerable to menstrual cycle changes in older women; women had less SWS and more awakenings and arousals in their luteal compared with the follicular phase [20]. Similarly, an in-home study using actigraphy found that in 163 late reproductive-age women (average age = 52), there was a moderate decline in SE (5%) and a decrease in TST (25 minutes) in the premenstrual week compared to the previous week [21]. This discrepancy might be due to different sleeping environment and longer observation duration compared to previous PSG studies; it is also possible that sleep may be affected more by the menstrual cycle with advancing age.

Objective findings of few changes in sleep continuity across the menstrual cycle in young women do not entirely match with subjective sleep assessments. In women across a wide age range, self-reported sleep quality ratings tend to be poorer during the premenstrual week and first few days of menstruation when estradiol and progesterone levels are low or declining [22, 23]. This subjective-objective discrepancy might be due to different sleeping environments and longer observation periods for self-report compared to PSG studies, as well as reflecting differences in what each construct is measuring. Variability between individuals in the relationship between sleep and menstrual cycle phase [24] likely also impacts results. Importantly, women who experience menstrual-related symptoms such as premenstrual mood changes or menstrual pain, are more likely to report poor sleep quality: ~70% of women report that their sleep is negatively impacted by menstrual symptoms, on average, 2.5 days every month [25].

Premenstrual Syndrome

Premenstrual syndrome (PMS) is characterized by emotional, behavioral, and physical symptoms in the premenstrual phase of the menstrual cycle, with resolution soon after the onset of menses. Up to 18% of women report premenstrual symptoms that are perceived as distressing and/or impair daily function [26]. Premenstrual dysphoric disorder (PMDD) is a severe form of PMS that occurs in 3% to 8% of women [26] and is classified as a depressive disorder [27]. Women with severe PMS/PMDD typically complain of sleep problems, as well as daytime sleepiness, fatigue, and inability to concentrate during the late luteal phase (for review, see [28]).

Laboratory-based PSG studies, however, have not identified clear patterns of sleep alterations in women with PMS/PMDD [13, 19]. For example, women with either severe PMS or PMDD reported poorer subjective sleep quality in their symptomatic late luteal (compared to the follicular) phase, but no corresponding worsening of PSG-measured sleep quality (e.g., SE, arousals, SOL) was found [14]. Worse self-reported sleep quality was associated with higher anxiety levels, suggesting that mood state may play a role in how severe PMS impacts sleep reports in the late luteal phase [14].

Although PSG evidence for a change in sleep from the follicular to the symptomatic late luteal phase is limited, trait-like differences in sleep architecture in both the follicular and late luteal phases have been reported in women with PMS/PMDD compared to healthy controls (see review [28]). In a study that measured sleep every third night across an entire menstrual cycle, women with PMDD and insomnia symptoms had more SWS than controls regardless of menstrual cycle phase [29]. Similarly, women with severe PMS/PMDD had greater SWS in both the follicular and late luteal phases compared to controls [14]. The greater SWS observed may be related to lower melatonin secretion in women with PMDD [29, 30]. Indeed, others have also reported differences in psychophysiological parameters that are evident outside of the symptomatic late luteal phase in women with PMDD compared to controls [31]. These "trait-like" differences may contribute to different symptom expressions in the late luteal phase in women with PMDD.

Dysmenorrhea

Dysmenorrhea, defined as painful menstrual cramps of uterine origin, is the most common gynecological condition among women of reproductive age, experienced in its severe form by approximately 10% to 25% of women [32]. Primary dysmenorrhea is menstrual pain without organic disease, while secondary dysmenorrhea is associated with conditions such as endometriosis and pelvic inflammatory disease. Painful menstrual cramps impact quality of life, mood, and sleep quality [32]. Women with primary dysmenorrhea are more likely to experience disturbed sleep when they experience pain during menstruation compared with pain-free phases of the menstrual cycle and compared with women who do not suffer menstrual pain [33]. The relationship between sleep and pain is bidirectional such that menstrual pain disrupts sleep and disturbed sleep may exacerbate pain [34]. Treating nocturnal pain with nonsteroidal anti-inflammatory drugs alleviates painful cramps and is associated with an improved sleep quality in women with primary dysmenorrhea [35, 36]. A recent study showed that melatonin was also effective at improving sleep and pain severity in women with primary dysmenorrhea [36].

In summary, aspects of sleep physiology and quality change across the menstrual cycle. Most notably, sleep spindle activity is increased when progesterone is present and body temperature is increased in the luteal phase; sleep spindles could function to maintain sleep continuity during this phase. Women are more likely to perceive poor sleep quality as well as daytime sleepiness leading up to and around menstruation, particularly if they suffer from significant premenstrual symptoms and/or painful menstrual cramps. Menstrual phase and presence of menstrual-related complaints should therefore be considered when assessing women's sleep complaints. It should also be kept in mind that sleep influences female reproductive function such that changes in sleep patterns or duration can alter menstrual cycle regularity and functioning [37].

PREGNANCY AND POSTPARTUM PERIODS

Pregnancy, childbirth, and the first postpartum year bring about some of the biggest changes to a woman's sleep and wake patterns. Poor and disrupted sleep during the perinatal transition has been associated with a range of negative mental and physical health outcomes. These include maternal mood disturbance and impaired daytime functioning [38–41], symptoms of, and higher risk for, perinatal depression and anxiety [42], risk of postpartum psychosis in vulnerable women [43, 44], gestational diabetes [45], prolonged labor and higher rates of cesarean delivery [46], preterm birth [47, 48] and other negative fetal outcomes (see a meta-analysis [49]), as well as more near-miss motor vehicle accidents [50].

Pregnancy and Childbirth

Pregnancy is accompanied by dramatic increase in many hormones (e.g., estrogen, progesterone, and prolactin) [51], which contribute to symptoms of fatigue and daytime sleepiness, morning sickness, nausea, increased urinary frequency, tender breasts, and mood changes [52–54]. A meta-analysis summarizing sleep quality data across pregnancy showed that 45.7% (36.5%, 55.2%) of women reported being a poor sleeper (score 5 or above) [55] based on the Pittsburgh Sleep Quality Index (PSQI) [56]. Studies that measured sleep via self-report, actigraphy, and PSG have all demonstrated that sleep is compromised during pregnancy and worsens as pregnancy progresses.

Daytime sleepiness, fatigue, and increased naps are reported as early as the first trimester of pregnancy [53, 57]. A longitudinal study measured sleep via self-report in 325 women during each trimester of pregnancy, and found night-time awakenings increased from the first trimester, and SE decreased throughout pregnancy; TST was elevated during the first trimester, slightly decreased during the second trimester, and reduced substantially during the third trimester [52]. Similarly, a cohort study of 2581 pregnant women (47% first-time mothers) across the first to the second trimester also showed decreased self-reported night-time sleep (30.7% vs 36.2% reported sleeping 7 hours, whereas 24.4% vs 14.7% reported sleeping 10 hours) [45].

From the second to the third trimester, reports of disrupted night-time sleep continue to rise, with meta-analysis showing aggregated PSQI scores increasing from 5.31 to 7.03 [55]. Sleep during late pregnancy is characterized by extended time to fall asleep and increased night-time awakenings, likely due to increased physical discomfort and urinary frequency as the fetus continues to grow. At 32 weeks of gestation, 60% women reported symptoms of insomnia [58]; as they approach the 40th week of pregnancy, the majority (75% to 98%) reported multiple night-time awakenings [52, 59, 60].

The worsening sleep pattern across pregnancy is supported by actigraphy studies that show night-time sleep deteriorates progressively throughout pregnancy, particularly during the last weeks of gestation [61, 62]. Studies using PSG add further insight. One of the few PSG studies examined changes in sleep from before pregnancy, across each trimester of pregnancy, and at 1 and 3 months postpartum [57, 63]. TST was highest during the first trimester (7.4 hours), followed by prepregnancy baseline and the third trimester (both 6.9 hours). Sleep efficiency decreased progressively across pregnancy, from 93% before pregnancy to 81% at 1 month postpartum, and SWS progressively decreased [57, 63]. For the third trimester, most PSG studies showed less SWS and REM sleep when compared with previous trimesters or nonpregnant controls [57, 64–68]. Along with greater stage 1 or 2 sleep [57, 65, 68], these changes point to lighter and less restorative sleep as pregnancy progresses.

The days leading up to childbirth and labor itself are usually associated with partial, sometimes total sleep deprivation. Women overwhelmingly report unable to sleep once contractions started [69]. In vulnerable women such as those with a history of bipolar disorder, this period of acute sleep deprivation could trigger episodes of severe psychiatric conditions such as mania and postpartum psychosis [43, 44].

Sleep occurs in 24-hour night–day cycles. As night-time sleep becomes compromised during pregnancy and childbirth, women may compensate by taking daytime naps. In fact, more than 75% of the women reported at least one nap each week in the third trimester [57, 60], which is consistent with findings on actigraphy [38, 70]. Working women who were less likely to nap reported sleeping 1 hour less in the last month of pregnancy [71].

Sleep Disorders During Pregnancy

The prevalence of some sleep disorders increases during pregnancy and may lead to further sleep fragmentation and increased daytime sleepiness among affected women. Sleep-disordered breathing (SDB) increases across pregnancy due to changes in the respiratory system, such as reduced pharyngeal dimensions, decreased nasal patency, and increased congestion and rhinitis [72–75]. Frequent snoring was reported by 7% to 11% of women prepregnancy but increased to 16% to 25% by the third trimester [76–79]. The few studies that longitudinally assessed objectively measured SDB across pregnancy showed consistent findings. Among 105 women (28% normal weight, 24% overweight, and 50% obese), the presence of SDB increased from 10.5% during the first trimester to 26.7% in the third trimester [80]. In 128 pregnant women with high risk for health conditions, rates for mild, moderate, and severe SDB increased from 12%, 6%, and 3% during early pregnancy, to 35%, 7%, and 5% in late pregnancy respectively [81]. Meta-analysis linked moderate to severe SDB during pregnancy to a range of negative maternal and fetal outcomes, such as risk for gestational diabetes, pregnancy-related hypertension, pre-eclampsia, preterm delivery, and low birth [82].

The prevalence rates of restless legs syndrome (RLS) are estimated to be 3% to 34% in pregnant populations [83, 84]. Although this rate varies due to diagnostic criteria and ethnic differences, most researchers agree that RLS is two to three times more common in pregnant compared to nonpregnant women [83]. Some studies showed that RLS had a mean onset around 6 months gestation [85], while others reported onset before the fifth month [86]. Prospective studies showed that rates of RLS increases as pregnancy progresses, peaking in the third trimester, and resolving shortly before delivery [83, 84, 86, 87]. Although the pathophysiology of RSL during pregnancy is not fully established, hormonal mechanisms, iron and folate metabolism, family history, depression, and multiparity were considered to play a role [83, 84, 87].

Postpartum Period

During the first few days after childbirth, sleep disruption is typically at its highest compared with all other stages of the perinatal transition. Some studies reported that caesarean delivery was associated with shorter TST and more frequent night-time awakenings than vaginal delivery, probably due to factors related to surgical recovery [88]. An actigraphy study found that night-time sleep duration and quality took a dive immediately after childbirth, but an improving and recovery trend was apparent on a day-to-day basis during the first week postpartum [70].

During the first postpartum month, both self-report and actigraphy studies showed that women experience more night-time awakenings and fragmented sleep, compared to the end of pregnancy and later postpartum months [89–93]. Napping or sleeping in are common ways to compensate for sleep disruptions during this period [71, 89–92]. Compared to the third trimester of pregnancy when naps were most likely to occur during early afternoon, naps during early postpartum periods were more likely to be distributed across late morning to early evening [70]. This, combined with more time awake at night, means that childbirth is followed by redistribution of sleep across 24-hour night and day.

Although sleep continues to improve gradually in subsequent months, due to the lack of longitudinal studies, it is currently not clear when or whether women's sleep fully return to prepregnancy levels. An actigraphy study showed that at 10 weeks postpartum, sleep patterns were similar to that in the third trimester of pregnancy, although sleep quality was still worse than matched nonpregnant controls [62]. This is consistent with findings on the PSG that despite improving trend in all aspects of sleep at 3 months postpartum, neither sleep quality nor quantity had yet returned to prepregnancy levels [57, 63].

INFANT BEHAVIORS

Actigraphy studies have shown that maternal sleep is closely associated with infant sleep–wake behaviors during the first 3 months postpartum [94, 95]. The number of self-report infant-related night-time awakenings, but not necessarily self-estimated total wake time, was associated with perceived sleep quality [96], suggesting that frequent and externally caused sleep disruption may be more distressing than reduction in sleep duration per se. Studies that have examined effects if feeding methods on objective sleep quality are mixed, finding either no difference in night-time sleep duration between feeding methods [71, 97] or that breastfeeding promoted longer night-time sleep duration [98, 99].

Night-time feeding and caretaking may have an even greater impact on new parents' sleep patterns when an infant is difficult to settle and soothe [100, 101]. In women seeking support for unsettled infant behaviors (e.g., persistent crying, resistance to settling, short sleep intervals, frequent awakenings), 96% scored as "poor sleeper" on the PSQI [102], and 47% reported significant insomnia symptoms [103].

FATIGUE, SLEEPINESS, AND PSYCHOMOTOR VIGILANCE

Disturbed sleep during the postpartum period could lead to impaired daytime functioning. Fatigue involves a sense of extreme tiredness or exhaustion and lessens individuals' capacity to function to their expectations [104, 105]. Sleepiness is the perceived likelihood of falling asleep when intending to be awake and is different from fatigue [106], although not always distinguished in studies.

Fatigue and daytime sleepiness are commonly reported postpartum. Between 40% and 60% of women report fatigue during the first 18 months postpartum [107, 108], with sleep disturbance being a major contributing factor [109]. Both longitudinal and cross-sectional studies have shown that for many women fatigue symptoms may persist for months into the postpartum period [71, 107, 110–112]. Although fatigue may be a symptom of postpartum depression [27], recent literature points to postpartum fatigue being a distinctive construct that is related to, but different from, postpartum depression symptoms in both community [113, 114] and help-seeking [40] women. Turning to sleepiness, one longitudinal study showed that it reduced from being above the clinical cut-off toward the higher end of the normal range from 6 to 18 weeks postpartum [93], suggesting that sleepiness may increase after childbirth but decline over time as maternal sleep disturbance gradually decreases.

The psychomotor vigilance task (PVT) measures sustained attention, an aspect of cognition that is sensitive to sleep loss [115]. Only two studies administered this task in the postpartum period. Healthy women between 2 to 13 weeks postpartum performed consistently slower and had more lapses on the PVT than matched controls [41, 116]. Over this early postpartum period, PVT performance gradually declined, even though sleep duration gradually increased, suggesting that adverse effects of sleep disturbance may be cumulative [116]. The other study measured PVT in women in later postpartum months and found that after a 5-day residential program for unsettled infant behaviors, PVT performance had small but statistically improvements in speed [117].

Sleep and Maternal Mood

Poorer self-reported sleep quality during early pregnancy predicted depressive symptoms in late pregnancy [118]. Shorter TST and longer SOL were associated with higher depressive symptoms during the first 3 months postpartum [94]. In women with prior depressive disorder who were not depressed during pregnancy, sleep complaints in the first 4 months postpartum were associated with a higher risk for depression recurrence [119]. Therefore, sleep complaints are not only relevant to concurrent mood, but might also be a risk factor for future mood problems, especially among vulnerable women.

When sleep is measured using actigraphy or PSG, the sleep–mood relationship has shown to be weaker [38, 120, 121]. Some aspects of sleep such as poor sleep continuity and efficiency [122, 123], variable sleep duration [124], and frequent napping [38] have been associated with worse mood in postpartum women.

In summary, pregnancy and childbirth pose major challenges to women's sleep and wake patterns: sleep disturbance increases as pregnancy progresses. Sleep disorders during pregnancy may not only be detrimental to the mother's health but are also a risk factor for adverse birth outcomes. While some sleep disturbance is an expected part of pregnancy, sleep should be evaluated in pregnant women when sleep disorders are suspected. Childbirth is associated with acute sleep deprivation. Even though sleep improves in the first few months postpartum, nighttime awakenings and reduced sleep quality continues well into the postpartum year. Recognizing, treating sleep disorders, and improving sleep quality during the perinatal transition is an emerging research area that has the potential to improve health and daytime functioning of countless women.

MENOPAUSAL TRANSITION

The natural menopausal transition typically starts in the late 40s, with the median age at the final menstrual period being 51.4 years [125]. This period is accompanied by substantial changes in endocrine physiology, such as decrease in estrogen and increases in follicle-stimulating hormone and testosterone, changes in menstrual cycles, skin conditions, and body temperature [126]. A range of symptoms have been reported during this period, such as hot flashes and/or night sweats, sleep disturbances, weight gain, headache, memory difficulties, sexual dysfunction [37]. These symptoms are not only distressing, bothersome, and reduce quality of life for midlife women personally, but are also associated with increased healthcare utilization and costs [127–129].

Changes in Sleep During the Menopausal Transition

Poor and disturbed sleep is not only commonly reported (33%–51%) [130–132] but is also among the most bothersome symptoms [133] during the menopausal transition (see review [134]). Meta-analysis of 24 cross-sectional studies found that compared to premenopause, the odds for reporting sleep disturbance are higher during perimenopause (1.60), postmenopause (1.67), and surgical menopause (2.17) [135].

Night-time awakening is the most common sleep complaint [136–139]. The Study of Women's Health Across the Nation (SWAN) followed up 3045 women and found an increase in the odds for difficulty staying asleep across the menopausal transition after adjusting for demographics and health-related factors [138]. Odds for reporting difficulty falling asleep also increased across the transition but decreased for early morning awakening from late perimenopause to postmenopause [138].

Polysomnography studies, however, have shown inconsistent findings on changes in sleep architecture during the menopausal transition. Some studies reported comparable sleep architecture between pre- and postmenopausal women [140–142], while other reported more SWS in peri- and postmenopausal women compared to premenopausal women [143–145]. Although more SWS may reflect better sleep, it could also reflect a recovery response to sleep deprivation, making it difficult to interpret these findings on SWS. Quantitative analysis of sleep EEG from the SWAN study also showed no menopause status related differences in PSG derived sleep variables; however, beta activity during sleep was higher in peri- and post-, compared to premenopausal women, suggesting higher cortical arousal, an effect partially accounted for by a higher frequency of self-reported hot flashes [140]. The only longitudinal study of changes in PSG measured sleep across the menopausal transition followed up 60 midlife women at a premeno-pausal baseline and again 6 years later [145]. This study reported less TST and more time awake after sleep onset (WASO) at the follow-up, after adjusting for vasomotor symptoms (VMS), body mass index, and mood [145].

Emerging evidence shows the importance of considering severity of sleep disturbance in midlife women; women in the menopausal transition who meet criteria for an insomnia disorder show a corresponding greater amount of PSG-defined sleep disturbance than age-matched women without sleep complaints [146]. Thus, reported sleep complaints are matched with PSG-measured sleep disturbances in midlife women with insomnia. Also, women with menopausal insomnia are more likely to have nocturnal hot flashes, which were a predictor of their nocturnal awakenings [146].

Vasomotor Symptoms and Sleep Disturbance

VMS include hot flashes (daytime occurrences) and night sweats (night-time occurrences), affecting up to 80% of women during the menopause transition [147]. Data from SWAN show that the median duration for VMS is 7.4 years, with symptoms persisting over 10 years in some women [148]. Each VMS occurrence ranges, on average, 1 to 5 minutes (but some up to 60 minutes), and starts with heat or warmth sensations in the upper body, accompanied by peripheral vasodilation, sweating, and elevated skin blood flow [149]. It is hypothesized that VMS result from disturbance of the temperature regulating system in the hypothalamus [147].

Self-reported VMS are consistently associated with worse self-reported sleep quality and chronic insomnia [138, 150–152]. Longitudinal data show that women with moderate-severe hot flashes are almost three times more likely to report frequent night-time awakenings compared with those without [153]. However, findings on the relationship between VMS and sleep are mixed when either VMS and/or sleep was measured using methods other than self-report. For example, when VMS was measured using self-report and sleep using actigraphy or PSG, earlier studies showed no relationship [141, 143], but later studies linked hot flashes to disrupted sleep [154–156]. When VMS were measured using skin con-ductance or skin temperature, their occurrences were linked to sleep disruption in some [154, 155, 157] but not all studies [141, 156, 158]. Discrepancies in findings may be related to how VMS were classified in association with awakenings [154], and differences between women in how VMS affects sleep.

Experimental design offers stronger causal inference compared to observa-tional studies discussed so far. Joffe and colleagues [155] experimentally induced hot flushes using gonadotropin-releasing hormone agonist leuprolide in healthy premenopausal women without hot flashes or sleep disturbances [155]. This study demonstrated a causal relationship between objectively recorded VMS and greater awakenings, WASO, and Stage 1 sleep on the PSG. Finally, the extent of hot flash impact on sleep varies between women: an analysis in perimenopausal women with VMS found that an awakening coincided with most (69%) hot flashes and that VMS were responsible for an average of 27% of PSG measured WASO, with wide variability in the degree of impact between women [154].

Sleep During the Menopausal Transition is Multifactorial

Taken together, studies show that VMS play an important role in mediating sleep disturbance that arises during the menopausal transition, but other factors are also likely to contribute. Data from SWAN suggested that the increase in sleep disturbance during the menopausal transition is partially related to changes in hormone levels [138]. It is also possible that some women are more susceptible to sleep problems during reproductive hormone transitions. For example, higher neuroticism, a dimension of personality, has been linked to menopause-associated insomnia [159], and those who suffer from premenstrual dysphoric disorder are more likely to develop postpartum and menopausal depression [160, 161] and are at increased risk for insomnia in the menopausal transition [159]. Aging related changes in sleep could also contribute to sleep disturbance during the menopausal transition. Compared to women in their 20s, poorer PSG sleep efficiency similar to that of postmenopausal women was reported in women in late reproductive stage (aged 45–51 years) [142]. Underrecognized and underdiagnosed sleep disorders such as sleep-disordered breathing, RLS, and periodic limb movement syndrome may also contribute to the age-related deterioration in women's sleep and become increasingly important to consider as women enter postmenopause. A study of over 100 women aged 44 to 56 who reported disturbed sleep found that 53% had sleep disorders, mainly sleep disordered breathing, RLS, or both [158]. In addition, co-morbid physical and psychiatric conditions, as well as pain disorders are also commonly associated with sleep complaints during the menopausal transition [162].

Importantly, the menopausal transition coincides with many psychosocial and personal challenges associated with midlife, such as changing family roles, loss of loved ones, changes and increasing work-related demands, health concerns, and concerns about ageing and retirement [163]. Life stressors could contribute to sleep disturbances [163, 164]. In midlife women, perceived stress and poor perceived health have been associated with sleep disturbances [139, 165], and those with more chronic stress exposure over a 9-year period also showed elevated WASO on PSG and risk for insomnia [166].

Some factors have shown to be protective against the sleep disturbances in the menopausal transition, for example, lower financial strain [167], higher education levels [151], greater marital satisfaction [168], and a moderate amount of exercise [169]. Although not examined in relation to sleep, self-compassion was found to reduce the negative impact of VMS on daily functioning and mood [170], and along with more positive attitudes to ageing, self-compassion was a strong predictor of perceived physical and mental health in midlife women [171]. This suggests that beyond physiological and sociodemographic factors, women's beliefs and attitudes play important roles in their overall experiences during the menopausal transition.

In summary, sleep disturbances are commonly reported during the menopause transition and are linked with the presence of nocturnal VMS. While PSG-measured sleep disturbance may not be evident in all women going through the menopausal transition, it is apparent in women with insomnia disorder developed in this context, with VMS being a probable contributing factor to their sleep disturbance. A multitude of other factors can contribute to sleep disturbance during the menopausal transition, with changes in reproductive hormones, aging, comorbid health conditions, sleep disordered breathing, stress, and a number of other biopsychosocial factors potentially playing a role. These factors should be considered in women presenting with sleep complaints during this life stage.

IMPLICATIONS AND INTERVENTIONS

Much of the sleep disturbance across women's lifespan discussed in this chapter are caused by physiological and external factors that are outside of one's control. However, this does not mean that sleep and sleep-related quality of life cannot be improved. Self-reported sleep is a strong predictor of mood disturbance suggesting that psychological factors exert strong influence on how women may be affected by sleep problems. In new mothers, sleep complaints were associated with aspects of cognitive appraisal that were closely linked to maternal distress such as negative expectations about the future and low perceived ability to cope with motherhood [172]. This finding is consistent with the finding that thoughts and beliefs about sleep as well as the world, which are modifiable through psychological intervention, play important roles in how objectively measured sleep affects mood [173].

Psychological interventions to specifically address sleep challenges in women are limited but growing. Although behavioral and education based intervention [174] did not improve maternal or infant sleep immediately after childbirth, cognitive behavioral therapy for insomnia (CBT-I) has been shown to improve sleep during both pregnancy [175] and postpartum periods [176] in women with insomnia. For women going through the menopausal transition and suffering from insomnia and hot flashes, CBT-I delivered via telephone was also effective for improving sleep [177, 178]. In light of high prevalence of other mental/physical conditions in women with sleep problems, clinical guidelines [179] suggests treating sleep problem as a comorbid condition in its own right, rather than a condition secondary to other mental/physical conditions for the benefit of overall well-being.

REFERENCES

1. Adan A, Natale V. Gender differences in morningness–eveningness preference. *Chronobiol Int*. 2002;19:709–720.
2. Ferrara M, De Gennaro L. How much sleep do we need? *Sleep Med Rev*. 2001;5:155–179.

3. Middelkoop HA, Smilde-van den Doel DA, Neven AK, Kamphuisen HA, Springer CP. Subjective sleep characteristics of 1,485 males and females aged 50-93: effects of sex and age, and factors related to self-evaluated quality of sleep. *J Gerontol A Biol Sci Med Sci.* 1996;51:M108–M115.

4. Groeger JA, Zijlstra FR, Dijk DJ. Sleep quantity, sleep difficulties and their perceived consequences in a representative sample of some 2000 British adults. *J Sleep Res.* 2004;13:359–371.

5. Manber R, Gress JL, Baker FC. Sex differences in sleep and sleep disorders: a focus on women's sleep. *Int J Sleep Disord.* 2006;1:7–15.

6. Johnson EO, Roth T, Schultz L, Breslau N. Epidemiology of DSM-IV insomnia in adolescence: lifetime prevalence, chronicity, and an emergent gender difference. *Pediatrics.* 2006;117:e247–e256.

7. Zhang B, Wing YK. Sex differences in insomnia: a meta-analysis. *Sleep.* 2006;29:85–93.

8. Mong JA, Baker FC, Mahoney MM, et al. Sleep, rhythms, and the endocrine brain: influence of sex and gonadal hormones. *J Neurosci.* 2011;31:16107–16116.

9. Mihm M, Gangooly S, Muttukrishna S. The normal menstrual cycle in women. *Anim Reprod Sci.* 2011;124:229–236.

10. Schwartz MD, Mong JA. Estradiol modulates recovery of REM sleep in a time-of-day-dependent manner. *Am J Physiol Regul Integr Comp Physiol.* 2013;305:R271–R280.

11. Driver HS, Dijk DJ, Werth E, Biedermann K, Borbély AA. Sleep and the sleep electroencephalogram across the menstrual cycle in young healthy women. *J Clin Endocrinol Metab.* 1996;81:728–735.

12. Driver HS, Werth E, Dijk DJ, Borbély AA. The menstrual cycle effects on sleep. *Sleep Med Clin.* 2008;3:1–11.

13. Baker FC, Kahan TL, Trinder J, Colrain IM. Sleep quality and the sleep electroencephalogram in women with severe premenstrual syndrome. *Sleep.* 2007;30:1283–1291.

14. Baker FC, Sassoon SA, Kahan T, et al. Perceived poor sleep quality in the absence of polysomnographic sleep disturbance in women with severe premenstrual syndrome. *J Sleep Res.* 2012;21:535–545.

15. Shechter A, Varin F, Boivin DB. Circadian variation of sleep during the follicular and luteal phases of the menstrual cycle. *Sleep.* 2010;33:647–656.

16. Belelli D, Lambert JJ. Neurosteroids: endogenous regulators of the GABA(A) receptor. *Nat Rev Neurosci.* 2005;6:565–575.

17. Plante DT, Goldstein MR. Medroxyprogesterone acetate is associated with increased sleep spindles during non-rapid eye movement sleep in women referred for polysomnography. *Psychoneuroendocrinology.* 2013;38:3160–3166.

18. Baker FC, Mitchell D, Driver HS. Oral contraceptives alter sleep and raise body temperature in young women. *Pflugers Arch.* 2001;442:729–737.

19. Shechter A, Boivin DB. Sleep, hormones, and circadian rhythms throughout the menstrual cycle in healthy women and women with premenstrual dysphoric disorder. *Int J Endocrinol.* 2010;2010:259345.

20. de Zambotti M, Willoughby AR, Sassoon SA, Colrain IM, Baker FC. Menstrual cycle-related variation in physiological sleep in women in the early menopausal transition. *J Clin Endocrinol Metab.* 2015;100:2918–2926.

21. Zheng H, Harlow SD, Kravitz HM, et al. Actigraphy-defined measures of sleep and movement across the menstrual cycle in midlife menstruating women: Study of Women's Health Across the Nation Sleep Study. *Menopause*. 2014;22(1):66–74.

22. Baker FC, Driver HS. Self-reported sleep across the menstrual cycle in young, healthy women. *J Psychosom Res*. 2004;56:239–243.

23. Kravitz HM, Janssen I, Santoro N, et al. Relationship of day-to-day reproductive hormone levels to sleep in midlife women. *Arch Intern Med*. 2005;165:2370–2376.

24. Van Reen E, Kiesner J. Individual differences in self-reported difficulty sleeping across the menstrual cycle. *Arch Womens Ment Health*. 2016;19:599–608.

25. National Sleep Foundation. Women and sleep poll. http://www.sleepfoundation. org. Published 1998. Accessed 2006.

26. Halbreich U. The diagnosis of premenstrual syndromes and premenstrual dysphoric disorder—clinical procedures and research perspectives. *Gynecol Endocrinol*. 2004;19:320–334.

27. American Psychiatric Association. Diagnostic and statistical manual of mental disorders (DSM-5®). Washington, DC: American Psychiatric Association; 2013.

28. Baker FC, Lamarche LJ, Iacovides S, Colrain IM. Sleep and menstrual-related disorders. *Sleep Med Clin*. 2008;3:25–35.

29. Shechter A, Lespérance P, Ng Ying Kin NM, Boivin DB. Nocturnal polysomnographic sleep across the menstrual cycle in premenstrual dysphoric disorder. *Sleep Med*. 2012;13:1071–1078.

30. Shechter A, Lespérance P, Ng Ying Kin NM, Boivin DB. Pilot investigation of the circadian plasma melatonin rhythm across the menstrual cycle in a small group of women with premenstrual dysphoric disorder. *PLOS ONE*. 2012;7:e51929.

31. Poromaa IS. Physiological correlates of premenstrual dysphoric disorder (PMDD). *Curr Top Behav Neurosci*. 2014;21:229–243.

32. Iacovides S, Avidon I, Baker FC. What we know about primary dysmenorrhea today: a critical review. *Hum Reprod Update*. 2015;21:762–778.

33. Baker FC, Driver HS, Rogers GG, Paiker J, Mitchell D. High nocturnal body temperatures and disturbed sleep in women with primary dysmenorrhea. *Am J Physiol*. 1999;277(6 Pt 1):E1013–E1021.

34. Lautenbacher S, Kundermann B, Krieg JC. Sleep deprivation and pain perception. *Sleep Med Rev*. 2005;10(5):357–369.

35. Iacovides S, Avidon I, Bentley A, Baker FC. Reduced quality of life when experiencing menstrual pain in women with primary dysmenorrhea. *Acta Obstet Gynecol Scand*. 2014;93:213–217.

36. Keshavarzi F, Mahmoudzadeh F, Brand S, et al. Both melatonin and meloxicam improved sleep and pain in females with primary dysmenorrhea-results from a double-blind cross-over intervention pilot study. *Arch Womens Ment Health*. 2018;21:601–609.

37. Baker FC, Lampio L, Saaresranta T, Polo-Kantola P. Sleep and sleep disorders in the menopausal transition. *Sleep Med Clin*. 2018;13:443–456.

38. Bei B, Milgrom J, Ericksen J, Trinder J. Subjective perception of sleep, but not its objective quality, is associated with immediate postpartum mood disturbances in healthy women. *Sleep*. 2010;33:531–538.

39. Coo Calcagni S, Bei B, Milgrom J, Trinder J. The relationship between sleep and mood in first-time and experienced mothers. *Behav Sleep Med*. 2012;10:167–179.

40. Wilson N, Wynter K, Fisher J, Bei B. Related but different: distinguishing post-partum depression and fatigue among women seeking help for unsettled infant behaviours. *BMC Psychiatry*. 2018;18:309.

41. Insana SP, Stacom EE, Montgomery-Downs HE. Actual and perceived sleep: associations with daytime functioning among postpartum women. *Physiol Behav*. 2011;102:234–238.

42. Swanson LM, Pickett SM, Flynn H, Armitage R. Relationships among depression, anxiety, and insomnia symptoms in perinatal women seeking mental health treatment. *J Womens Health*. 2011;20:553–558.

43. Sharma V, Mazmanian D. Sleep loss and postpartum psychosis. *Bipolar Disord*. 2003;5:98–105.

44. Lewis KJS, Di Florio A, Forty L, et al. Mania triggered by sleep loss and risk of postpartum psychosis in women with bipolar disorder. *J Affect Disord*. 2018;225:624–629.

45. Rawal S, Hinkle SN, Zhu Y, Albert PS, Zhang C. A longitudinal study of sleep duration in pregnancy and subsequent risk of gestational diabetes: findings from a prospective, multiracial cohort. *Am J Obstet Gynecol*. 2017;216:399.e1–399.e8.

46. Lee KA, Gay CL. Sleep in late pregnancy predicts length of labor and type of delivery. *Am J Obstet Gynecol*. 2004;191:2041–2046.

47. Okun ML, Schetter CD, Glynn LM. Poor sleep quality is associated with preterm birth. *Sleep*. 2011;34:1493–1498.

48. Felder JN, Baer RJ, Rand L, Jelliffe-Pawlowski LL, Prather AA. Sleep disorder diagnosis during pregnancy and risk of preterm birth. *Obstet Gynecol*. 2017;130:573–581.

49. Warland J, Dorrian J, Morrison JL, O'Brien LM. Maternal sleep during pregnancy and poor fetal outcomes: a scoping review of the literature with meta-analysis. *Sleep Med Rev*. 2018;41:197–219.

50. Malish S, Arastu F, O'Brien LM. A preliminary study of new parents, sleep disruption, and driving: a population at risk? *Matern Child Health J*. 2016;20:290–297.

51. Cunningham F, Leveno K, Bloom S, Spong CY, Dashe J. *Williams Obstetrics*. 24th ed. New York, NY: McGraw-Hill; 2014.

52. Hedman C, Pohjasvaara T, Tolonen U, Suhonen-Malm AS, Myllylä VV. Effects of pregnancy on mothers' sleep. *Sleep Med*. 2002;3:37–42.

53. Mindell JA, Jacobson BJ. Sleep disturbances during pregnancy. *J Obstet Gynecol Neonatal Nurs*. 2000;29:590–597.

54. Lee KA, Zaffke ME. Longitudinal changes in fatigue and energy during pregnancy and the postpartum period. *J Obstet Gynecol Neonatal Nurs*. 1999;28:183–191.

55. Sedov ID, Cameron EE, Madigan S, Tomfohr-Madsen LM. Sleep quality during pregnancy: a meta-analysis. *Sleep Med Rev*. 2018;38:168–176.

56. Buysse DJ, Reynolds CF, Monk TH, Berman SR, Kupfer DJ. The Pittsburgh Sleep Quality Index: a new instrument for psychiatric practice and research. *Psychiatry Res*. 1989;28:193–213.

57. Lee KA, Zaffke ME, McEnany G. Parity and sleep patterns during and after pregnancy. *Obstet Gynecol*. 2000;95:14–18.

58. Sivertsen B., Hysing M., Dørheim S.K., Eberhard-Gran M. Trajectories of maternal sleep problems before and after childbirth: a longitudinal population-based study. *BMC Pregnancy Childbirth*. 2015;15:129.

59. Baratte-Beebe KR, Lee K. Sources of midsleep awakenings in childbearing women. *Clin Nurs Res*. 1999;8:386–397.

60. Neau J-P, Texier B, Ingrand P. Sleep and vigilance disorders in pregnancy. *Eur Neurol*. 2009;62:23–29.

61. Beebe KR, Lee KA. Sleep disturbance in late pregnancy and early labor. *J Perinat Neonatal Nurs*. 2007;21:103–108.

62. Matsumoto K, Shinkoda H, Kang MJ, Seo YJ. Longitudinal study of mothers' sleep-wake behaviors and circadian time patterns from late pregnancy to postpartum—monitoring of wrist actigraphy and sleep logs. *Biol Rhythm Res*. 2003;34: 265–278.

63. Lee KA, McEnany G, Zaffke ME. REM sleep and mood state in childbearing women: sleepy or weepy? *Sleep*. 2000;23:877–885.

64. Karacan I, Williams RL, Hursch CJ, McCaulley M, Heine MW. Some implications of the sleep patterns of pregnancy for postpartum emotional disturbances. *Br J Psychiatry*. 1969;115:929–935.

65. Wilson DL, Barnes M, Ellett L, Permezel M, Jackson M, Crowe SF. Decreased sleep efficiency, increased wake after sleep onset and increased cortical arousals in late pregnancy. *Aust N Z J Obstet Gynaecol*. 2011;51:38–46.

66. Brunner DP, Münch M, Biedermann K, Huch R, Huch A, Borbély AA. Changes in sleep and sleep electroencephalogram during pregnancy. *Sleep*. 1994;17:576–582.

67. Hertz G, Fast A, Feinsilver SH, Albertario CL, Schulman H, Fein AM. Sleep in normal late pregnancy. *Sleep*. 1992;15:246–251.

68. Izci-Balserak B, Keenan BT, Corbitt C, Staley B, Perlis M, Pien GW. Changes in sleep characteristics and breathing parameters during sleep in early and late pregnancy. *J Clin Sleep Med*. 2018;14:1161–1168.

69. Kennedy HP, Gardiner A, Gay C, Lee KA. Negotiating sleep: a qualitative study of new mothers. *J Perinat Neonatal Nurs*. 2007;21:114–122.

70. Bei B, Coo Calcagni S, Milgrom J, Trinder J. Day-to-day alteration of 24-hour sleep pattern immediately before and after giving birth: 24-hour sleep before and after childbirth. *Sleep Biol Rhythms*. 2012;10:212–221.

71. Gay CL, Lee KA, Lee S-Y. Sleep patterns and fatigue in new mothers and fathers. *Biol Res Nurs*. 2004;5:311–318.

72. Bende M, Gredmark T. Nasal stuffiness during pregnancy. *Laryngoscope*. 1999;109(7 Pt 1):1108–1110.

73. Pilkington S, Carli F, Dakin MJ, et al. Increase in Mallampati score during pregnancy. *Br J Anaesth*. 1995;74:638–642.

74. Hegewald MJ, Crapo RO. Respiratory physiology in pregnancy. *Clin Chest Med*. 2011;32:1–13.

75. Dzieciolowska-Baran E, Teul-Swiniarska I, Gawlikowska-Sroka A, Poziomkowska-Gesicka I, Zietek Z. Rhinitis as a cause of respiratory disorders during pregnancy. In: Pokorski M, ed. *Respiratory regulation—clinical advances*. Dordrecht, The Netherlands: Springer; 2013:213–220.

76. Facco FL, Kramer J, Ho KH, Zee PC, Grobman WA. Sleep disturbances in pregnancy. *Obstet Gynecol*. 2010;115:77–83.

77. O'Brien LM, Bullough AS, Owusu JT, et al. Pregnancy-onset habitual snoring, gestational hypertension, and preeclampsia: prospective cohort study. *Am J Obstet Gynecol*. 2012;207:487.e1–9.

78. Sarberg M, Svanborg E, Wiréhn A-B, Josefsson A. Snoring during pregnancy and its relation to sleepiness and pregnancy outcome—a prospective study. *BMC Pregnancy Childbirth.* 2014;14:15.

79. Bourjeily G, Raker CA, Chalhoub M, Miller MA. Pregnancy and fetal outcomes of symptoms of sleep-disordered breathing. *Eur Respir J.* 2010;36:849–855.

80. Pien GW, Pack AI, Jackson N, Maislin G, Macones GA, Schwab RJ. Risk factors for sleep-disordered breathing in pregnancy. *Thorax.* 2014;69:371–377.

81. Facco FL, Ouyang DW, Zee PC, Grobman WA. Sleep disordered breathing in a high-risk cohort prevalence and severity across pregnancy. *Am J Perinatol.* 2014;31:899–904.

82. Ding X-X, Wu Y-L, Xu S-J, et al. A systematic review and quantitative assessment of sleep-disordered breathing during pregnancy and perinatal outcomes. *Sleep Breath.* 2014;18:703–713.

83. Srivanitchapoom P, Pandey S, Hallett M. Restless legs syndrome and pregnancy: a review. *Parkinsonism Relat Disord.* 2014;20:716–722.

84. Manconi M, Ulfberg J, Berger K, et al. When gender matters: restless legs syndrome. Report of the "RLS and woman" workshop endorsed by the European RLS Study Group. *Sleep Med Rev.* 2012;16:297–307.

85. Manconi M, Govoni V, De Vito A, et al. Restless legs syndrome and pregnancy. *Neurology.* 2004;63:1065–1069.

86. Hübner A, Krafft A, Gadient S, Werth E, Zimmermann R, Bassetti CL. Characteristics and determinants of restless legs syndrome in pregnancy: a prospective study. *Neurology.* 2013;80:738–742.

87. Lee KA, Zaffke ME, Baratte-Beebe K. Restless legs syndrome and sleep disturbance during pregnancy: the role of folate and iron. *J Womens Health Gend Based Med.* 2001;10:335–341.

88. Lee S-Y, Lee KA. Early postpartum sleep and fatigue for mothers after cesarean delivery compared with vaginal delivery: an exploratory study. *J Perinat Neonatal Nurs.* 2007;21:109–113.

89. Nishihara K, Horiuchi S. Changes in sleep patterns of young women from late pregnancy to postpartum: relationships to their infants' movements. *Percept Mot Skills.* 1998;87(3 Pt 1):1043–1056.

90. Signal TL, Gander PH, Sangalli MR, Travier N, Firestone RT, Tuohy JF. Sleep duration and quality in healthy nulliparous and multiparous women across pregnancy and post-partum. *Aust N Z J Obstet Gynaecol.* 2007;47:16–22.

91. Swain AM, O'Hara MW, Starr KR, Gorman LL. A prospective study of sleep, mood, and cognitive function in postpartum and nonpostpartum women. *Obstet Gynecol.* 1997;90:381–386.

92. Wolfson AR, Crowley SJ, Anwer U, Bassett JL. Changes in sleep patterns and depressive symptoms in first-time mothers: last trimester to 1-year postpartum. *Behav Sleep Med.* 2003;1:54–67.

93. Filtness AJ, MacKenzie J, Armstrong K. Longitudinal change in sleep and daytime sleepiness in postpartum women. *PLOS ONE.* 2014;9:e103513.

94. Goyal D, Gay CL, Lee KA. Patterns of sleep disruption and depressive symptoms in new mothers. *J Perinat Neonatal Nurs.* 2007;21:123–129.

95. Horiuchi S, Nishihara K. Analyses of mothers' sleep logs in postpartum periods. *Psychiatry Clin Neurosci.* 1999;53:137–139.

96. Gress JL, Chambers AS, Ong JC, Tikotzky L, Okada R, Manber R. Maternal subjective sleep quality and nighttime infant care. *J Reprod Infant Psychol.* 2010;28:384–391.

97. Montgomery-Downs HE, Clawges HM, Santy EE. Infant feeding methods and maternal sleep and daytime functioning. *Pediatrics.* 2010;126:e1562–e1568.

98. Doan T, Gardiner A, Gay CL, Lee KA. Breast-feeding increases sleep duration of new parents. *J Perinat Neonatal Nurs.* 2007;21:200–206.

99. Doan T, Gay CL, Kennedy HP, Newman J, Lee KA. Nighttime breastfeeding behavior is associated with more nocturnal sleep among first-time mothers at one month postpartum. *J Clin Sleep Med.* 2014;10:313–319.

100. Dennis C-L, Ross L. Relationships among infant sleep patterns, maternal fatigue, and development of depressive symptomatology. *Birth.* 2005;32:187–193.

101. Hiscock H, Wake M. Infant sleep problems and postnatal depression: a community-based study. *Pediatrics.* 2001;107:1317–1322.

102. Wynter K, Wilson N, Thean P, Bei B, Fisher J. Psychological and sleep-related functioning among women with unsettled infants in Victoria, Australia: a cross-sectional study. *J Reprod Infant Psychol.* 2019;37(4):413–428.

103. Wilson N, Wynter K, Anderson C, Rajaratnam SMW, Fisher J, Bei B. More than depression: A multi-dimensional assessment of postpartum distress symptoms before and after a residential early parenting program. *BMC Psychiatry.* 2019;48:19.

104. Aaronson LS, Teel CS, Cassmeyer V, et al. Defining and measuring fatigue. *Image J Nurs Sch.* 1999;31:45–50.

105. Milligan R, Lenz ER, Parks PL, Pugh LC, Kitzman H. Postpartum fatigue: clarifying a concept. *Res Theory Nurs Pract.* 1996;10:279–291.

106. Shen J, Barbera J, Shapiro CM. Distinguishing sleepiness and fatigue: focus on definition and measurement. *Sleep Med Rev.* 2006;10:63–76.

107. Parks PL, Lenz ER, Milligan RA, Han HR. What happens when fatigue lingers for 18 months after delivery? *J Obstet Gynecol Neonatal Nurs.* 1999;28:87–93.

108. McGovern P, Dowd B, Gjerdingen D, et al. Mothers' health and work-related factors at 11 weeks postpartum. *Ann Fam Med.* 2007;5:519–527.

109. Rychnovsky J, Hunter LP. The relationship between sleep characteristics and fatigue in healthy postpartum women. *Womens Health Issues.* 2009;19:38–44.

110. Giallo R, Gartland D, Woolhouse H, Brown S. "I didn't know it was possible to feel that tired": exploring the complex bidirectional associations between maternal depressive symptoms and fatigue in a prospective pregnancy cohort study. *Arch Womens Ment Health.* 2016;19:25–34.

111. Gardner DL. Fatigue in postpartum women. *Appl Nurs Res.* 1991;4:57–62.

112. Tsuchiya M, Mori E, Iwata H, et al. Fragmented sleep and fatigue during postpartum hospitalization in older primiparous women. *Nurs Health Sci.* 2015;17:71–76.

113. Giallo R, Wade C, Cooklin A, Rose N. Assessment of maternal fatigue and depression in the postpartum period: support for two separate constructs. *J Reprod Infant Psychol.* 2011;29:69–80.

114. Giallo R, Gartland D, Woolhouse H, Brown S. Differentiating maternal fatigue and depressive symptoms at six months and four years post partum: considerations for assessment, diagnosis and intervention. *Midwifery.* 2015;31:316–322.

115. Dinges DF, Powell JW. Microcomputer analyses of performance on a portable, simple visual RT task during sustained operations. *Behav Res Methods Instrum Comput.* 1985;17:652–655.

116. Insana SP, Williams KB, Montgomery-Downs HE. Sleep disturbance and neurobehavioral performance among postpartum women. *Sleep*. 2013;36:73–81.

117. Wilson N, Wynter K, Anderson C, Rajaratnam SMW, Fisher J, Bei B. Postpartum fatigue, daytime sleepiness, and psychomotor vigilance are modifiable through a brief residential early parenting program. *Sleep Med*. 2019;59:33–41.

118. Skouteris H, Germano C, Wertheim EH, Paxton SJ, Milgrom J. Sleep quality and depression during pregnancy: a prospective study. *J Sleep Res*. 2008;17:217–220.

119. Okun ML, Luther J, Prather AA, Perel JM, Wisniewski S, Wisner KL. Changes in sleep quality, but not hormones predict time to postpartum depression recurrence. *J Affect Disord*. 2011;130:378–384.

120. Dørheim SK, Bondevik GT, Eberhard-Gran M, Bjorvatn B. Subjective and objective sleep among depressed and non-depressed postnatal women. *Acta Psychiatr Scand*. 2009;119:128–136.

121. Okun ML, Kline CE, Roberts JM, Wettlaufer B, Glover K, Hall M. Prevalence of sleep deficiency in early gestation and its associations with stress and depressive symptoms. *J Womens Health*. 2013;22:1028–1037.

122. Park EM, Meltzer-Brody S, Stickgold R. Poor sleep maintenance and subjective sleep quality are associated with postpartum maternal depression symptom severity. *Arch Womens Ment Health*. 2013;16:539–547.

123. Krawczak EM, Minuzzi L, Simpson W, Hidalgo MP, Frey BN. Sleep, daily activity rhythms and postpartum mood: a longitudinal study across the perinatal period. *Chronobiol Int*. 2016;33:791–801.

124. Tsai S-Y, Thomas KA. Sleep disturbances and depressive symptoms in healthy postpartum women: a pilot study. *Res Nurs Health*. 2012;35:314–323.

125. Santoro N. The menopausal transition. *Am J Med*. 2005;118(12 Suppl 2):8–13.

126. Roberts H, Hickey M. Managing the menopause: An update. *Maturitas*. 2016;86:53–58.

127. Bolge SC, Balkrishnan R, Kannan H, Seal B, Drake CL. Burden associated with chronic sleep maintenance insomnia characterized by nighttime awakenings among women with menopausal symptoms. *Menopause*. 2010;17:80–86.

128. Kleinman NL, Rohrbacker NJ, Bushmakin AG, Whiteley J, Lynch WD, Shah SN. Direct and indirect costs of women diagnosed with menopause symptoms. *J Occup Environ Med*. 2013;55:465–470.

129. Whiteley J, DiBonaventura MD, Wagner J-S, Alvir J, Shah S. The impact of menopausal symptoms on quality of life, productivity, and economic outcomes. *J Womens Health*. 2013;22:983–990.

130. Joffe H, Massler A, Sharkey KM. Evaluation and management of sleep disturbance during the menopause transition. *Semin Reprod Med*. 2010;28:404–421.

131. Polo-Kantola P. Dealing with Menopausal Sleep Disturbances. *Sleep Med Clin*. 2008;3:121–131.

132. Shaver JL, Zenk SN. Sleep disturbance in menopause. *J Womens Health Gend Based Med*. 2000;9:109–118.

133. Ford K, Sowers M, Crutchfield M, Wilson A, Jannausch M. A longitudinal study of the predictors of prevalence and severity of symptoms commonly associated with menopause. *Menopause*. 2005;12:308–317.

134. Baker FC, de Zambotti M, Colrain IM, Bei B. Sleep problems during the menopausal transition: prevalence, impact, and management challenges. *Nat Sci Sleep*. 2018;10:73–95.

135. Xu Q, Lang CP. Examining the relationship between subjective sleep disturbance and menopause: a systematic review and meta-analysis. *Menopause*.
2014;21:1301–1318.

136. Cheng M-H, Hsu C-Y, Wang S-J, Lee S-J, Wang P-H, Fuh J-L. The relationship
of self-reported sleep disturbance, mood, and menopause in a community study.
Menopause. 2008;15:958–962.

137. Shin C, Lee S, Lee T, et al. Prevalence of insomnia and its relationship to menopausal
status in middle-aged Korean women. *Psychiatry Clin Neurosci*. 2005;59:395–402.

138. Kravitz HM, Zhao X, Bromberger JT, et al. Sleep disturbance during the menopausal transition in a multi-ethnic community sample of women. *Sleep*. 2008;31:
979–990.

139. Woods NF, Mitchell ES. Sleep symptoms during the menopausal transition and
early postmenopause: observations from the Seattle Midlife Women's Health Study.
Sleep. 2010;33:539–549.

140. Campbell IG, Bromberger JT, Buysse DJ, et al. Evaluation of the association of menopausal status with delta and beta EEG activity during sleep. *Sleep*.
2011;34:1561–1568.

141. Freedman RR, Roehrs TA. Lack of sleep disturbance from menopausal hot flashes.
Fertil Steril. 2004;82:138–144.

142. Kalleinen N, Polo-Kantola P, Himanen S-L, et al. Sleep and the menopause—do
postmenopausal women experience worse sleep than premenopausal women?
Menopause Int. 2008;14:97–104.

143. Young T, Rabago D, Zgierska A, Austin D, Laurel F. Objective and subjective sleep
quality in premenopausal, perimenopausal, and postmenopausal women in the
Wisconsin Sleep Cohort Study. *Sleep*. 2003;26:667–672.

144. Hachul H, Frange C, Bezerra AG, et al. The effect of menopause on objective sleep
parameters: data from an epidemiologic study in São Paulo, Brazil. *Maturitas*.
2015;80:170–178.

145. Lampio L, Polo-Kantola P, Himanen S-L, et al. Sleep during menopausal transition: a 6-year follow-up. *Sleep*. 2017;40(7):zsx090.

146. Baker FC, Willoughby AR, Sassoon SA, Colrain IM, de Zambotti M. Insomnia in
women approaching menopause: beyond perception. *Psychoneuroendocrinology*.
2015;60:96–104.

147. Archer DF, Sturdee DW, Baber R, et al. Menopausal hot flushes and night
sweats: where are we now? *Climacteric*. 2011;14:515–528.

148. Avis NE, Crawford SL, Greendale G, et al. Duration of menopausal vasomotor
symptoms over the menopause transition. *JAMA Intern Med*. 2015;175:531–539.

149. Freedman RR. Menopausal hot flashes: mechanisms, endocrinology, treatment. *J
Steroid Biochem Mol Biol*. 2014;142:115–120.

150. Kravitz HM, Ganz PA, Bromberger J, Powell LH, Sutton-Tyrrell K, Meyer PM.
Sleep difficulty in women at midlife: a community survey of sleep and the menopausal transition. *Menopause*. 2003;10:19–28.

151. Blumel JE, Caño A, Mezones-Holguín E, et al. A multinational study of sleep
disorders during female mid-life. *Maturitas*. 2012;72:359–366.

152. Ohayon MM. Severe hot flashes are associated with chronic insomnia. *Arch Intern
Med*. 2006;166:1262–1268.

153. Kravitz HM, Joffe H. Sleep during the perimenopause: a SWAN story. *Obstet
Gynecol Clin North Am*. 2011;38:567–586.

154. de Zambotti M, Colrain IM, Javitz HS, Baker FC. Magnitude of the impact of hot flashes on sleep in perimenopausal women. *Fertil Steril.* 2014;102:1708–15.e1.
155. Joffe H, White DP, Crawford SL, et al. Adverse effects of induced hot flashes on objectively recorded and subjectively reported sleep. *Menopause.* 2013;20(9):905–914.
156. Thurston RC, Santoro N, Matthews KA. Are vasomotor symptoms associated with sleep characteristics among symptomatic midlife women? Comparisons of self-report and objective measures. *Menopause.* 2012;19:742–748.
157. Savard M-H, Savard J, Caplette-Gingras A, Ivers H, Bastien C. Relationship between objectively recorded hot flashes and sleep disturbances among breast cancer patients: investigating hot flash characteristics other than frequency. *Menopause.* 2013;20:997–1005.
158. Freedman RR, Roehrs TA. Sleep disturbance in menopause. *Menopause.* 2007;14:826–829.
159. Sassoon SA, de Zambotti M, Colrain IM, Baker FC. Association between personality traits and DSM-IV diagnosis of insomnia in peri- and postmenopausal women. *Menopause.* 2014;21:1–10.
160. Freeman EW, Sammel MD, Lin H, Nelson DB. Associations of hormones and menopausal status with depressed mood in women with no history of depression. *Arch Gen Psychiatry.* 2006;63:375–382.
161. Yonkers KA. The association between premenstrual dysphoric disorder and other mood disorders. *J Clin Psychiatry.* 1997;58(Suppl 15):19–25.
162. Ameratunga D, Goldin J, Hickey M. Sleep disturbance in menopause. *Intern Med J.* 2012;42:742–747.
163. Darling CA, Coccia C, Senatore N. Women in midlife: stress, health and life satisfaction. *Stress Health.* 2012;28:31–40.
164. Cuadros JL, Fernández-Alonso AM, Cuadros-Celorrio AM, et al. Perceived stress, insomnia and related factors in women around the menopause. *Maturitas.* 2012;72:367–372.
165. Vaari T, Engblom J, Helenius H, Erkkola R, Polo-Kantola P. Survey of sleep problems in 3421 women aged 41–55 years. *Menopause Int.* 2008;14:78–82.
166. Hall MH, Casement MD, Troxel WM, et al. Chronic stress is prospectively associated with sleep in midlife women: The SWAN Sleep Study. *Sleep.* 2015;38:1645–1654.
167. Hall MH, Matthews KA, Kravitz HM, et al. Race and financial strain are independent correlates of sleep in midlife women: the SWAN sleep study. *Sleep.* 2009;32:73–82.
168. Troxel WM, Buysse DJ, Matthews KA, et al. Marital/cohabitation status and history in relation to sleep in midlife women. *Sleep.* 2010;33:973–981.
169. Morse CD, Klingman KJ, Jacob BL, Kodali L. Exercise and insomnia risk in middle-aged women. *J Nurse Pract.* 2019;15(3):236–240.e2
170. Brown L, Bryant C, Brown VM, Bei B, Judd FK. Self-compassion weakens the association between hot flushes and night sweats and daily life functioning and depression. *Maturitas.* 2014;78:298–303.
171. Brown L, Bryant C, Brown V, Bei B, Judd F. Self-compassion, attitudes to ageing and indicators of health and well-being among midlife women. *Aging Ment Health.* 2016;20:1035–1043.

172. Coo S, Milgrom J, Kuppens P, Cox P, Trinder J. Exploring the association between maternal mood and self-reports of sleep during the perinatal period. *J Obstetr, Gynecol Neonat Nurs.* 2014;43(4):465–477.

173. Bei B, Wiley JF, Allen NB, Trinder J. A cognitive vulnerability model on sleep and mood in adolescents under naturalistically restricted and extended sleep opportunities. *Sleep.* 2015;38:453–461.

174. Stremler R, Hodnett E, Kenton L, et al. Effect of behavioural-educational intervention on sleep for primiparous women and their infants in early postpartum: multisite randomised controlled trial. *BMJ.* 2013;346:f1164.

175. Manber R, Bei B, Simpson N, et al. Cognitive behavioral therapy for prenatal insomnia: a randomized controlled trial. *Obstet Gynecol.* 2019;133(5):911–919.

176. Swanson LM, Flynn H, Adams-Mundy JD, Armitage R, Arnedt JT. An open pilot of cognitive-behavioral therapy for insomnia in women with postpartum depression. *Behav Sleep Med.* 2013;11:297–307.

177. McCurry SM, Guthrie KA, Morin CM, et al. Telephone-based cognitive behavioral therapy for insomnia in perimenopausal and postmenopausal women with vasomotor symptoms: a MsFLASH randomized clinical trial. *JAMA Intern Med.* 2016;176:913–920.

178. Drake CL, Kalmbach DA, Arnedt JT, et al. Treating chronic insomnia in postmenopausal women: a randomized clinical trial comparing cognitive-behavioral therapy for insomnia, sleep restriction therapy, and sleep hygiene education. *Sleep.* 2019;42:zsy217.

179. Schutte-Rodin S, Broch L, Buysse D, Dorsey C, Sateia M. Clinical guideline for the evaluation and management of chronic insomnia in adults. *J Clin Sleep Med.* 2008;4:487–504.

PART III

Sleep Disturbances, Disorders, and Treatments

14

Consequences of Poor or Inadequate Sleep

CRYSTAL L. YATES AND SIOBHAN BANKS ■

INTRODUCTION

Despite the National Sleep Foundation noting that adults need between 7 and 9 hours, recent reports show that 15% of American adults report sleeping less than 6 hours per night [1]. In fact, the 2005–2008 National Health and Nutrition Examination Survey (NHANES) indicated that 35% to 40% of the adult population in the United States do not get enough sleep [1]. Sleep is a biological necessity, playing an essential role in maintaining cognitive performance, physiological processes, emotion regulation, and quality of life [2]. Furthermore, inadequate sleep impacts individuals' health and wellbeing at the individual, organizational, and community levels. An Australian study reported inadequate sleep in Australia cost $45.21 billion during the 2016–2017 financial year [3]. This figure included $5.22 billion for reduced employment, $0.61 billion for premature death, $1.73 billion for absenteeism, and $27.33 billion for reduced well-being.

There are many reasons why sleep may be restricted or of poor quality, including that it is a product of the environment in which we live and lack of knowledge about the importance of sleep. Common reasons for inadequate sleep are—work commitments, long and irregular working hours (shift work), health issues, sleep disorders, transmeridian travel, busy social lives, young children, and consumption of media. This chapter will discuss the consequences of inadequate sleep on performance, cognition, mood, and health, with a particular focus on shift workers.

CONSEQUENCES OF INADEQUATE SLEEP ON PERFORMANCE/MOOD

Multiple studies have shown the detrimental effect of sleep loss on a range of cognitive performance tasks, from simple reaction time and cognitive processing to decision making and driving performance [4–10]. Worsened performance associated with sleep loss may be a result of periods of microsleep, a transient physiologic sleep lasting 3 to 14 seconds [11]. Restricting sleep to 6 hours or less per night over 2 weeks has been shown to result in subjective sleepiness, fatigue, and impaired mood equal to cognitive deficits seen after 2 full nights of no sleep at all [8].

Increased sleepiness and decreased alertness can be dangerous in the workplace, particularly when completing safety-critical tasks. Sleepiness leads to increased errors, incidents, and accident risk across a broad range of industries, including but not limited to healthcare, police, and transport [12]. Critically, in nearly every industry the danger can extend past the individual level, leading to public safety issues in the form of mechanical errors [13], medical errors including medication administration [12], and failure to intercept errors made by others [14].

Performance Impairment When at Work

When it comes to the impact of sleep loss and poor-quality sleep in the work place, a particularly vulnerable portion of the public are those that work at night. Human error is an important contributing factor in many workplace accidents, particularly when working at night [15]. To a large extent, this is related to the impact of night shift on sleep and circadian rhythms. Variations in performance across the day parallel circadian variation in body temperature [16, 17] (also see Chapter 4 of this volume). Night-shift work requires the individual to work during the circadian nadir, which, combined with sleep deficit, heightened sleepiness and decreased alertness, culminates in our observing the poorest performance during the early morning hours [18]. Night workers report increased sleepiness compared to day workers, on both subjective scales (including standard, validated scales such as the Stanford Sleepiness Scale, Karolinska Sleepiness Scale, and Visual Analogue Scale) [19, 20] and objective measures including sleep latency tests, where workers are asked to sit semirecumbent in a chair and their time taken to fall asleep is measured [20, 21]. In addition to impairments shown in the workplace, increased sleepiness and decreased alertness can result in dangerous driving on the roads during the commute home, affecting the safety of both the individual and the wider community [12, 22].

In addition, night workers are required to sleep during the day. They are not the only ones; many students stay up all night in preparation for exams, and social activities may keep people up through the night, meaning that they must then catch up on lost sleep during the day. Through evolution, organisms have developed a regulatory system corresponding to the 24-hour light/dark period, resulting from the Earth rotating around its axis [23]. For humans, this has resulted in physiology geared for sleep at night and wake during the day. Sleep is optimal at our temperature minimum, which is usually around the fourth or fifth hour, during the second half of, or toward the end of, the sleep period [24]. This allows the circadian drive for wake to be lowest after the homeostatic sleep drive has been extinguished during the first part of the sleep period. Sleep after the night shift is usually initiated 1 hour after finishing the shift [25]. Initiating sleep at this time corresponds with the rise of the circadian process, which promotes wakefulness making sleep onset difficult [26]. A number of external factors also influence the quality and duration of sleep during the day, including family commitments, and a nonideal sleeping environment during the day (increased noise and light) [27, 28]. Consequently, daytime sleep results in decreased sleep duration, by approximately 2 to 4 hours following night shift compared day workers [29, 30].

In addition to reduced sleep duration, sleep quality is also reduced in the daytime. Sleep quality can be estimated using both subjective (e.g., sleep diaries, Pittsburgh Sleep Quality Assessment (also see Chapter 23 of this volume) and objective (e.g., electroencephalography; also see Chapter 22 of this volume) measures. Electroencephalography (EEG) uses electrical activity to identify time spent in each of the two distinct sleep states, rapid eye movement (REM) and non-REM, which includes stages N1, N2 and N3 (or non-REM stages 1–4; also see Chapter 1 of this volume). For shift workers, daytime sleep results in decreased sleep duration and disrupted sleep architecture, particularly time spent in stage 2 and REM sleep [31]. In addition, daytime sleep also results in increased time taken to fall asleep (sleep onset latency), and increased number of awakenings after sleep onset (wake after sleep onset), further decreasing overall sleep quality [32].

Driving Performance

As previously noted, sleepiness and decreased alertness can also result in dangerous drivers of heavy vehicles and other road users, which can affect the safety of both individuals and the wider community [22, 33]. In fact, inadequate sleep significantly impacts driving performance [34, 35], with an estimated 23% of all motor vehicle accidents caused by lack of sleep. Similar to drugs and alcohol, the effects of sleep loss on driving performance are well noted; however, unlike roadside drug and alcohol testing that has helped reduce the number of impaired drivers on the roads, to date there is no quantifiable roadside test for driver fatigue and sleepiness. This is despite Lamond and Dawson [36] showing that performance impairment following extended wake of approximately 20 to 25 hours is equivalent to or greater than those observed at levels of alcohol intoxication deemed unacceptable when driving, working, and/or operating dangerous equipment (i.e., blood alcohol concentration 0.10%).

Cognitive Performance in the Classroom

Sleep loss not only affects performance in the workplace. Students can also be impacted by poor sleep quality and quantity. In fact, sleep quality and quantity affect students' learning capacity and academic performance [37], resulting in lower cognitive performance on neurobehavioral tests [38] (also see Chapter 7 of this volume). Sleep loss also detrimentally impacts declarative (spoken information) and procedural (motor skills) learning in students. Interestingly, studies looking at the impacts of early start times on school-aged children have found that early start times are associated with decreased sleep duration, an increased risk of worsened academic performance and academic effort than those with later start times [39] (also see Chapter 10 of this volume).

Sleep deprivation is common among college students, particularly around examination periods where sleep deprivation can extend to 24 to 48 hours [40]. Sleep deprived participants in studies of this population perform significantly worse, while rating their performance significantly higher than nondeprived participants, suggesting that students are not aware of the negative implications of sleep deprivation on their academic performance [40].

Mood and Psychological Well-Being

In addition to the detrimental effects of sleep restriction on cognitive performance, sleep deprivation increases self-reported negative mood states [41], with sleep loss leading to increased ratings of self-reported stress [42]. In addition, a recent adolescent study (with 29,510 participants) examined the relationship between bullying and sleep quality; these authors found that poorer subjective sleep quality was related to higher sadness, poorer physical health ratings, and higher anxiety [43]. This study suggested that promoting better sleep is recommended in future antibullying strategies.

Individual Differences in Response to Sleep Loss

While the detrimental effects of poor-quality sleep and short sleep duration have been shown, a significant interindividual variability in the responses to sleep loss and disturbance has been observed in multiple studies [41, 44–46]. Some individuals display minimal impairment during sleep loss (Figure 14.1A), while others are particularly vulnerable (Figure 14.1C) [47]. Studies conducted to further understand this concept have shown that interindividual variation cannot be explained by age, sex, baseline performance prior to sleep loss, or sleep need [47]. A number of possible genetic contributors have been considered, including PERIOD3 VNTR (PER3) and ADORA2A polymorphisms [48, 49].

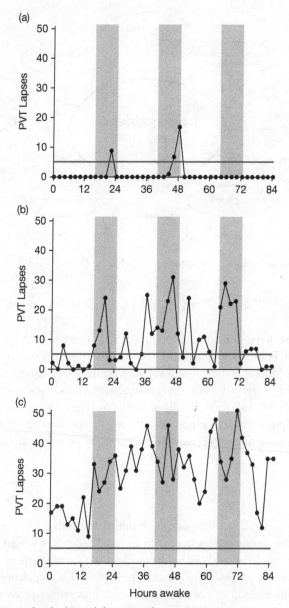

Figure 14.1 Inter-individual variability in performance on the psychomotor vigilance tasks during extended wake.

SOURCE: Modified from Basner M, Dinges DF. Maximizing sensitivity of the psychomotor vigilance test (PVT) to sleep loss. *Sleep*. 2011;34(5):581–591.

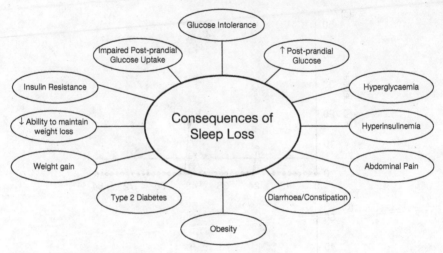

Figure 14.2 Physiological consequences of sleep loss.

CONSEQUENCES OF INADEQUATE SLEEP ON HEALTH

Many studies have linked not getting enough sleep with serious health consequences. Poor quality sleep and sleep loss have been linked to an increase in mortality risk [50, 51] and sleeping less than 6 hours on average per night has been associated with many physiological consequences, including obesity [52], type 2 diabetes [53], and cardiovascular disease [54–56] (Figure 14.2). Furthermore, inadequate sleep can impact immune health, which can result in an increased risk of developing inflammatory disease [57], cancer [58], and infectious disease [59].

Obesity

Many studies have shown that sleep duration is inversely related to obesity risk, with short sleep duration associated with an increased risk of weight gain [60–63]. A positive energy balance via either reduced energy expenditure or increased energy intake is one proposed mechanism to explain this association. First, short sleep duration results in increased fatigue, which may reduce physical activity (reducing energy expenditure) [64]. Second, short sleep duration results in increased wake time and hormonal changes that may affect hunger/appetite, which can lead to increases in food intake [65]. Third, during wake there is an increased utilization of central glucose [66], as a reflection of the higher energy demand of the brain.

Metabolism

Several epidemiological studies have demonstrated an association between short sleep duration and diabetes mellitus [62, 67–69]. This is likely due to the effect of sleep deprivation on physiological processes including endocrine and metabolic systems [70]. Laboratory studies have shown that sleep deprivation leads to impaired metabolism including decreased glucose tolerance [71, 72] and decreased insulin sensitivity [73] in humans. Sleep restriction for 5 nights with 4 hours in bed each night results in an amplified postprandial response compared to baseline, as shown in Figure 14.3 [74]. This study also reported increased afternoon cortisol and reduced sex hormone binding globulin, consistent with development of insulin resistance. This evidence suggests that, with recurring short periods of sleep restriction, these acute changes in metabolism raise the risk of developing metabolic syndrome [75], obesity [76], and type 2 diabetes [53].

Hunger and Food Intake

Short sleep duration results in increased wake time and hormonal changes that may affect hunger and/or appetite, resulting in possible increases in food intake (i.e., increasing total energy intake) [65]. Short sleep duration is also associated with low fruit and vegetable consumption, high fat diet, and high-frequency fast-food consumption [77]. Imaki, Hatanaka, and Ogawa [78] also reported a decreased vegetable intake in short sleepers, along with a disruption in habitual dietary patterns including increased frequency of snacking and dining out.

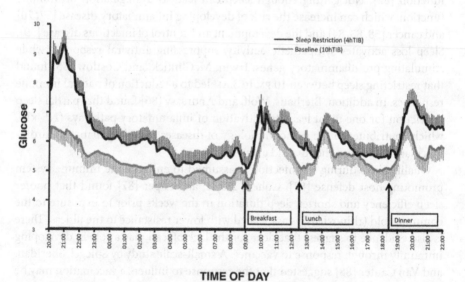

TIME OF DAY

Figure 14.3 Twenty-four-hour profile interstitial glucose (mmol/L) on baseline (grey bar) compared to after five nights of sleep restriction of 4-hour time in bed (black bar).
SOURCE: Modified from Reynolds AC, Dorrian J, Liu PY, et al. Impact of five nights of sleep restriction on glucose metabolism, leptin and testosterone in young adult men. PLOS ONE. 2012;7(7):e41218.

A number of studies have reported an association between sleep loss and hunger and appetite [65, 79, 80]. In laboratory conditions, Schmid and Hallschmid [80] compared hunger ratings following varied sleep durations, with subjective ratings of hunger markedly stronger after total sleep deprivation than after either 7 hours sleep or 4.5 hours sleep. In the same study, ghrelin (a hormone involved with stimulating food intake) increased with increasing sleep restriction, while leptin (a hormone involved in suppressing food intake) did not change. Furthermore, a population-based longitudinal study of 1024 participants reported that short sleep duration (less than 5 hours) was associated with increased ghrelin and decreased leptin [65]. A higher body mass index was reported in those with inadequate, short sleep compared to those who slept approximately 8 hours. The dietary intake of participants in that study were not reported; however, Kilkus, Booth, and Bromley [81] assessed dietary behavior and its association with sleep, showing that poor sleep quality, even after controlling for sleep duration, increases hunger and emotional eating. Together, these findings support the suggestion that sleep loss and poor-quality sleep impair endocrine regulation of energy homeostasis, which may be an underlying mechanism in the prevalence of obesity and diabetes in sleep restricted individuals [80].

Immune Response

Adequate sleep quality and duration are necessary to ensure appropriate immune function [82]. Not getting enough sleep can lead to dysregulation of immune function, which can increase the risk of developing inflammatory disease [57, 70] and cancer [58, 83, 84] and the development and control of infectious disease [59]. Sleep loss activates sympathetic activity, suppressing antiviral responses while stimulating proinflammatory genes. Irwin, McClintick, and Costlow [85] found that restricting sleep between 10 PM to 3 AM led to a reduction of natural immune responses. In addition, Bierhaus, Wolf, and Andrassy [86] found that partial sleep restriction for one night leads to activation of inflammatory pathways (NF-κB), which contributes to the pathophysiology of diseases including diabetes, cardiovascular disease and rheumatoid arthritis.

Quality sleep during an infection is assumed to enhance the immune system promoting host defense [82]. Cohen, Doyle, and Alper [87] found that poorer sleep efficiency and shorter sleep duration in the weeks prior to exposure to the common cold (rhinovirus) is associated with lower resistance to the illness. There is also evidence to suggest that sleep, or the lack of, can play a role in developing immunity through response to vaccines. A small-scale study by Spiegel, Sheridan, and Van Cauter [88] suggested that the response to influenza vaccination may be impaired in individuals with chronic partial sleep restriction. A subsequent study has suggested this may be due to the role of sleep in facilitating the transfer of antigenic information, using the time the body is asleep to foster adaptive immune responses resulting in improved immunological memory [89]. This cumulative evidence provides a plausible explanation to connect sleep loss with the risk of infectious and inflammatory disease.

CONCLUSION

Sleep is essential for healthy functioning. However, sleep deprivation is increasingly common in today's 24/7 society. Inadequate sleep results in impaired cognitive performance that can lead to an increased risk for accidents and injuries. There are large individual differences in cognitive impairment as a result of sleep loss, which may have a genetic basis. Sleep loss also impairs metabolic, endocrine, and immune function, increasing the risk of metabolic diseases such as obesity and type 2 diabetes, as well as longer recovery time from illness.

REFERENCES

1. Centers for Disease Control and Prevention. Effect of short sleep duration on daily activities—United States, 2005–2008, in *MMWR*. 2011;60(8):239–242.
2. Hirshkowitz M, Whiton K, Albert SM, et al. National Sleep Foundation's sleep time duration recommendations: Methodology and results summary. *Sleep Health.* 2015;1:40–43.
3. Hillman D, Mitchell S, Streatfeild J, Burns C, Bruck D, Pezzullo L. The economic cost of inadequate sleep. *Sleep.* 2018;41(8):zsy083.
4. Herscovitch J, Stuss D, Broughton R. Changes in cognitive processing following short-term cumulative partial sleep deprivation and recovery oversleeping. *J Clin Exper Neuropsychol.* 1980;2:301–319.
5. Tietzel AJ, Lack LC. The short-term benefits of brief and long naps following nocturnal sleep restriction. *Sleep.* 2001;24:293–300.
6. Belenky G, Wesensten NJ, Thorne DR, et al. Patterns of performance degradation and restoration during sleep restriction and subsequent recovery: a sleep dose-response study. *J Sleep Res* 2003;12:1–12.
7. Dinges DF, Kribbs NB. Performing while sleepy: Effects of experimentally-induced sleepiness. In Monk TS, ed. *Human Performance and Cognition. Sleep, Sleepiness and Performance.* Oxford, UK: Wiley; 1991:97–128.
8. Van Dongen HP, Maislin G, Mullington JM, Dinges DF. The cumulative cost of additional wakefulness: Dose-response effects on neurobehavioral functions and sleep physiology from chronic sleep restriction and total sleep deprivation. *Sleep.* 2003;26:117–126.
9. Gupta CC, Dorrian J, Grant CL, et al. It's not just what you eat but when: The impact of eating a meal during simulated shift work on driving performance. *Chronobiol Int.* 2017;34:66–77.
10. Banks S, Van Dongen HP, Maislin G, Dinges DF. Neurobehavioral dynamics following chronic sleep restriction: dose–response effects of one night for recovery. *Sleep.* 2010;33:1013–1026.

11. Chokroverty S. Sleep deprivation and sleepiness. In: Chokroverty S, ed. *Sleep Disorders Medicine.* 3rd ed. Philadelphia, PA: Saunders; 2009:22–28.
12. Dorrian J, Lamond N, Van Den Heuvel C, Pincombe J, Rogers AE, Dawson D. A pilot study of the safety implications of Australian nurses' sleep and work hours. *Chronobiol Int.* 2006;23:1149–1163.
13. Mitler MM, Carskadon MA, Czeisier CA, Dement WC, Dinges DF, Graeber RCJS. Catastrophes, sleep, and public policy: consensus report. 1988;11:100–109.
14. Dorrian J, Roach GD, Fletcher A, Dawson D. The effects of fatigue on train handling during speed restrictions. *Transport Res Part F.* 2006;9:243–257.
15. Harrington JM. Health effects of shift work and extended hours of work. *Occ Environ Med.* 2001;58:68–72.
16. Colquhoun WP. *Biological Rhythms and Human Performance.* London, UK: Academic Press; 1971.
17. Kleitman N, Jackson DP. Body temperature and performance under different routines. *J Appl Physiol* 1950;3:309–328.
18. Akerstedt T. Psychological and psychophysiological effects of shift work. *Scand J Work Environ Health.* 1990;16:67–73.
19. Folkard S, Monk TH, Lobban MC. Short and long-term adjustment of circadian rhythms in "permanent" night nurses. *Ergonomics.* 1978;21:785–799.
20. Torsvall L, Akerstedt T, Gillander K, Knutsson A. Sleep on the night shift: 24-hour EEG monitoring of spontaneous sleep/wake behavior. *Psychophysiology.* 1989;26:352–358.
21. Kecklund G, Åkerstedt T. Sleepiness in long distance truck driving: an ambulatory EEG study of night driving. *Ergonomics.* 1993;36:1007–1017.
22. Gold DR, Rogacz S, Bock N, et al. Rotating shift work, sleep, and accidents related to sleepiness in hospital nurses. *Am J Health Nations Health.* 1992;82:1011–1014.
23. Herichova I. Changes of physiological functions induced by shift work. *Endocr Reg.* 2013;47:159–170.
24. Kräuchi K, Deboer T. Body temperature, sleep, and hibernation. In Kryger M, Roth T, Dement W, ed. Principles and Practice of Sleep Medicine, 5th ed. Philadelphia, PA: Saunders; 2010;323–334.
25. Knauth P, Rutenfranz J. Duration of sleep related to the type of shift work. *Adv Biosci* 1981;30:161–168.
26. Dijk DJ, Czeisler CA. Contribution of the circadian pacemaker and the sleep homeostat to sleep propensity, sleep structure, electroencephalographic slow waves, and sleep spindle activity in humans. *J Neurosci* 1995;15:3526–2538.
27. Monk TH. Shift work: basic principles. In: Kryger M, Roth T, Dement W, ed. *Principles and Practice of Sleep Medicine.* 4th ed. Philadelphia, PA: Saunders; 2005:673–679.
28. Monk TH, Wagner JA. Social factors can outweigh biological ones in determining night shift safety. *Hum Factors.* 1989;31:721–724.
29. Åkerstedt T. Work hours, sleepiness and the underlying mechanisms. *J Sleep Res.* 1995;4:15–22.
30. Pilcher JJ, Lambert BJ, Huffcutt AI. Differential effects of permanent and rotating shifts on self-report sleep length: a meta-analytic review. *Sleep.* 2000;23:155–163.
31. Akerstedt T. Shift work and disturbed sleep/wakefulness. *Occ Med.* 2003;53:89–94.

32. Tilley AJ, Wilkinson R, Warren P, Watson B, Drud M. The sleep and performance of shift workers. *Hum Factors.* 1982;24:629–641.

33. Dorrian J, Tolley C, Lamond N, et al. Sleep and errors in a group of Australian hospital nurses at work and during the commute. *Appl Ergon.* 2008;39:605–613.

34. Ftouni S, Sletten TL, Howard M, et al. Objective and subjective measures of sleepiness, and their associations with on-road driving events in shift workers. *J Sleep Res.* 2013;22:58–69.

35. Banks S, Catcheside P, Lack L, Grunstein RR, Mcevoy RD. Low levels of alcohol impair driving simulator performance and reduce perception of crash risk in partially sleep deprived subjects. *Sleep.* 2004;27:1063–1067.

36. Lamond N, Dawson D. Quantifying the performance impairment associated with fatigue. *J Sleep Res*1999;8:255–262.

37. Curcio G, Ferrara M, De Gennaro L. Sleep loss, learning capacity and academic performance. *Sleep Med Rev* 2006;10:323–337.

38. Touchette E, Petit D, Séguin JR, Boivin M, Tremblay RE, Montplaisir JY. Associations between sleep duration patterns and behavioral/cognitive functioning at school entry. *Sleep.* 2007;30:1213–1219.

39. Lewin DS, Wang G, Chen YI, et al. Variable school start times and middle school student's sleep health and academic performance. *J Adolesc Health.* 2017;61:205–211.

40. Pilcher JJ, Walters AS. How sleep deprivation affects psychological variables related to college students' cognitive performance. *J Am College Health.* 1997;46:121–126.

41. Durmer JS, Dinges DF. Neurocognitive consequences of sleep deprivation. *Semin Neurol.* 2005;25(1):117–1129.

42. Dinges DF, Pack F, Williams K, et al. Cumulative sleepiness, mood disturbance, and psychomotor vigilance performance decrements during a week of sleep restricted to 4–5 hours per night. *Sleep.* 1997;20:267–277.

43. Agostini A, Lushington K, Dorrian J. The relationships between bullying, sleep, and health in a large adolescent sample. *Sleep Biol Rhyth.* 2019;17:173–182.

44. Dorrian J, Dinges DF. Sleep deprivation and its effects on cognitive performance. In: Dorrian J, Dinges DF, eds. *Encyclopedia of Sleep Medicine.* Chichester, UK: Wiley; 2005:139–144.

45. Kleitman N. *Sleep and Wakefulness.* Chicago, IL: University of Chicago Press; 1963.

46. Doran SM, Van Dongen HP, Dinges DF. Sustained attention performance during sleep deprivation: Evidence of state instability. *Arch Italien de Biol.* 2001;139:253–267.

47. Van Dongen HP, Baynard MD, Maislin G, Dinges DF. Systematic interindividual differences in neurobehavioral impairment from sleep loss: evidence of trait-like differential vulnerability. *Sleep.* 2004;27:423–433.

48. Goel N, Banks S, Mignot E, Dinges DF. Per3 polymorphism predicts cumulative sleep homeostatic but not neurobehavioral changes to chronic partial sleep deprivation. *PLOS ONE* 2009;4:e5874.

49. Rupp TL, Wesensten NJ, Newman R, Balkin TJ. Per 3 and adora 2 a polymorphisms impact neurobehavioral performance during sleep restriction. *J Sleep Res.*2013;22:160–165.

50. Kripke DF, Garfinkel L, Wingard DL, Klauber MR, Marler MR. Mortality associated with sleep duration and insomnia. *Arch Gen Psychiatr.* 2002;59:131–136.

51. Hublin C, Partinen M, Koskenvuo M, Kaprio J. Sleep and mortality: a population-based 22-year follow-up study. *Sleep.* 2007;30:1245–1253.

52. Gangwisch J, Malaspina D, Boden-Albala B, Heymsfield S. Inadequate sleep as a risk factor for obesity: Analyses of the NHANES I. *Sleep.* 2005;28:1289–1296.

53. Cappuccio FP, D'elia L, Strazzullo P, Miller MA. Quantity and quality of sleep and incidence of type 2 diabetes a systematic review and meta-analysis. *Diabetes Care.* 2010;33:414–420.

54. Ayas NT, White DP, Manson JE, et al. A prospective study of sleep duration and coronary heart disease in women. *JAMA Intern Med.* 2003;163:205–209.

55. Hoevenaar-Blom MP, Spijkerman AM, Kromhout D, Van Den Berg JF, Verschuren W. Sleep duration and sleep quality in relation to 12-year cardiovascular disease incidence: the Morgen Study. *Sleep.* 2011;34:1487–1492.

56. Altman NG, Izci-Balserak B, Schopfer E, et al. Sleep duration versus sleep insufficiency as predictors of cardiometabolic health outcomes. *Sleep Med.* 2012;13:1261–1270.

57. Crofford LJ, Kalogeras KT, Mastorakos G, et al. Circadian relationships between interleukin (IL)-6 and hypothalamic-pituitary-adrenal axis hormones: failure of il-6 to cause sustained hypercortisolism in patients with early untreated rheumatoid arthritis. *J Clin Endocrinol Metab.* 1997;82:1279–1283.

58. Savard J, Miller SM, Mills M, et al. Association between subjective sleep quality and depression on immunocompetence in low-income women at risk for cervical cancer. *Psychosom Med.* 1999;61:496–507.

59. Everson CA. Sustained sleep deprivation impairs host defense. *Am J Physiol* 1993;265:R1148–R1154.

60. Patel SR, Hu FB. Short sleep duration and weight gain: a systematic review. *Obesity* 2008;16:643–653.

61. Buxton OM, Pavlova M, Reid EW, Wang W, Simonson DC, Adler GK. Sleep restriction for 1 week reduces insulin sensitivity in healthy men. *Diabetes.* 2010;59:2126–2133.

62. Shankar A, Syamala S, Kalidindi S. Insufficient rest or sleep and its relation to cardiovascular disease, diabetes and obesity in a national, multiethnic sample. *PLOS ONE.* 2010;5:e14189.

63. Klingenberg L, Sjödin A, Holmbäck U, Astrup A, Chaput JP. Short sleep duration and its association with energy metabolism. *Obesity Rev.* 2012;13:565–577.

64. Van Cauter E, Knutson KL. Sleep and the epidemic of obesity in children and adults. *Eur J Endocrinol* 2008;159:S59–S66.

65. Taheri S, Lin L, Austin D, Young T, Mignot E. Short sleep duration is associated with reduced leptin, elevated ghrelin, and increased body mass index. *PLOS Med.* 2004;1:e62.

66. Knutson KL. Impact of sleep and sleep loss on glucose homeostasis and appetite regulation. *Sleep Med Clin.*2007;2:187–197.

67. Buxton OM, Marcelli E. Short and long sleep are positively associated with obesity, diabetes, hypertension, and cardiovascular disease among adults in the united states. *Soc Sci Med.* 2010;71:1027–1036.

68. Kita T, Yoshioka E, Satoh H, et al. Short sleep duration and poor sleep quality increase the risk of diabetes in Japanese workers with no family history of diabetes. *Diabetes Care.* 2012;35:313–318.

69. Vishnu A, Shankar A, Kalidindi S. Examination of the association between insufficient sleep and cardiovascular disease and diabetes by race/ethnicity. *Int Endocrinol.* 2011;2011:789358.
70. Mullington JM, Haack M, Toth M, Serrador JM, Meier-Ewert HK. Cardiovascular, inflammatory, and metabolic consequences of sleep deprivation. *Progress in Cardiovascular Diseases* 2009;51:294–302.
71. Grant CL, Coates AM, Dorrian J, et al. The impact of caffeine consumption during 50 hr of extended wakefulness on glucose metabolism, self-reported hunger and mood state. *J Sleep Res.* 2018;27:e12681.
72. Wehrens SM, Hampton SM, Finn RE, Skene DJ. Effect of total sleep deprivation on postprandial metabolic and insulin responses in shift workers and non-shift workers. *Journal of Endocrinology* 2010;206:205–215.
73. Gonzalez-Ortiz M, Martinez-Abundis E, Balcazar-Munoz B, Pascoe-Gonzalez S. Effect of sleep deprivation on insulin sensitivity and cortisol concentration in healthy subjects. *Diabetes Nutr Metab.* 2000;13:80–83.
74. Reynolds AC, Dorrian J, Liu PY, et al. Impact of five nights of sleep restriction on glucose metabolism, leptin and testosterone in young adult men. *PLOS ONE* 2012;7:e41218.
75. Reiter RJ, Tan D-X, Korkmaz A, Ma S. Obesity and metabolic syndrome: Association with chronodisruption, sleep deprivation, and melatonin suppression. *Ann Med.* 2012;44:564–577.
76. Cappuccio FP, Taggart FM, Kandala N, et al. Meta-analysis of short sleep duration and obesity in children and adults. *Sleep.* 2008;31:619.
77. Stamatakis KA, Brownson RC. Sleep duration and obesity-related risk factors in the rural Midwest. *Prevent Med.* 2008;46:439–444.
78. Imaki M, Hatanaka Y, Ogawa Y, Yoshida Y, Tanada S. An epidemiological study on relationship between the hours of sleep and life style factors in Japanese factory workers. *J Physiol Anthropol App Hum Sci.* 2002;21:115–120.
79. Spiegel K, Tasali E, Penev P, Van Cauter E. Brief communication: sleep curtailment in healthy young men is associated with decreased leptin levels, elevated ghrelin levels, and increased hunger and appetite. *Ann Intern Med.* 2004;141:846–850.
80. Schmid SM, Hallschmid M, Jauch-Chara K, Born J, Schultes B. A single night of sleep deprivation increases ghrelin levels and feelings of hunger in normal-weight healthy men. *J Sleep Res* 2008;17:331–334.
81. Kilkus JM, Booth JN, Bromley LE, Darukhanavala AP, Imperial JG, Penev PD. Sleep and eating behavior in adults at risk for type 2 diabetes. *Obesity.* 2012;20:112–117.
82. Besedovsky L, Lange T, Haack MJPR. The sleep-immune crosstalk in health and disease. *Physiological Reviews* 2019;99:1325–1380.
83. Sigurdardottir LG, Valdimarsdottir UA, Fall K, et al. Circadian disruption, sleep loss, and prostate cancer risk: a systematic review of epidemiologic studies. *Cancer Epidemiol Prevent Biomark.* 2012;21:1002–1011.
84. Bovbjerg DH. Circadian disruption and cancer: sleep and immune regulation. *Brain Behav Immun.* 2003;17:48–50.
85. Irwin MR, Mcclintick J, Costlow C, Fortner M, White J, Gillin JC. Partial night sleep deprivation reduces natural killer and cellular immune responses in humans. *FASEB J.* 1996;10:643–653.

86. Bierhaus A, Wolf J, Andrassy M, et al. A mechanism converting psychosocial stress into mononuclear cell activation. *P Natl Acad Sci.* 2003;100:1920–1925.
87. Cohen S, Doyle WJ, Alper CM, Janicki-Deverts D, Turner RB. Sleep habits and susceptibility to the common cold. *JAMA Intern Med.* 2009;169:62–67.
88. Spiegel K, Sheridan JF, Van Cauter E. Effect of sleep deprivation on response to immunization. *JAMA.* 2002;288:1471–1472.
89. Lange T, Dimitrov S, Bollinger T, Diekelmann S, Born J. Sleep after vaccination boosts immunological memory. *J Immunol.* 2011;187:283–290.

15

Circadian Rhythm Disorders

SABRA M. ABBOTT ∎

INTRODUCTION

We live in a 24-hour environment, and many of our behaviors are shaped by the daily rising and setting of the sun. Humans are diurnal and are best adapted to be awake and active during the day and resting at night, while nocturnal animals like rats and mice are active at night and rest during the day. The general term used to define these rhythms is "circadian" or "about a day." This chapter will focus on the biology underlying these circadian rhythms, followed by a discussion of the sleep disorders that result when an individual's circadian rhythm is no longer appropriately aligned with the surrounding environment.

Circadian rhythms (also see Chapter 4 of this volume) were first identified in nature in plants, with Jean-Jacques d'Ortous de Mairan noting that the mimosa plant would open its leaves during the day and close them at night [1]. In the first documented circadian experiment, it was noted that these patterns continued, even when the plant was placed in constant darkness, suggesting the presence of an endogenous time-keeping mechanism [1]. Several early human experiments placed humans in time-free environments and then monitored their rhythms to document the presence of endogenous rhythms. In one of the earliest experiments, Nathaniel Kleitman spent a week in Mammoth Cave following a self-imposed 28-hour sleep–wake cycle, with a goal of monitoring core body temperature. His results demonstrated that despite a non-24 sleep–wake pattern, core body temperature followed a near-24-hour pattern [2]. Later, more detailed studies conducted by Jurgen Aschoff in a converted German bunker in which individuals were allowed to live for several days in a time-free environment further demonstrated the endogenous nature of biological rhythms, including patterns of activity, body temperature, and urine excretion [3].

In the early 1970s, the primary circadian pacemaker for mammals was identified—the suprachiasmatic nucleus (SCN). This small set of paired nuclei are located in the hypothalamus, directly above the optic chiasm. When this area was lesioned in rats, the daily rhythm of drinking behavior was abolished [4]. Later studies in hamsters demonstrated that rhythms could be restored to a lesioned animal by placing an SCN from a rhythm animal into the brain of an arrhythmic animal [5].

The SCN maintains its intrinsic rhythmicity through a complex transcription–translation feedback loop. The primary components consist of two sets of core clock genes, making up a positive loop (*Clock* and *Bmal1*) and a negative loop (*Period* and *Cryptochrome*). In the positive loop, CLOCK and BMAL1 proteins dimerize and activate the transcription of *Period* and *Cryptochrome*. In the negative loop, PER and CRY proteins, in turn, build up to high enough levels where they can eventually feedback and inhibit their own transcription [6]. While the SCN serves as the primary circadian pacemaker, these same core clock genes are also present in many other tissues throughout the body, and the relative coordination of these transcription–translation feedback loops are important for overall health [7].

The circadian clock can be reset, or entrained, by many environmental signals. The two signals we most frequently take advantage of clinically are light and melatonin. These stimuli are both capable of resetting the internal clock in a time-of-day-dependent manner. To understand the predicted response to these stimuli, it is helpful to think of circadian resetting as a response to error signals. Light is normally present during the day, so exposure to light at times that an individual would normally expect to see it generally has little effect on the circadian clock. However, light exposure in the early evening can be interpreted as a signal that day length is longer than predicted. As a result, the following day the onset of activity will move later, a phenomenon referred to as a phase delay. Conversely, light exposure in the early morning, can be interpreted as a sign that dawn is occurring earlier than predicted, so the following day behaviors will move earlier, referred to as a phase advance [8]. Melatonin, on the other hand, is a hormone that we have low levels of during the daytime, with levels beginning to rise shortly before bedtime, remaining high overnight, and then dropping off the following morning. As such, melatonin exposure in the early evening, prior to the natural rise, can cause phase advances, while melatonin exposure in the morning can cause phase delays [9]. Clinically, we can take advantage of these time-of-day-dependent responses to move the clock earlier or later as needed.

CIRCADIAN RHYTHM SLEEP–WAKE DISORDERS

In the sleep clinic, we encounter several examples of disorders that can develop when the endogenous circadian rhythm is no longer appropriately aligned with the external environment, referred to as the circadian rhythm sleep–wake disorders. These disorders can be primarily due to intrinsic factors, as seen in delayed sleep–wake phase disorder (DSWPD), advanced sleep–wake phase disorder (ASWPD), irregular sleep–wake rhythm disorder (ISWRD), and non-24-hour sleep–wake rhythm disorder (N24SWD), or they can be due to primarily extrinsic factors, as seen with shift work disorder (SWD) and jet lag disorder. In general, diagnosis of these disorders relies primarily on the use of sleep logs or devices called actigraphy (also see Chapter 21 of this volume) which track movement, to demonstrate the overall patterns of rest and activity. In many cases, further support for the diagnosis can come from the use of chronotype questionnaires, which determine a patient's circadian preferences, and/or measures of other markers of circadian timing, such as melatonin. However, these measures are not required for the diagnosis of a circadian rhythm sleep–wake disorder.

DELAYED SLEEP–WAKE PHASE DISORDER

In DSWPD, individuals fall asleep and wake up later than desired. They will frequently present to the sleep clinic with complaints of insomnia; 10% to 22% of patients complaining of insomnia are demonstrated to be going to bed too early with respect to their circadian time [10]. However, they differ from a typical patient with insomnia in that once they fall asleep, they are typically able to stay asleep, often having difficulty waking up despite multiple alarms. In fact, many patients with DSWPD first present to the sleep clinic around the time that they start their first job that requires them to follow a conventional schedule, arriving for work between 7 and 9 AM. Unlike during college, when they could compensate for their sleep disorder by avoiding early morning classes and sleeping with their preferred delayed schedule (see Chapter 10), in the real world this sleep schedule becomes much more challenging to maintain in the context of a conventional work day.

DSWPD Diagnosis

To diagnose DSWPD, one must establish evidence of a stable delay in the sleep–wake schedule, demonstrated through either sleep logs or activity monitoring for at least 1 week, but preferably two weeks. Representative activity data from a patient with DSWPD is shown in Figure 15.1. In addition, other markers of circadian preference and timing, such as questionnaires regarding preferred chronotype, or measures of the timing of biological markers such as melatonin can also be useful, though are not required [11].

The causes of DSWPD are likely multifactorial and still not fully elucidated. There is some evidence that individuals with DSWPD have a longer than average intrinsic period, or tau [12, 13]. As a result, the daily resetting light signal may be strong enough to keep them from moving progressively later each day (as we will describe later relation to the disorder N24SWD); however, this light signal is only able to entrain them with a delayed phase angle with respect to the environmental light–dark schedule. Recent genetic studies have identified at least one family with DSWPD in which a mutation in CRY1 was associated with a delayed phenotype [14]. This is a gain of function mutation that results

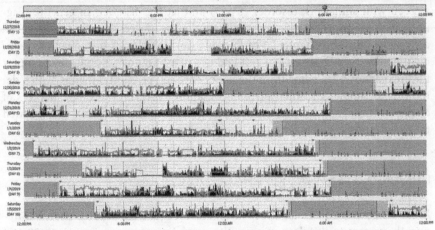

Figure 15.1 Actigraphy sample from a patient with delayed sleep–wake phase disorder. Black vertical lines indicate activity, yellow line indicates light exposure, and blue shaded boxes indicate sleep. During this recording period, this individual was generally able to follow her preferred schedule, falling asleep between 4 and 6 AM and waking up between 1 and 4 PM. She was required to wake up much earlier than usual on day 3, resulting in her falling asleep earlier than usual on day 4 (around midnight) but then she quickly returned to her prior patterns.

in an overall lengthening of the circadian period. A second possibility is that individuals with DSWPD are exposed to either too much light during the biological evening, causing further delays, or to not enough morning advancing light [15,16]. Finally, it is possible that individuals with DSWPD are either overly sensitive to the delaying effects of evening light or insensitive to the advancing effects of morning light [17].

DSWPD Treatment

The treatment of DSWPD depends primarily on the use of timed light and melatonin. According to the most recent guidelines issued by the American Academy of Sleep Medicine (AASM), the primary recommendation for the treatment of adults with DSWPD is to administer timed treatment with evening melatonin. While the only published randomized placebo controlled trial administered melatonin at a fixed time, between 7 and 9 PM [18], from a practical perspective we have found that circadian-based dosing (i.e., administering treatment based on the current circadian timing of the individual) is often more effective. A more recent randomized placebo controlled trial demonstrated that administering 0.5 mg of melatonin 1 hour prior to the desired bedtime, along with instructions to go to bed at the desired time, successfully advanced the timing of sleep—but not the timing of melatonin onset—in treated individuals [19].

Theoretically, timed light could also be used to produce phase advances in circadian timing. While the most recent AASM guidelines were not able to identify any large randomized controlled trials to support the use of bright light therapy in the treatment of DSWPD, in clinical practice we do often find this to be effective. A typical treatment regimen will consist of strategic avoidance of bright light in the hours prior to bedtime, combined with bright light exposure in the biological morning (i.e., right after the natural wake time).

ADVANCED SLEEP–WAKE PHASE DISORDER

In ASWPD, individuals fall asleep and wake up earlier than their desired time, often falling asleep between 6 and 8 PM, and waking up between 2 and 4 AM. Patients often present with complaints of an inability to maintain sleep. They also will frequently have daytime sleepiness, as they are able to push themselves to stay up later, but are unable to sleep in, so consequently they end up sleep deprived. The prevalence of ASWPD is thought to be 0.25% to 7%, depending on the population studied, with the highest rates among older men [20]. Part of this is related to the fact that falling asleep and waking up earlier than average is often less debilitating than falling asleep and waking up later than average, in terms of being able to successfully make it to work and school on time. As a result, there may be significantly more individuals who exhibit an advanced circadian phase, but do not consider it to be a disorder.

ASWPD Diagnosis

To diagnose ASWPD, current recommendations are to obtain at least 1 week, but preferably 2 weeks, of sleep diaries and/or actigraphy, which demonstrate the advance in sleep-wake behaviors [11]. In addition, standardized chronotype questionnaires and circadian phase markers such as the timing of melatonin onset can be obtained to support the diagnosis.

In terms of the etiology of the disorder, there have been several familial cases of ASWPD, which provide insight into the underlying mechanism. Mutations have been demonstrated in PER2 [21, 22], PER3 [23], and CRY2 [24]. In all cases of familial ASWPD in which a genetic mutation has been identified, the mutation acts on the core transcription–translation feedback loop, resulting in the entire process progressing faster than 24 hours. As a result, the daily exposure to light is enough to keep the individual from progressively getting earlier each day, but not enough to maintain a sleep–wake schedule at conventional times. In addition to genetic mutations that shorten individuals' free-running periods, it is also theoretically possible that these individuals exhibit decreased sensitivity to the phase delaying effects of evening light or increased sensitivity to the phase advancing effects of morning light; however, there is currently no data available to support this hypothesis.

ASWPD Treatment

There are currently very few clinical trials evaluating treatment options for ASWPD. However, there are limited data that evening bright light (at least 4,000 lux) administered for 2 hours immediately before bedtime can be effective in causing circadian delays [25]. While it is theoretically possible that early morning melatonin could also be an effective treatment, by further delaying the circadian clock [26], there are currently no data to support the use of this treatment (and, anecdotally, when this has been tried in clinic patients, they often dislike the sedating effects of the early morning melatonin, so do not continue the treatment).

IRREGULAR SLEEP–WAKE RHYTHM DISORDER

In the two disorders described previously, DSWPD and ASWPD, sleep–wake patterns occur fairly predictably in a single consolidated bout, simply not at the preferred time for the individual. However, with ISWRD, sleep occurs in multiple shorter bouts, distributed across the 24-hour period. Typically, individuals must exhibit at least three discrete sleep periods, to distinguish them from someone who simply has variable bed/wake times and also takes a single long nap during the day. In addition, the total sleep time obtained within a 24-hour window should be within the normal range of daily sleep time.

ISWRD Diagnosis

To diagnose this disorder, the recommendations are to obtain either sleep logs (provided by the patient or caretaker) and/or actigraphy for at least 1 week, but preferably 2 weeks [11].

Classically, ISWRD has been described in adults with neurodegenerative disease and children with neurodevelopmental disorders. Presumably the underlying mechanism relates to a weakening of the neuronal timekeeping mechanisms, often in conjunction with an environment that lacks strong daily time cues, including light, activity, feeding patterns, and social interactions [27]. In many cases these individuals have been demonstrated to have abnormal circadian rhythms of core body temperature [28]. In addition to the previously described populations, this disorder can also be encountered in other individuals with chronic illness who may spend large amounts of their day bedbound from pain or lack of energy. As a result, they may sleep and wake in small bouts both day and night, rather than achieving a consolidated period of rest and activity.

ISWRD Treatment

The treatment of ISWRD focuses on strengthening the available time cues for these individuals. According to the AASM guidelines, there is evidence in support of the use of bright light therapy for ISWRD in the elderly. Typically, light intensity ranged from 2,500 to 5,000 lux, for 1 to 2 hours in the morning [29]. In children and adolescents, timed melatonin therapy appears to be effective, with a recommended dose of 2 to 10 mg given 1 hour prior to bedtime. In adults with dementia, using melatonin alone appears to not be effective and can actually impair daytime mood and function [29]. Several studies have shown promising data for mixed-modality therapy, where individuals are treated with a combination of light, activity, and scheduled sleep–wake times [30]; however, there is still not enough data in support of this treatment option for it to be considered a treatment guideline at this point.

NON-24-HOUR SLEEP–WAKE RHYTHM DISORDER

In N24SWD, patients exhibit a sleep–wake schedule that is typically slightly longer than 24 hours. Sleep complaints can vary, depending on where they are in this cycle, with symptoms of either insomnia and/or excessive daytime sleepiness when their schedule has shifted out of phase with the environment that later transitions to normal sleep when they are falling asleep at night and waking up during the day.

N24SWD Diagnosis

While some patients are aware of exhibiting this particular pattern, others do not recognize it until their sleep patterns are tracked over several weeks. As such, the diagnosis of this disorder depends on obtaining sleep logs and/or actigraphy for at least 2 weeks, although preferably longer, as patients can sometimes fluctuate between a pattern of sleeping at night and a pattern of rotating around the clock [11]. An example sleep log from a patient with N24SWD is presented in Figure 15.2.

The underlying cause of N24SWD is believed to stem from the fact that at baseline, most humans have a daily rhythm that is slightly longer than 24 hours. For most people, daily exposure to environmental time cues can be enough to help them to maintain a 24-hour schedule. The strongest of these time cues is light, but these cues can also come from other rhythmic behaviors, including activity, meal timing, and social interactions. Individuals who are lacking exposure to these strong time cues may then follow their intrinsic rhythm of >24 hours, rather than a rhythm that is aligned with the 24-hour environment. As light is the strongest of these time cues, this disorder was first identified in individuals who were blind. Interestingly, not all blind individuals who lack light perception develop N24SWD, speaking to the fact that other time cues besides light may be effective. More recently, a second group of individuals with N24SWD have been identified who are not blind, raising this question of what additional factors may contribute to the development of this disorder. Many of these individuals start out with severe DSWPD, with bedtimes as late as 4 to 6 AM, but their schedule then moves progressively later, until eventually they are following a non-24hour schedule. There are some data showing that these individuals have an intrinsic period that is significantly longer than 24 hours [13]. In addition, there is the

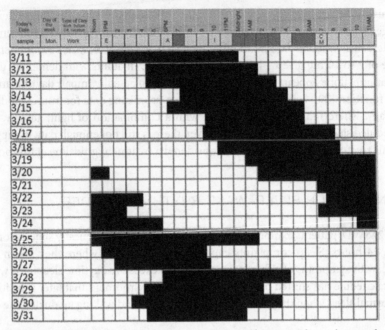

Figure 15.2 Example sleep log from a sighted patient with non–24-hour sleep–wake disorder. Black bars indicate the time periods of sleep. Sleep–wake times exhibit a gradual daily delay, with an overall daily pattern that is greater than 24 hours.

theoretical possibility that while these individuals have normal image-forming vision, they may have impaired circadian light perception.

N24SWD Treatment

The general principle underlying the treatment of these individuals is to maximize exposure to the time cues to which they are able to respond. For blind individuals, the primary focus has been on the use of supplemental melatonin. While the earliest studies used relatively large doses (10 mg) administered 1 hour prior to bedtime [31], more recent studies have shown that doses as low as 0.5mg can be effective [32]. The treatment of sighted individuals with N24SWD is more complicated, with fewer clear guidelines. However, a recently published case series provided a treatment algorithm consisting of a combination of evening melatonin and morning light therapy to try to prevent these individuals from progressively moving their schedule later [33].

SHIFT WORK DISORDER

In our increasingly 24/7 society, we have a growing need for an available work-force at all hours of the day. While some individuals can manage working a nontraditional schedule without difficulty, many others struggle to maintain a schedule of working during times when they would normally be sleeping and sleeping during times when they would normally be working.

Shift Work Disorder Diagnosis

To meet the diagnostic criteria for SWD, individuals must have sleep complaints of at least 3 months in duration, that are associated with a requirement to work during times that they would normally be sleeping. As with the other circadian rhythm disorders, the diagnosis is confirmed by obtaining sleep logs and/or activity monitoring for at least 14 days [11].

There is growing evidence that chronic exposure to the sleep and circadian disruption associated with shift work can be detrimental to human health. Some of the earliest and strongest evidence for this connection came from studies looking at the association between shift work exposure and breast cancer. In cohort and case-control studies of shift workers in multiple countries, strong evidence emerged for an increased risk for breast cancer associated with cumulative shift work exposure [34]. Based on these data, in 2007 the World Health Organization declared shift work to be a probable carcinogen. Shift work has also been associated with increased risk for other diseases, including diabetes, heart disease, obesity, and stroke. While the underlying cause of these associations are still being elucidated, it is thought that they result from a combination of circadian dysregulation (i.e., lack of alignment of the circadian system with the environment, and of central and peripheral circadian oscillators with each other), sleep restriction, and melatonin suppression [35].

SWD Treatment

Treatment of SWD focuses both on optimizing alertness and performance while at work and improving sleep during time off. Under ideal conditions, one would simply completely adjust their schedule to fit their work requirements. This would mean maintaining a nocturnal schedule both on workdays and on days off. Efforts are made to optimize sleep, by avoiding bright light exposure on the commute home from work and utilizing blackout curtains and white noise machines to create an optimal environment for sleep. Melatonin may be taken at sleep onset both to assist with falling asleep and with adjusting the body to the shifted schedule. To optimize work performance, bright light exposure at the beginning of the shift can be beneficial. Careful use of caffeine (i.e., not too late in the shift) and short naps can also be beneficial. If these interventions are not effective, prescription stimulant medications may also be utilized [36].

However, even with the previously described interventions, rigorously maintaining this schedule is generally challenging, as the demands of caring for a family, the desire to socialize with nonshift-working friends, and the need to complete errands at locations that are not open 24 hours/day necessitate being awake during the day. As such, one recommendation is to maintain what is called a compromise phase position, in which individuals go to bed slightly earlier on their day off (e.g., 3 AM instead of 8 AM), which will still allow them to be awake for some portion of the day, but they won't have to completely invert their schedule between their work days and free days [37]. Another novel solution that has been proposed recently is to have employers adapt work schedules based on the circadian preference of their employees. Under the design, people who are "night owls" work more evening/night shifts, while those who are "early birds" work more early morning and day shifts. While this does require more planning, in a pilot study of this intervention, adapting such a schedule resulted in improved sleep and subjective well-being among employees [38].

JET LAG DISORDER

With the advent of transcontinental travel by airplane, a new disorder was essentially created. Even under ideal conditions, the body is generally not able to adjust timing by more than an hour each day. As a result, jet lag disorder can develop under any conditions where an individual travels by plane across two or more time zones. The typical complaints of difficulty falling and staying asleep that are encountered in the other circadian disorders can be experienced, and individuals also may experience other physical symptoms such as gastrointestinal upset [11]. These symptoms are thought to result when peripheral clocks such as those found in the digestive system struggle to adjust to the new time zone and may be temporarily out of synch with both the external environment and each other.

When traveling westward, the internal clock needs to delay, or move later. These travelers generally will experience sleepiness in the early evening and early morning awakenings. They are generally advised to seek light in the evening and avoid light in the morning. A low dose of melatonin (0.5 mg) may be beneficial for early morning awakenings. For eastward travel, the opposite problem occurs, with difficulty falling asleep and morning sleepiness. In this case, light exposure shortly after the time that they would normally awaken, and a low dose of melatonin at bedtime can be beneficial [36]. However, it is important to keep in mind that specific treatment times are dependent on the number of time zones crossed. There are numerous online jet lag calculators available that can assist with determining optimal times for light and melatonin to best adapt to the new time zone.

CONCLUSION

Circadian rhythms are ubiquitous across nearly all species studied. The role of these rhythms is to allow proper alignment of our daily behaviors and physiologic processes with the surrounding environment. When these processes are disrupted, it can be to the detriment of both overall health and our ability to function in society. In the Circadian Medicine clinic, we encounter a wide variety of disorders of circadian timing. The proper diagnosis and treatment of these disorders can significantly improve overall health and well-being.

REFERENCES

1. Moore-Ede MC, Sulzman FM, Fuller CA. *The clocks that time us: physiology of the circadian timing system.* Cambridge, MA: Harvard University Press; 1982.
2. Kleitman N. *Sleep and Wakefulness.* Chicago, IL: University of Chicago Press; 1963.
3. Aschoff J. Circadian rhythms in man. *Science.* 1965;148:1427–1432.
4. Stephan FK, Zucker I. Circadian rhythms in drinking behavior and locomotor activity of rats are eliminated by hypothalamic lesions. *Proc Natl Acad Sci USA.* 1972;69:1583–1586.
5. DeCoursey PJ, Buggy J. Circadian rhythmicity after neural transplant to hamster third ventricle: specificity of suprachiasmatic nuclei. *Brain Res.* 1989;500:263–275.
6. Andreani TS, Itoh TQ, Yildirim E, Hwangbo DS, Allada R. Genetics of circadian rhythms. *Sleep Med Clin.* 2015;10:413–421.
7. Honma S. The mammalian circadian system: a hierarchical multi-oscillator structure for generating circadian rhythm. *J Physiol Sci.* 2018;68:207–219.
8. Ruger M, St Hilaire MA, Brainard GC, et al. Human phase response curve to a single 6.5 h pulse of short-wavelength light. *J Physiol.* 2013;591:353–363.
9. Burgess HJ, Revell VL, Molina TA, Eastman CI. Human phase response curves to three days of daily melatonin: 0.5 mg versus 3.0 mg. *J Clin Endocrinol Metab.* 2010;95:3325–3331.
10. Flynn-Evans EE, Shekleton JA, Miller B, et al. Circadian phase and phase angle disorders in primary insomnia. *Sleep.* 2017;40:zsx163.
11. American Academy of Sleep Medicine. *The International Classification of Sleep Disorders: Diagnostic and Coding Manual.* 2nd ed. Darien, IL: American Academy of Sleep Medicine; 2014.
12. Micic G, de Bruyn A, Lovato N, et al. The endogenous circadian temperature period length (tau) in delayed sleep phase disorder compared to good sleepers. *J Sleep Res* 2013;22:617–624.
13. Micic G, Lovato N, Gradisar M, Burgess HJ, Ferguson SA, Lack L. Circadian melatonin and temperature taus in delayed sleep–wake phase disorder and non-24-hour sleep-wake rhythm disorder patients: an ultradian constant routine study. *J Biol Rhythms.* 2016;31:387–405.
14. Patke A, Murphy PJ, Onat OE, et al. Mutation of the human circadian clock gene CRY1 in familial delayed sleep phase disorder. *Cell.* 2017;169:203–215.
15. Joo EY, Abbott SM, Reid KJ, et al. Timing of light exposure and activity in adults with delayed sleep-wake phase disorder. *Sleep Med.* 2017;32:259–265.
16. Wilson JT, Reid KJ, Braun RI, Abbott SM, Zee PC. Habitual light exposure relative to circadian timing in delayed sleep-wake phase disorder. *Sleep.* 2018;41:zsy166.
17. Watson LA, Phillips AJK, Hosken IT, et al. Increased sensitivity of the circadian system to light in delayed sleep-wake phase disorder. *J Physiol.* 2018;596:6249–6261.
18. Rahman SA, Kayumov L, Shapiro CM. Antidepressant action of melatonin in the treatment of Delayed Sleep Phase Syndrome. *Sleep Med.* 2010;11:131–136.

19. Sletten TL, Magee M, Murray JM, et al. Efficacy of melatonin with behavioural sleep-wake scheduling for delayed sleep–wake phase disorder: a double-blind, randomised clinical trial. *PLOS Med.* 2018;15:e1002587.

20. Paine SJ, Fink J, Gander PH, Warman GR. Identifying advanced and delayed sleep phase disorders in the general population: a national survey of New Zealand adults. *Chronobiol Int.* 2014;31:627–636.

21. Vanselow K, Vanselow JT, Westermark PO, et al. Differential effects of PER2 phosphorylation: molecular basis for the human familial advanced sleep phase syndrome (FASPS). *Genes Dev.* 2006;20:2660–2672.

22. Toh KL, Jones CR, He Y, et al. An hPer2 phosphorylation site mutation in familial advanced sleep phase syndrome. *Science.* 2001;291:1040–1043.

23. Zhang L, Hirano A, Hsu PK, et al. A PERIOD3 variant causes a circadian phenotype and is associated with a seasonal mood trait. *Proc Natl Acad Sci USA.* 2016;113:e1536–1544.

24. Hirano A, Shi G, Jones CR, et al. A Cryptochrome 2 mutation yields advanced sleep phase in humans. *Elife* 2016;5:e16695.

25. Campbell SS, Dawson D, Anderson MW. Alleviation of sleep maintenance insomnia with timed exposure to bright light. *J Am Geriatr Soc.* 1993;41:829–836.

26. Zee PC. Melatonin for the treatment of advanced sleep phase disorder. *Sleep.* 2008;31:923.

27. Abbott SM, Zee PC. Irregular sleep–wake rhythm disorder. *Sleep Med Clin.* 2015;10:517–522.

28. Okawa M, Mishima K, Hishikawa Y, Hozumi S, Hori H, Takahashi K. Circadian rhythm disorders in sleep–waking and body temperature in elderly patients with dementia and their treatment. *Sleep.* 1991;14:478–485.

29. Auger RR, Burgess HJ, Emens JS, Deriy LV, Thomas SM, Sharkey KM. Clinical practice guideline for the treatment of intrinsic circadian rhythm sleep-wake disorders: advanced sleep–wake phase disorder (ASWPD), delayed sleep-wake phase disorder (DSWPD), non-24-hour sleep-wake rhythm disorder (N24SWD), and irregular sleep-wake rhythm disorder (ISWRD). An update for 2015: an American Academy of Sleep Medicine Clinical Practice Guideline. *J Clin Sleep Med* 2015;11:1199–1236.

30. Zhou QP, Jung L, Richards KC. The management of sleep and circadian disturbance in patients with dementia. *Curr Neurol Neurosci Rep.* 2012;12:193–204.

31. Sack RL, Brandes RW, Kendall AR, Lewy AJ. Entrainment of free-running circadian rhythms by melatonin in blind people. *N Engl J Med.* 2000;343:1070–1077.

32. Hack LM, Lockley SW, Arendt J, Skene DJ. The effects of low-dose 0.5-mg melatonin on the free-running circadian rhythms of blind subjects. *J Biol Rhythms.* 2003;18:420–429.

33. Malkani RG, Abbott SM, Reid KJ, Zee PC. Diagnostic and treatment challenges of sighted non-24-hour sleep-wake disorder. *J Clin Sleep Med.* 2018;14:603–613.

34. Megdal SP, Kroenke CH, Laden F, Pukkala E, Schernhammer ES. Night work and breast cancer risk: a systematic review and meta-analysis. *Eur J Cancer.* 2005;41:2023–2032.

35. Kecklund G, Axelsson J. Health consequences of shift work and insufficient sleep. *BMJ.* 2016;355:i5210.

36. Reid KJ, Abbott SM. Jet lag and shift work disorder. *Sleep Med Clin.* 2015;10:523–535.

37. Smith MR, Fogg LF, Eastman CI. Practical interventions to promote circadian adaptation to permanent night shift work: study 4. *J Biol Rhythms* 2009;24:161–172.
38. Vetter C, Fischer D, Matera JL, Roenneberg T. Aligning work and circadian time in shift workers improves sleep and reduces circadian disruption. *Curr Biol* 2015;25:907–911.

16

Pediatric Sleep Disorders

KEVIN GIPSON AND RAFAEL PELAYO ■

INTRODUCTION

Sleep researcher Allan Rechtschaffen once said, "If sleep does not serve an absolutely vital function, then it is the biggest mistake evolution has ever made." Parents intuitively understand the vital importance of sleep to their children's well-being (and the parents' sanity!). A 2014 National Sleep Foundation "Sleep in the Modern Family" survey of more than 1000 families found that the vast majority of parents and caregivers feel that sleep is important to their child's mood, well-being, behavior, and school performance [1] (we wonder about the parents who that responded to the survey that they did not think sleep was important for their child). Perhaps the inverse can also be inferred: when a child is not sleeping well, their parents may worry about the child's ability to develop, thrive, and, ultimately, compete. In this same cohort of parents and caregivers, 75 to 17% worried that their child's sleep quality was "poor"; this proportion increased as children transitioned into adolescence [1]. About 5% to 10% of parents and caregivers report thinking their child has a sleep problem, and most say that they would like to change something about their child's sleep [2].

Those fortunate enough to have secure, happy childhoods might look back at this as a time when we slept very well. We all intuitively recognize that, when undisrupted by social or physiologic problems, there is something particularly special about the sleep of a young child. When a child's sleep is disordered, however, the entire family suffers. This occurs first because of lack of sleep and then, should sleep disorders persist, often from the worry that the child's learning, behavior, and development might be disrupted by the sleep problem. Parents work hard to ensure safe and secure sleep for their children, often at the cost of their own sleep, and most parents rate their child's sleep quality a being better than their own [2]. A child's poor sleep can disrupt a parent's daytime function at their jobs, threatening their income or even careers.

Older children have significantly worse quality sleep, as rated by parents and caregivers, compared with younger children [1]. In a survey of adolescents, only 41% endorsed the statement, "I had a good night's sleep" during most nights of the week [3]. There are real, life-and-death consequences of disordered sleep in the adolescent population. A 2006 survey found that 51% of adolescent drivers self-reported at least one episode of drowsy driving, with a startling 5% acknowledging that they had "nodded off" or even fallen asleep while driving within the past year [3]. In this same population, 25% reported being in a motor vehicle collision, which they attributed to their drowsiness while driving [3]. As we like to say at the Stanford Sleep Medicine Center and in our undergraduate Sleep and Dreams course at Stanford University: "Drowsiness is Red Alert." Our goal is for young drivers to identify and acknowledge when they are sleepy and then to either not drive or get off the road. In this age of pervasive ride-share apps, there is no reason for a young person to get behind the wheel when they are sleepy.

Pediatric sleep disorders are common (Table 16.1) but quite treatable, and early intervention can have potentially enormous impacts on a child's future health and development. In this chapter, we will outline the various sleep disorders that may emerge during childhood.

Table 16.1 PREVALENCE OF PEDIATRIC SLEEP DISORDERS IN THE PRIMARY CARE PEDIATRICS POPULATION

Sleep Disorder	Estimated Prevalence in Children and Adolescents
Bruxism	5%–35%
Circadian rhythm disorder	5%–10%
Hypersomnia	Unknown
Infant apnea	25%–84% (preterm), <0.5%–2% (term)
Insomnia	5%–20%
Narcolepsy	Unknown
Nocturnal enuresis	15%–20% (5 years), 1%–2% (≥15 y)[a]
Parasomnias	14%–37%
Periodic limb movement disorder/restless leg syndrome	2%–8%
SDB	1%–3% for OSA, 5%–27% for primary snoring

OSA, obstructive sleep apnea; SDB, sleep-disordered breathing.

[a]See Schmidt B. Methylxanthine therapy for apnea of prematurity: evaluation of treatment benefits and risks at age 5 years in the International Caffeine for Apnea of Prematurity (CAP) trial. *Neonatology.* 2005;88:208–13; White DP. Central sleep apnea: improvement with acetazolamide therapy. *Arch Intern Med.* 1982;142:1816–1819.

SOURCE: Adapted from Meltzer LJ, Johnson C, Crosette J, Ramos M, Mindell JA. *Pediatrics.* 2010;125(6):e1410–e1418.

BEHAVIORALLY INSUFFICIENT SLEEP AND INSOMNIA

Behaviorally Insufficient Sleep

There's a common saying: "I slept like a baby." However, if you have a young child or have friends or family who are new parents, you'll know that a newborn baby's sleep can be seemingly fitful and brief. A newborn often starts off sleeping for only 2 hours or so at a time, waking frequently to feed. Although the sleep of infants is naturally somewhat fragmented, by 2 to 12 months of age a fairly consistent pattern is established, with most children beginning to sleep consistently through the night by around age 9 months [4].

Sleep needs change with age, with children requiring progressively less total sleep time (TST) as they enter adolescence and young adulthood. However, many children in the United States do not get sufficient sleep. As children progress through adolescence, their bedtimes are progressively pushed while their wake times stay anchored at around 6:30 AM [3], as required by a school system which rarely takes adolescent sleep needs into sufficient consideration. Homework also frequently contributes to insufficient sleep, with up to 28% of children reporting that this interferes with their ability to get a good night's sleep [2]. In our experiences with speaking to school groups, the percentage of parents and students blaming homework for interfering with their sleep is much higher. As a consequence, around 45% of adolescents get less than 8t hours of sleep on school nights [3]. Lack of sleep has also been identified as an independent risk factor for suicidality among adolescents [5].

Insomnia

Insomnia is a complex disorder characterized, in a very broad sense, as difficulty initiating and/or maintaining sleep and which results in some difficulty with daytime function and/or dissatisfaction with one's sleep [6]. The majority of children and adolescents fall asleep within 20 minutes of "lights out" [2]; however, when sleep onset is prolonged, a disorder of sleep initiation may be contributing. About 46% of children wake at night, possibly signaling a sleep maintenance problem [1]. Insomnia may manifest differently in children and adolescents than it does in adults, often as bedtime resistance, waking throughout the night, and an inability to sleep without the close attention of the parent [6]. Children with prolonged issues with insomnia may develop attentional and behavioral problems, particularly in the school setting.

Behavioral insomnia in childhood, due to either inappropriate sleep associations or ineffective parental limit-setting, is estimated to occur among as many as 10% to 30% of children, and the prevalence rate is likely higher in children who are not neurotypical [6]. Up to 46% of adolescents have some difficulty each week with either initiating or maintaining sleep, with 20% of adolescents reporting this on a near-nightly basis [3]. Insomnia appears to be more common in girls after puberty [6].

Physiologic problems such as obstructive sleep apnea (OSA) and gastroesophageal reflux can also frustrate sleep initiation and maintenance. Patients with chronic respiratory diseases such as asthma or cystic fibrosis may also have difficulties with sleep, related to persistent cough.

In regards to parental insomnia, nearly half of parents report worsening of their own sleep quality after having children [2]. Most parents and caregivers of preschool and school-aged children report being awakened by their child at least once weekly [2].

Generally, when a young child's sleep is discontinuous, there is a problem of the stability of sleep associations. Sleep and its initiation are a physiologically driven process, but learned behaviors deeply color and shape it. Suppose you went to sleep as you usually might, resting your head on your pillow, and then awoke later in the night to find yourself in the kitchen. Would you find this comforting or disturbing? Would you go right back to sleep under the kitchen table? In the same way, children who are soothed to sleep in their parent's arms and then placed in a crib may have difficulty reinitiating sleep after normal nocturnal awakenings, when they find themselves in a completely different situation.

Sleep is not monolithic, but cyclical. We all awaken briefly and intermittently throughout the night, with ephemeral "microarousals" occurring as frequently as 10 times per hour as we move through the various stages of sleep. In most cases, we don't remember these moments of brief consciousness. The associations that a child makes at bedtime, including their parents' presence, the sleeping area (be it a parent's arms, the parent's bed, a crib), and other environmental features play an important role in a child's subsequent ability to maintain or reestablish sleep throughout the night. With unpredictable sleep associations, the normal, brief awakenings that occur in sleep are, as a consequence, prolonged as the child seeks out the comforting sleep associations upon which they've come to rely.

Parents usually play a major role in their child's sleep initiation at night. In one survey of parents and caregivers in the United States, 46% responded that they put their infant to bed while still awake, whereas 76% to 84% did so with their toddlers [2]. Many parents remain in the child's bedroom until they have fallen asleep. When the child invariably awakens later in the evening, they could have a sense of displacement and perhaps even fear when they find their parent absent, whereas if they'd fallen asleep alone everything would seem normal when they awaken later. When night-time awakenings do occur in younger children, the majority of parents and caregivers will go to the child to attend to them in some way; although practices vary, around 30% to 40% of parents and caregivers stay with their toddler or school-aged children until they have fallen back to sleep [2]. Around 10% to 20% of parents and caregivers bring their children to the parents' bed, which can potentially further complicate sleep association problems [2]. Thus, enabling children to build the skill of falling asleep on their own is critical and comprises an important parenting task during early childhood.

Limit-Setting Sleep Disorder

A core task of childhood is to continuously work to find the shape and structure of the world, pushing boundaries and exerting independence by degrees. Thus, parenting a young child can be challenging. Maintaining appropriate boundaries around bedtimes and sleep is a parenting task requiring constant vigilance, and in many cases, we see, this can be a nidus of stress for families.

Young children want to be with their parents. Being awake and hanging out with parents is fun, and for many families the evenings represent the precious little time they have to spend together after busy days at work and school. Bedtime may present a challenge for children insofar as this is when, in most cases, they are separated from their parents.

Parents and caregivers report significant resistance to bedtime in around 15% to 30% of children across age ranges [2]. When families are unable to maintain consistent bedtime routines, either because of parenting philosophy or external pressures including socioeconomic factors (e.g., room-sharing is more prevalent in economically disadvantaged populations in the United States), a child's natural inclination to push boundaries and resist bedtime can spiral into dysregulation.

Consistent timing of evening activities, including mealtimes and a wind-down routine, are important for fostering the stability of a child's sleep initiation. However, only about 50% of families maintain consistent schedules for these activities during the week [1]. Similarly, "anchoring" of wake times can be vitally important for stabilizing a child or adolescent's sleep, and this, too, is only maintained by around 50% of families, with the usual trend being permissiveness around "sleeping in" on weekends. There is also often a disjunction between what parent think their children need in terms of sleep duration, and what their children actually get, with as much as a 14% difference in idealized versus actual sleep times; this discrepancy is even worse in adolescents [1].

As screen-based technology has become more readily affordable, tablets and cell phones now frequently end up in children's bedrooms. Up to 39% of children have an electronic device (e.g., television, computer, tablet) left on in their bedroom overnight [1]. As much as 47% of families permit their children to watch television or videos to wind down before bed [1]. Rules and limit-setting are particularly important for adolescents; however, rules around bedtimes and the use of technology in the bedroom are inconsistently articulated and enforced by parents [1]. Up to 43% of parents and caregivers report that their teenagers "read or sent electronic communications after initially going to sleep" (p. 8) [1]. While the impact of screen and light exposure on sleep and the circadian rhythm is not yet fully characterized, it is clear that the use of stimulating media at (and after) bedtime contributes meaningfully to lost sleep time and insomnia. With adolescents a nightly fight over electronic use may be counterproductive, since it is difficult to sleep when we are angry. Ideally, if an individual understands the reasons for reducing exposure to electronics close to bedtime, they can voluntarily modify their behavior.

DELAYED SLEEP–WAKE PHASE DISORDER

Delayed sleep–wake phase disorder (DSWPD) is among the most common sleep disorders among adolescents, perhaps second only to behaviorally induced insufficient sleep syndrome. DSWPD was first described in 1981 among a group of young adults with an atypical depression characterized by difficulty falling asleep. This was in contrast to trouble staying asleep or early morning awakenings seen in more typical forms of depression. The impaired mood of these young adults did not respond to antidepressant medication. However, when their sleep patterns were corrected by realigning their biological clocks, their mood greatly improved [7]. In adolescents, behavioral disruptions in sleep initiation may lead to a sleep-phase delay. DSWPD is the commonest circadian rhythm disorder in adolescents, with a prevalence of 7% to 16% [6]. These patients usually have very different wake up times on weekend compared to weekdays. TST is usually of normal, age-appropriate duration when late start times are permitted by the child's school schedule, but in many cases these children undercut their TST to conform to school schedules, resulting in chronically insufficient sleep. As we learn more about the normal patterns of sleep in adolescents, it is clear that the current status quo of school start times and other societal expectations around sleep need to be re-evaluated.

The management of DSWPD is tailored to the individual and may involve a combination of behavioral and medical treatments. In the behavioral sleep medicine clinic, patients are guided in shifting their sleep patterns gradually to the desired sleep schedule—hopefully one that is compatible not only with social norms or the exigencies of school and work, but also their intrinsic sleep schedule, or chronotype. In some cases, the use of melatonin 1 hour prior to the desired bedtime or early-morning light exposure can assist in shifting the sleep schedule [8].

PARASOMNIAS IN CHILDREN

The parasomnias are a fascinating group of sleep disorders, defined as undesirable behaviors or experiences that emerge during sleep and that result in a disruption of sleep, psychosocial problems or emotional distress, and even injury [6]. In children, parasomnias generally have a benign course, as long as the family environment is supportive and appropriate safety measures are in place.

Sleepwalking

Sleepwalking, or somnambulism, is a nonrapid eye movement (NREM) parasomnia that usually occurs during the first third of the night. The behaviors exhibited during these episodes can be quite complex, but the child will generally be disoriented and will not remember their dream content if interrupted. The prevalence of sleepwalking in preschool and school-aged children is not well-characterized, ranging somewhere between 1% and 29%, and seems rather common [6]. Sleepwalking may run in families. With proper safety precautions in place, such as ensuring that the child is not sleeping in the top bunk and does not have easy access to windows or stairwells, sleepwalking is generally a benign phenomenon. The peak prevalence is in adolescents. In people prone to sleepwalking, it can be more likely to occur when they are sleep deprived, have had a recent febrile illness, or are under acute stress. Sleepwalking is a common parasomnia among college students.

Nightmares

Nightmares are also quite common, occurring in up to 75% of children. However, while occasional nightmares are a normal human experience, nightmare disorder is characterized by persistent, dysphoric dream content, which causes a disruption of sleep and daytime mood and/or function. This is seen in as much as 8% of the general population and may be associated with real-life trauma and psychosocial stressors. In contrast to sleep terrors, older children will remember and be able to articulate the dream content once they are fully awake.

Sleep Terrors

Perhaps the most disturbing to parents, sleep terrors are a not uncommon parasomnia of childhood, occurring in 1% to 6% of children. Like other disorders of arousal from NREM sleep, sleep terrors characteristically occur in the first third of the night, usually heralded by a "blood-curdling" scream. Parents naturally run to attend to the child, but find them utterly inconsolable, resistant to usual soothing from the parents, and often with a distant look in their eyes. The child may exhibit signs of autonomic arousal and fear, such as sweating and tachycardia. As sleep terrors arise from NREM sleep, patients who have sleep terrors often also exhibit sleepwalking. The child may take a good while to calm after these events and will have no memory of the fearful dream content.

Confusional Arousals

Confusional arousals result from a disruption of NREM stage 3, wherein a child awakens and exhibits signs of confusion, such as looking around, without leaving the bed. In contrast to sleep terrors, the child is not frightened or inconsolable during these episodes, and in most instances, they can generally return to sleep on their own without parental intervention.

Sleep Paralysis

Sleep paralysis is a potentially frightening parasomnia, most likely related to a disruption of normal rapid eye movement (REM) sleep, wherein a person awakens during the night but experiences an inability to move. These episodes can be very distressing, not only because the sensation of near-paralysis is frightening but also because these events can be attended by dream-like imagery often including "shadowy figures." An important aspect of REM sleep is a loss of the normal muscle tone of the arms and legs, a phenomenon called REM "atonia." This probably plays a protective role: By being effectively "paralyzed" during dreaming, you are protected from injuring yourself or others by enacting your dreams. A disruption of REM sleep with an incomplete resolution of atonia could be the genesis of these events. The mean age of onset for sleep paralysis is somewhere between 14 to 17 years of age [6].

Bed-Wetting

Sleep enuresis, or bed-wetting, is seen in 14% of preschoolers and 4% of school-aged children [2]. Primary nocturnal enuresis is defined as bed-wetting at least twice a week for at least 3 months in a child who is older than 5 years of age who has never been consistently dry at night. In contrast, secondary enuresis occurs in children who have been continent at night for at least 6 months. While nocturnal enuresis is a fairly common issue that is best treated with behavioral interventions, such as night-time fluid restriction and bed-wetting alarms, ruling-out sleep-disordered breathing (SDB) is an important consideration in these cases.

Bruxism

Bruxism consists of repetitive jaw movements in sleep such as teeth-grinding and jaw clenching. This can lead to jaw pain and headache in children and, in severe or persistent, cases can cause significant wear or damage to the teeth. Bruxism can be associated with respiratory-related arousals and airflow limitation, so its presence should also prompt and evaluation for SDB. Bruxism may also be exacerbated by daytime stressors.

Nocturnal Seizures

It is important to differentiate the various parasomnias from nocturnal seizures, which can mimic even complex behaviors such as sleepwalking. A detailed history of the events, including eliciting from the parents whether there were signs of tonic or clonic movements, can help the clinician differentiate typical parasomnias and sleep behaviors from seizure. However, when there is doubt, it is reasonable to perform a nocturnal electroencephalogram or sleep study with added sensors, or a "seizure montage" to formally evaluate for seizure activity.

SLEEP-DISORDERED BREATHING IN CHILDREN

Many parents worry about their children's night-time breathing. Around 8% to 19% of parents report snoring in their children, 5% to 11% report difficult breathing at night, and a further 1% to 2% have observed overt pauses in their child's breathing during sleep [2]. When children have difficulty breathing at night, this can lead to sleep fragmentation and nonrestorative sleep. Chronic severe SDB can act as a physiologic stressor and may contribute to cardiovascular and metabolic disease. In childhood, problems with breathing during sleep tend to manifest primarily as behavioral symptoms, including inattention and irritability. As children transition to adolescence, daytime sleepiness and fatigue become more prevalent. The early identification and treatment of SDB in children is vitally important, as the developing brain is thought to be particularly sensitive to disruption of the normal sleep architecture, and to the low oxygen levels that may attend severe SDB. Multiple studies have linked SDB to cognitive problems in children; however, it may be possible to mitigate or reverse this effect with appropriate treatment [9]. Further, disrupted breathing during sleep can be a major cause of distress for parents [10].

In the clinic, it is important to screen children and adolescents for signs and symptoms of SDB, as parents will often not bring these concerns forward during routine well-child visits. This includes asking questions about both the child and parents' perception of the child's sleep and a physical exam informed by an understanding of the oropharyngeal airway and its development, as described in the following discussion. An in-lab polysomnogram (PSG) is the gold-standard test for the diagnosis of SDB in children, when warranted by a compelling history and physical exam. The standard pediatric PSG is comprised of a number of different physiologic measurements, including continuous recording of the patient's airflow and respiratory effort, oxygen and CO_2 levels, electroencephalography, body position and movement, and several other variables. Using this information, the clinician can assess the architecture of a child's sleep and can characterize any apneas, which are pauses in breathing as long as at least two of the patient's normal breath cycles, and hypopneas, which are significant reductions in airflow that lead to arousals or oxygen problems (Figure 16.1). This analysis results in both quantitative metrics for describing a child's sleep, including the apnea hypopnea index and the oxygen desaturation index, and also qualitative descriptions of the overall sleep architecture and the presence of any sleep fragmentation. In children and adolescents, an apnea hypopnea index >1 event per hour is considered indicative of sleep apnea. The decision to treat, and which treatment modality is chosen, remains a purely a clinical judgement.

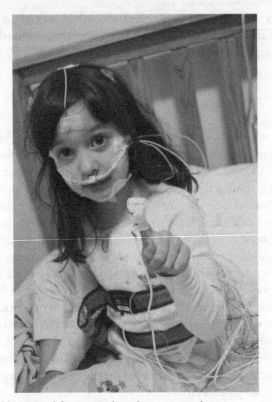

Figure 16.1 Child prepared for overnight polysomnography.

Obstructive Sleep Apnea

When we sleep, our upper airway muscle tone relaxes, and our breathing generally becomes slower and shallow. In patients with OSA, there is some anatomic problem which blocks or severely diminishes airflow into the lungs. This loss of airflow can lead to arousals of the brain and disruption of sleep and to hypoxemia. In children, this is usually related to hypertrophy of the tonsils and adenoids. The prevalence of OSA in children is estimated to be around 1% to 5%; however, this number could be increasing in the context of the current childhood obesity epidemic [6].

A thorough patient history is important for screening children and adolescents for OSA in the general pediatric clinic. Parents often can report snoring or even labored breathing in their children when prompted. However, because the predominant mode of OSA in children is hypopneas, essentially very shallow breathing, parents may often be unaware of any problems in their child's breathing during sleep. Stertorous breathing is a common concern for parents of young children and is often related to upper respiratory infections with nasal congestion. Snoring is worrisome for OSA when it is present for ≥3 days per week outside of upper respiratory infections. Children with significant obstructive airway anatomy often sleep prone with their neck hyperextended, and this can be a helpful clue when taking a history [9]. The use of clinical scales to assess a patient's sleepiness in various contexts, such as the Epworth Sleepiness Scale for Children and Adolescents, can be useful in screening patients, but it should be remembered that sleepiness is not usually a manifestation of OSA in the young patient [11]. Morning headache related to CO_2 retention is occasionally reported by children and adolescents with nocturnal hypoventilation. A child's past medical history, including a history of prematurity or asthma, can suggest increased susceptibility to SDB. Pediatric obesity is an independent risk factor for OSA in children. A focused physical exam includes assessment of the tonsils, palate, dentition, and the nasal passages for signs of narrowing and crowding, which predisposes children to OSA. Mouth-breathing is a maladaptive breathing pattern which can strongly suggest anatomical issues. While obesity contributes to OSA in older children, infants with significant SDB may present with failure to thrive as the work of nocturnal breathing may "burn" excessive calories. In older children, secondary nocturnal enuresis, defined as night-time incontinence after at least 6 months of night-time dryness, may indicate SDB [12].

Treatment for Obstructive Sleep Apnea in Children

For most children with OSA, adenotonsillectomy (AT) should be considered as a first-line intervention [13]. AT is usually safe and well-tolerated by children and results in both quantitative and qualitative improvements in a child's sleep. Children with severe OSA,\ and those with very narrow oropharyngeal airways are at risk for having residual OSA after AT; children with severe OSA, or with obesity or a history of cardiac abnormalities, should be monitored inpatient postoperatively, as they may have and increased risk of cardiorespiratory issues following AT [14].

In some cases, patients will have residual sleep apnea after first-line interventions such as AT and palatal expansion. This can be present immediately or can emerged gradually over time. Adenoidal tissue may reaccumulate in up to 25% of patients over time [15]. In refractory cases, a trial of positive airway pressure therapy is reasonable. In some patients, nasal steroids combined with montelukast, a leukotriene receptor antagonist, may improve nasal breathing by reducing tissue inflammation in the nasal passages and adenoids. Patients with severe nocturnal hypoventilation may benefit from supplemental oxygen therapy which, while not correcting the underlying ventilatory problem, may mitigate a patient's exposure to nocturnal hypoxemia. In complex cases, drug-induced sleep endoscopy can be performed by an otolaryngologist to better understand a patient's airway anatomy and dynamics, and may permit the surgeon to identify the precise level of obstruction in cases where significant OSA persists after AT [16]. Imaging studies, including 3D reconstruction computed tomography, may be useful in complex cases. When hypoventilation is suspected on PSG, an early-morning blood gas should be obtained to assess for nocturnal CO_2 retention.

Central Sleep Apnea

The automatic control of breathing is a complex process that involves both the brainstem centers of respiratory patterning and peripheral and central chemoreceptors and mechanoreceptors [17]. Central sleep apnea (CSA) is a cessation or severe diminution of airflow due to dysregulation of the central respiratory drive. Clinically, CSA is most commonly seen in newborns and infants, likely borne of an immaturity of the brain's control of respiration.

When CSA is a consideration, the physical exam should include a basic neurological evaluation, including an assessment of tone in infants, and a fundal exam in older children. In this evaluation, the critical task is excluding intracranial or brainstem abnormalities, which impinge on the centers of respiratory control in the medulla and pons, and evaluating for early signs of neuromuscular disease. On PSG, the hallmark of CSA in children is the absence of respiratory effort for the duration of two breath cycles. Neuroimaging may be warranted when a brainstem lesion is considered.

Sudden infant death syndrome (SIDS) has, rightfully, seized the attention of parents nationwide, although significant gains have been made in attenuating the dangers of SIDS by way of the "back to sleep" campaign. The relationship of immature control of breathing to brief resolved unexplained event (formerly called apparent life-threatening events) and SIDS remains unclear. Fortunately, the "Back to Sleep" campaign to educate parents about safe infant sleeping practices including, critically, placing infants to sleep on their backs in a safe crib has dramatically reduced the incidence of these awful events. Any clinical encounter with a newborn or young infant should include discussing safe sleeping practices with the parents.

Significant or symptomatic central apneas requiring some sort of intervention occur in <0.5% of full-term newborns [6]. Within the first 6 months of life, up to 2% of infants may exhibit at least one apneic event, and these are frequently observed by parents [18]. Periodic breathing is a particularly common neonatal respiratory pattern consisting of 5- to 10-second pauses in breathing followed by 10 to 15 seconds of compensatory tachypnea.

PSG should be considered in patients with a non-reassuring history, particularly in those children with report of apparent central apneas that are especially prolonged or accompanied by color change or other signs of respiratory distress. Apnea of prematurity is commonly seen in infants born too early and may result in apneas in excess of 20 seconds. Older children with CSA may report morning headache or waking at night with a sensation of "drowning." Congenital central hypoventilation syndrome (CCHS) is a very rare disease associated with a mutation of the gene *PHOX2B*. CCHS typically presents in infancy, with affected babies exhibiting often markedly shallow breathing and even apnea and cyanosis during sleep despite an absence of respiratory distress (i.e., no retractions, nasal flaring, or other signs of increased work of breathing). These children may have diffuse autonomic dysfunction, but the commonest manifestation is marked hypoventilation or even apnea during sleep. A nocturnal ventilatory support requirement is common in these patients, although dysregulation of breathing can manifest in the day as well. CCHS should be excluded by genetic testing for *PHOX2B in* children with severe CSA in the neonatal period.

Apnea of prematurity is safely, and usually effectively, treated with oral caffeine [19]. Patients with idiopathic CSA may benefit from the use of the carbonic anhydrase inhibitor or supplemental oxygen, but evidence is limited [20]. Patients with refractory CSA or CCHS may require management with nocturnal ventilation. It is critical to rule out brainstem involvement which could contribute to CSA, such as Chiari I malformation, as these patients might benefit from neurosurgical evaluation and possible surgical decompression.

SDB in Special Populations

OSA is common in children with a history of prematurity, chronic lung diseases including bronchopulmonary dysplasia, and in children with some syndromes including trisomy 21 and Piere–Robin sequence. Children with craniofacial disorders are especially at risk for obstructive breathing patterns in their sleep and are best cared for in a multidisciplinary setting where they have access to otolaryngologists and oromaxillofacial surgeons in addition to their sleep physician [21]. Emerging treatments in pediatric syndromes and craniofacial disorders, including hypoglossal nerve stimulation and mandibular distraction osteogenesis are presently being studied [22, 23]. In neuromuscular diseases, the respiratory "pump"—comprised of the diaphragm and accessory muscles of respiration—may be impaired, causing insufficient nocturnal ventilation [24]. Sleep disturbances in the context of neuromuscular disease may herald decline in lung function. Children with sickle cell disease are also at increased risk for SDB, and nocturnal oxygen desaturations may contribute to acute chest and pain crises [25]. Rett syndrome is associated with CSA. OSA disproportionately impacts children from socioeconomically disadvantaged backgrounds [26].

RESTLESS LEGS SYNDROME AND PERIODIC LIMB MOVEMENTS

Restless legs syndrome (RLS) is a relatively uncommon sleep-related disorder of childhood, although it becomes more prevalent as patients enter adolescence. The prevalence in children has been estimated at 2% to 4% in some studies, with moderate to severe RLS symptoms seen in as many as 0.5% to 1% of children [6]. RLS is usually characterized as an uncomfortable, "creepy crawly" sensation in the legs (and sometimes arms) which usually begins following a period of relative inactivity in the evening, and is improved or relieved by movement [6]. This sensation can be fairly distressing to patients, and frequently disrupts sleep initiation. Periodic limb movements (PLMs), in contrast, are a polysomnographic finding that must be linked to patient symptoms, as often PLMs observed on PSG are not associated with a disruption of sleep. It can be hard to disentangle RLS and PLM symptoms from the more common "growing pains" that children tend to report around age 3 to 4 years. A potential mimicker of RLS, growing pains is a soreness in the legs that can bother children at bedtime or even awake them from sleep. Approximately 3% to 6% of children report growing pains to their parents, and 4% to 5% of children report less specific "uncomfortable" sensations in their legs [2].

DISORDERS OF HYPERSOMNOLENCE

Hypersomnolence, or excessive daytime sleepiness, is both an extremely disabling problem for patients and often a difficult clinical problem for the sleep practitioner. Up to 16% of children are known by their parents to fall asleep in class [1]. We have a saying here at Stanford: "You can be bored in class, but never sleepy." When children and adolescents are falling asleep in class, it is a warning sign of a sleep disorder. When behavioral drivers of insufficient sleep and physiologic issues such as OSA are ruled out, less common causes of excessive daytime sleepiness should be evaluated.

Narcolepsy and Idiopathic Hypersomnia

Narcolepsy is a rare disorder which likely has its genesis in childhood. Narcolepsy type 1 (NT1) is an autoimmune condition which results in disruption of the normal production of hypocretin (orexin), a wakefulness-promoting molecule, resulting in marked daytime sleepiness. Cataplexy, a hallmark feature of NT1, is characterized as brief episodes of bilateral weakness in the jaw, neck, or limbs, most commonly triggered by strong positive emotion such as hilarious laughter [6]. Cataplectic events have been translated into the public consciousness as "sleep attacks," although true sleep attacks are rare, and most narcoleptics remain quite awake during cataplexy. Narcolepsy with cataplexy may be detected as early as 4 years of age, according to case reports, but usually first manifests in adolescence. A likely autoimmune process, NT1 is thought in many cases to be triggered by viral illness, so screening for precipitating illnesses in the past can be informative. Diagnosis of narcolepsy is still achieved using the multiple sleep latency test, a serial "nap test" designed to detect short sleep onset latency and the presence of short-onset REM periods, a feature of abnormal sleep architecture that is characteristic of narcolepsy. To be valid, the daytime multiple sleep latency test should be preceded by an overnight PSG to ensure that the patient is well-rested. Adjunctive diagnostic tools include serum testing for leukocyte antigen HLA DQB1*0602, a strong genetic marker for NT1, and assaying cerebrospinal fluid hypocretin levels.

NT1 is treated with a combination of supportive measures, including strategic napping, and pharmacologic agents, including stimulant medications and sodium oxybate. A number of other promising new treatments for disorder are on the horizon. Narcolepsy type 2—also called narcolepsy without cataplexy, or idiopathic hypersomnia—is similarly diagnosed and managed. At this time, however, there is no established role for the use of sodium oxybate, and there is no clear genetic etiology for this disorder of persistent daytime sleepiness.

Kleine–Levin Syndrome

Kleine–Levin syndrome (KLS) is a disorder of periodic, relapsing–remitting hypersomnolence that is often accompanied by marked cognitive and psychiatric/behavioral disturbances. Patients with KLS may sleep for periods of several days to weeks, waking only intermittently to use the restroom or eat [6]. If awakened by the parents, these patients are often irritable and confused, and many report a derealized or dream-like perception of their environment. This rare disorder usually manifests in early adolescence, and while currently treatable only with supportive care, including ensuring safe sleeping spaces and parental education, it typically spontaneously resolves over a period of about 14 years [6].

NORMAL SLEEP OCCURRENCES SOMETIMES CONFUSED WITH SLEEP DISORDERS

Often, sleep clinicians care for the "worried well": parents or children who have concerns about occurrences that, after a careful evaluation in sleep clinic or lab, turn out to be normal sleep behaviors or phenomena. Providing appropriate reassurance is an often-important role of the sleep clinic, as worries about sleep can, themselves, lead to distress for parents and children and disruption of family dynamics and even sleep itself.

Sleep-Talking

Sleep-talking is a fairly common occurrence in children, with around 11% of preschoolers and school-aged children exhibiting this behavior according to parent and caregiver reports [2]. It is thought to arise from both REM and NREM sleep. The speech may or may not be comprehensible, but there is generally no indication of emotional distress in the child. The speech content is rarely sensible, is often fragmentary, and is usually related to concrete happenings in the dream. In settings where the child shares a room with parents or siblings, sleep-talking could be disruptive to other members of the family, but is generally neither a problem for, nor remembered by, the sleep-talker themselves. Less commonly, sleep-talking can be associated with confusional arousals.

Hypnagogic and Hypnopompic Hallucinations

Hypnagogic and hypnopompic hallucinations, a sort of "bleed-over" of dream content into the liminal space between sleep and wakefulness, can be quite distressing to children. Hypnagogic hallucinations occur when one is falling asleep, and hypnopompic hallucinations occur with arousals from sleep. The hallucinations are often auditory but can include visual phenomena. These sleep-related hallucinations can be associated with narcolepsy or sleep paralysis and may be more common in settings of sleep deprivation but are normal in a child or adolescent with otherwise appropriate sleep schedules and quality.

Body-Rocking and Head-Banging

These rhythmic, repetitive behaviors generally occur at bedtime during drowsy N1 stage sleep and may be a sort of self-soothing behavior. Often these same behaviors will manifest in children during quiet activities while awake. In the vast majority of cases, these behaviors do not result in injury and are not necessarily associated with any developmental or intellectual problem. Parents, who are usually the ones bothered by this phenomenon, should be reassured.

Hypnic Jerks

Hypnic jerks are sudden and momentary contractions of muscles in the body that can occur when one falls asleep [6]. These can be uncomfortable, often felt by patients as a falling or even an "electric" sensation. Interestingly, it is believed that this experience is probably related to the transition from wakefulness into drowsy, N1 phase sleep. As with hypnagogic/hypnopompic hallucinations and sleep paralysis, it is important to ensure that patients experiencing frequent myoclonic jerk are not suffering from insufficient sleep.

CONCLUSIONS

Sleep is central to a child's development and well-being. Children and adolescents need to feel safe and secure to sleep well. For many children and their families, this important sense of security is eroded by socioeconomic factors that may be largely out of their control. Where we can, clinicians must work to ensure that the very young have safe and loving environments in which to sleep, and that adolescents do not suffer from insufficient sleep due to financial exigencies of their families or from overly intensive school demands. When sleep is disordered, it is critical to identify the physiologic or behavioral drivers of the problem so that medical interventions can be made. The stakes are high, as we are learning: As sleep matures as a scientific field, it is becoming increasingly evident that sleep

Box 16.1

WILLIAM CHARLES DEMENT, MD, PHD

William "Bill" Dement, MD, PhD, began teaching Sleep and Dreams at Stanford University in 1970. This was the first undergraduate course offered at the university level devoted to teaching students about the importance of sleep. The course became immediately popular with hundreds of students registering for the first time it was offered. The course has remained popular all this time. It is not uncommon for incoming students to tell Dr. Dement that their parents took his class. Now they sometimes tell him their grandparents took his class. "Drowsiness is Red Alert!" became the class motto to help them learn the dangers of drowsy driving. Students shout it out if they are caught falling asleep in class (and get bonus points).

Dr. Dement created the acronyms REM and NREM sleep as part of his early work on dreaming in the 1950s. He is lauded as the father of sleep medicine for his formative contributions to the science of sleep and the clinical practice of sleep medicine. He founded the world's first sleep medicine clinic in 1970 at Stanford. His work is foundational to the field of sleep research and medicine. He was instrumental in the establishment of the specialty of sleep medicine and was in the founding of the American Academy of Sleep Medicine in 1975. He served as its president for 12 years. While his scientific and clinical accomplishments touch virtually every aspect of sleep science and medicine, perhaps his most enduring contribution to the public health has been his tireless advocacy work relating to the dangers of sleep deprivation. He has undoubtedly saved countless lives with his important work educating students, lawmakers, and the general public.

disruptions during childhood and adolescence are associated with significant cognitive, behavioral, and health problems. Sleep disorders in childhood are common and potentially very disruptive but, happily, are eminently treatable.

ACKNOWLEDGMENTS

We acknowledge the great William C. Dement, MD, PhD (Box 16.1). There would not be a need for a college textbook if he had not pioneered teaching sleep science to undergraduate students at Stanford starting in 1970.

REFERENCES

1. 2014 Sleep in America Poll—Sleep in the Modern Family. *Sleep Health*. 2015;1:e13.
2. 2004 Sleep in America Poll—Children and Sleep. *Sleep Health*. 2015;1:e3.
3. 2006 Sleep in America Poll—Teens and Sleep. *Sleep Health*. 2015;1:e5.

4. Mindell JA, Owens JA. *A Clinical Guide to Pediatric Sleep: Diagnosis and Management of Sleep Problems*. Philadelphia, PA: Lippincott Williams & Wilkins; 2015.

5. Chiu H-Y, Lee H-C, Chen P-Y, Lai Y-F, Tu Y-K. Associations between sleep duration and suicidality in adolescents: a systematic review and dose-response meta-analysis. *Sleep Med Rev.* 2018;42:119–126.

6. American Academy of Sleep Medicine. *International Classification of Sleep Disorders*. 3rd ed. Darien, IL: American Academy of Sleep Medicine. 2014.

7. Weitzman ED, Czeisler CA, Coleman RM, et al. Delayed sleep phase syndrome. A chronobiological disorder with sleep-onset insomnia. *Arch Gen Psychiatr.* 1981;38:737–746.

8. Kothare SV, Quattrucci Scott R, eds. *Sleep Disorders in Adolescents*. New York, NY: Springer International; 2017.

9. Marcus CL, Brooks LJ, Draper KA, et al. Diagnosis and management of childhood obstructive sleep apnea syndrome. *Pediatrics.* 2012;130:576–584.

10. Bhargava S. Diagnosis and management of common sleep problems in children. *Pediatr Rev.* 2011;32:91–99.

11. Janssen KC, Phillipson S, O'Connor J, Johns MW. Validation of the Epworth Sleepiness Scale for children and adolescents using Rasch analysis. *Sleep Med.* 2017;33:30–35.

12. El-Mitwalli A, Bediwy AS, Zaher AA, Belal T, Saleh AB. Sleep apnea in children with refractory monosymptomatic nocturnal enuresis. *Nat Sci Sleep.* 2014;6:37–42.

13. Marcus CL, Moore RH, Rosen CL, et al. A randomized trial of adenotonsillectomy for childhood sleep apnea. *N Engl J Med.* 2013;368:2366–2376.

14. Lavin JM, Shah RK. Postoperative complications in obese children undergoing adenotonsillectomy. *Int J Pediatr Otorhinolaryngol.* 2015;79:1732–1735.

15. Kim SY, Lee WH, Rhee CS, Lee CH, Kim JW. Regrowth of the adenoids after coblation adenoidectomy: cephalometric analysis. *Laryngoscope.* 2013;123:2567–2572.

16. Wilcox LJ, Bergeron M, Reghunathan S, Ishman SL. An updated review of pediatric drug-induced sleep endoscopy. *Laryngoscope Investig Otolaryngol.* 2017;2:423–231.

17. Hernandez AB, Patil SP. Pathophysiology of central sleep apneas. *Sleep Breath.* 2016;20:467–482.

18. Parmelee A, Stern E, Harris M. Maturation of respiration in prematures and young infants. *Neuropediatrics.* 2008;3:294–304.

19. Schmidt B. Methylxanthine therapy for apnea of prematurity: evaluation of treatment benefits and risks at age 5 years in the International Caffeine for Apnea of Prematurity (CAP) trial. *Neonatology.* 2005;88:208–213.

20. White DP. Central sleep apnea: improvement with acetazolamide therapy. *Arch Intern Med.* 1982;142:1816–1819.

21. Cielo CM, Marcus CL. Obstructive sleep apnoea in children with craniofacial syndromes. *Paediatr Resp Rev.* 2015;16:189–196.

22. Diercks GR, Wentland C, Keamy D, et al. Hypoglossal nerve stimulation in adolescents with down syndrome and obstructive sleep apnea. *JAMA Otolaryngol Head Neck Surg.* 2017;144:37–42.

23. Steinbacher DM, Kaban LB, Troulis MJ. Mandibular advancement by distraction osteogenesis for tracheostomy-dependent children with severe micrognathia. *J Oral Maxillofac Surg.* 2005;63:1072–1079.

24. Bushby K, Finkel R, Birnkrant DJ, et al. Diagnosis and management of Duchenne muscular dystrophy, part 2: implementation of multidisciplinary care. *Lancet Neurol.* 2010;9:177–189.
25. Kaleyias J, Mostofi N, Grant M, et al. Severity of obstructive sleep apnea in children with sickle cell disease. *J Pediatr Hematol/Oncol.* 2008;30:659–665.
26. Spilsbury JC, Storfer-Isser A, Kirchner HL, et al. Neighborhood disadvantage as a risk factor for pediatric obstructive sleep apnea. *J Pediatr.* 2006;149:342–347.

17

Sleep-Related Breathing Disorders

KEREN ARMONI DOMANY AND RIVA TAUMAN ∎

INTRODUCTION

The class of sleep-related breathing disorders encompasses a range of conditions characterized by abnormal breathing during sleep. All of these conditions are characterized by partial or complete cessation of breathing that occurs repetitively throughout the night, resulting in daytime sleepiness or fatigue, quality-of-life impairment, and long-term consequences. According to the third edition of the *International Classification of Sleep Disorders*, there are four major types of sleep-related breathing disorders that can occur separately or overlap with each other. The full listing and diagnoses are in Table 17.1 [1]. In this chapter, we will review the most common sleep-related breathing disorders in adults and in children.

OBSTRUCTIVE SLEEP APNEA

Obstructive Sleep Apnea, Adults

Obstructive sleep apnea (OSA) is a relatively common disorder that is increasingly being recognized due to the obesity epidemic, as well as greater public and physician awareness. OSA refers to repetitive full or partial obstruction of the upper airway during sleep that is accompanied by intermittent hypoxia, alveolar hypoventilation, sleep fragmentation, and increased work of breathing. The muscles of the throat intermittently relax and block the airway during sleep, and an obvious sign of snoring frequently occurs. If the condition is associated with symptoms, it is called OSA syndrome. The estimated prevalence of OSA in North America is approximately 10% to 15% in females and 20% to 30% in males [2, 3].

Table 17.1 Sleep-Related Breathing Disorders

Sleep-Related Breathing Disorders

Obstructive sleep apnea	1. Adults
	2. Pediatrics
Central sleep apnea	1. Central sleep apnea with Cheyne-Stokes breathing
	2. Central sleep apnea due to a medical disorder without Cheyne-Stokes breathing
	3. Central sleep apnea due to high altitude periodic breathing
	4. Central sleep apnea due to a medication or substance
	5. Primary central sleep apnea
	6. Primary central sleep apnea of infancy
	7. Primary central sleep apnea of prematurity
	8. Treatment-emergent central sleep apnea (complex)
Sleep-related hypoventilation disorders	Obesity hypoventilation syndrome
	Congenital central alveolar hypoventilation syndrome
	Late-onset central hypoventilation with hypothalamic dysfunction
	Idiopathic central alveolar hypoventilation
	Sleep-related hypoventilation due to a medication or substance
	Sleep-related hypoventilation due to a medical disorder
Sleep-related hypoxemia disorder	(Stand-alone diagnosis)

OSA Definition and Diagnosis

OSA is characterized by episodes of upper airway occlusion: these are referred to as apneas if the airway is completely occluded, and hypopneas if the occlusion is partial. An obstructive apnea or hypopnea is defined pragmatically as the cessation or decrease in airflow despite continued breathing efforts. At their termination, apneas/hypopneas are often, but not always, associated with a drop in blood oxygen saturation and/or a change in the electroencephalographic signal, indicative of arousal. These arousals to not usually lead to a complete awakening and the patient remains unaware of them.

Laboratory-based polysomnography (PSG), or sleep study, is the first-line diagnostic test. However, due to low availability and high economic burden, home sleep apnea testing is an acceptable alternative for those who are suspected to have OSA without any major comorbidity (e.g., congestive heart failure or chronic lung disease). The formal diagnosis of OSA syndrome is based upon a combination of abnormal sleep study plus daytime signs or symptoms of disturbed sleep. Based on PSG, the number of respiratory events including apneas and hypopneas are scored throughout the night. The most accepted approach to diagnosing and determining the severity of OSA is based on the American Academy of Sleep Medicine (AASM) guidelines [4]. According to the AASM, the apnea hypopnea index (AHI) is used to define the total number of events per hour. The severity classification used most commonly is as follows: mild OSA (AHI = 5–14), moderate OSA (AHI = 15–30), and severe OSA (AHI ≥ 30).

Risk Factors

Age—The risk for OSA increases from young adulthood, reaching a plateau at age 60 [2, 5, 6].

Gender—OSA is two to three times more common in males, while the gap narrows beginning at menopause [7].

Obesity—Prevalence of OSA progressively increases as the body mass index increases; one study even showed that a 10% increase in weight is associated with a sixfold increase in risk of incident OSA [8].

Race—Risk is higher among African Americans [9, 10]. Asians have a similar prevalence of OSA compared to those in the United States, despite the lower rate of obesity in Asia; this finding is probably due to Asians' typical craniofacial anatomy placing them at increased risk.

Craniofacial and upper airway—Abnormalities such as hypertrophy (enlargement) of adenoid and tonsil tissues (mostly in the pediatric population) or maxillary and mandibular hypoplasia.

Medical conditions—Conditions such as pregnancy, hypothyroidism, congestive heart failure, and end-stage renal disease all increase risk for OSA.

Other factors—Including smoking, nasal congestion, family history of OSA, and medications.

Pathophysiology

OSA is characterized by recurrent obstruction of the pharyngeal airway during sleep (Figure 17.1), which can lead to abnormal blood exchange with intermittent hypoxemia and hypercapnia and sleep fragmentation. The most well-established contributor to OSA is the anatomical factor, with blockage most often occurring at the velopharyngeal and/or oropharyngeal airway. However, in recent years, it has been established that nonanatomical factors also contribute to OSA. Reduced upper muscle activity during sleep, increased arousal threshold, and unstable ventilatory control are nonanatomical factors that contribute to OSA. In addition, the underlying pathophysiology may vary by age, with younger patients more likely to have alterations in ventilatory control and older patients more likely to have predominant upper airway collapsibility. A developing approach suggests that there are several major phenotypes of OSA; hence, personalized medicine defining the specific phenotype might help in identifying the most appropriate treatment for each individual. However, the implications of this approach in clinical practice is yet to be determined.

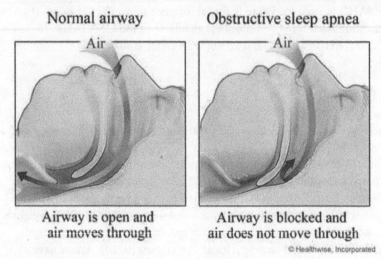

Figure 17.1 Normal airway and airway impacted by obstructive sleep apnea.

Clinical Manifestation

Snoring and unrefreshing sleep, nocturnal gasping or choking, sleepiness during the day, and mood changes (mostly in women) are all common clinical manifestation of OSA. Additional symptoms include restless sleep, fatigue, poor concentration, dry mouth during sleep or upon awakening, nocturia, and morning headaches. On physical examination, clinicians may observe obesity, crowded oropharyngeal airway, increased neck circumference, enlarged tonsils, and elevated blood pressure hypertension.

Complications and Adverse Outcomes

Adults with OSA are at increased risk for adverse clinical outcomes ranging from decreased alertness and quality of life to cardiovascular morbidities and mortality.

A broad range of cardiovascular morbidities are associated with OSA, although usually with moderate to severe OSA. These include systemic hypertension, pulmonary arterial hypertension, coronary artery disease, cardiac arrhythmias, heart failure, and stroke.

Patients with OSA have an increased prevalence of insulin resistance, type-2 diabetes [11–13], incident diabetes, and even diabetic complications [14]. In patients with metabolic syndrome, OSA has been associated with higher levels of glucose and triglyceride as well as markers of inflammation, arterial stiffness, and atherosclerosis. These findings suggest that OSA may exacerbate the cardiometabolic risk attributed to obesity and metabolic syndrome [15].

Intermittent nocturnal hypoxia due to OSA may contribute to the development and severity of nonalcoholic fatty liver disease, particularly in those with severe OSA [16, 17].

Adults with OSA have an approximately twofold increased incidence of depression compared with matched controls without OSA; this risk is higher in women than men [18–20]. An association between OSA and sexual dysfunction has also been found.

Patients with OSA may be at greater risk for perioperative complications. Hence, it is important to diagnose OSA in surgery patients and to alert both their surgeon and anesthesiologists.

Motor vehicle crashes are two to three times more common among patients with OSA compared to those without OSA [21]. Therefore, patients should be warned about the consequences of daytime sleepiness, including the risks of motor vehicle accidents from driving while sleepy, which can be caused by untreated OSA [22]. Successful OSA treatment has been shown to improve driving simulator performance and to decrease motor vehicle crashes.

Patients with untreated, severe OSA have a two- to threefold increased risk of all-cause mortality compared with patients without OSA. This association is more pronounced in men than in women and in younger patients compared with older patients [23, 24].

Management

OSA is a chronic disease that requires long-term, multidisciplinary, and sometimes challenging management. The goals of therapy are to reduce or eliminate apneas, hypopneas, and oxyhemoglobin desaturation during sleep and thereby improve sleep quality, daytime function, and long-term outcomes. Potential benefits of successful OSA treatment include improved quality of life, improved systemic blood pressure control, reduced motor vehicle crashes, reduced healthcare utilization and costs, and possibly decreased cardiovascular morbidity and mortality.

First-line treatments in adults are both weight loss (for obese patients) and continuous positive airway pressure (PAP) therapy which have been shown to improve outcomes in several randomized clinical trials [25–28]. Continuous PAP is a noninvasive method of ventilation which provides distending pressure to maintain an open airway. It delivers PAP at a level that remains constant throughout the respiratory cycle. Continuous PAP involves the use of nasal or full-face mask (called an "interface") that is securely attached with a headgear. Another mode is bilevel PAP [29]. Bilevel PAP delivers an inspiratory PAP and expiratory PAP according to preset values.

The main challenge with both continuous and bilevel PAP is patient adherence [16, 30, 31]. It is estimated that 29% to 83% of patients are nonadherent, meaning that they use their PAP therapy ≤4 hours per night [30, 31]. Several types of intervention have been developed to help promote PAP use, including improving device side effects, scheduled follow-up to evaluate downloaded PAP use, and behavioral therapy.

Alternative therapies for selected patients with OSA include oral appliances, upper airway surgery, and hypoglossal nerve stimulation [32]. Hence, the management of a patient with OSA is challenging and requires a multidisciplinary approach. Overall, OSA is a serious disease that requires a low index of suspicion for diagnosis and affects many aspects of the individual's life and causes a wide spectrum of adverse consequences if left untreated.

OBSTRUCTIVE SLEEP APNEA, PEDIATRICS

Similar to adults, pediatric OSA is characterized by episodes of complete or partial upper airway obstruction during sleep, often resulting in abnormal gas exchange and fragmented sleep. Less common than among adults, OSA occurs in 1% to 5% of children at any age, but is most common among those between ages 2 to 6 years [33]. However, habitual snoring, the hallmark symptom of OSA, is present in 10% of children. Untreated OSA is associated with learning and behavioral problems, cardiovascular complications, and impaired growth, including failure to thrive [34–36]. Early diagnosis and treatment of OSA may decrease morbidity. Nevertheless, diagnosis is frequently delayed.

Risk Factors

The major risk factor in children is *hypertrophy of adenoid and tonsils* in otherwise healthy children. Figure 17.2 demonstrates the commonly used tonsils size

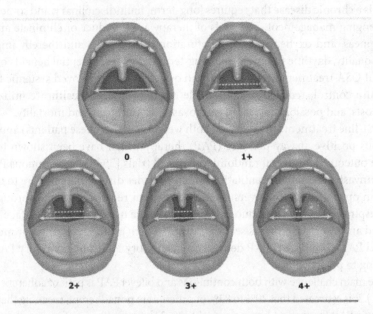

Figure 17.2 Tonsil size is usually scored on a scale from zero to 4 where zero tonsils are entirely within the tonsillar pillar, status post tonsillectomy; 1+ tonsils occupy <25% of the lateral dimension of the oropharynx (solid yellow arrow); 2+ tonsils occupy 26% to 50% of the lateral dimension of the oropharynx; 3+ tonsils occupy 51% to 75% of the lateral dimension of the oropharynx; and 4+ tonsils occupy >75% of the lateral dimension of the oropharynx.

scoring system. Obesity is another important risk factor for OSA at all ages but is particularly prominent among adolescents. Other risk factors include craniofacial and neuromuscular disorders such as Down, Crouzon and Apert syndromes, Pierre Robin sequence, and cerebral palsy. The mechanism in such cases are either reduced upper airway size, impaired neural control of the upper airway, or increase collapsibility of the upper airway.

Clinical Manifestations

Night-time symptoms include snoring, labored breathing, parent-witnessed apneas, mouth breathing, and restless sleeps. Daytime symptoms include mouth breathing, growth impairment, and poor school functioning. The long-term consequences of untreated OSA in children are learning and behavioral problems (which mimic attention deficit hyperactivity disorder), systemic hypertension, accelerated atherosclerosis, altered cardiac morphology, impaired growth (including failure to thrive), and increased healthcare utilization [37].

Diagnosis

Overnight PSG is the gold standard for the diagnosis of OSA [33]. In contrast to adults, home sleep tests are still not validated in children. The pediatric PSG criteria also differ from those for adults. In children, PSG is considered normal when the obstructive AHI is <1 per hour; obstructive AHI 1 to 5 per hour of sleep is considered mild OSA; 5 to 10 is considered moderate OSA; and severe OSA is typically associated with an AHI >10 per hour of sleep [4].

Treatment

In pediatrics, the decision to treat and choice of treatment depends upon OSA severity, as well as the age of the child, associated symptoms, comorbidities, and risk factors such as obesity or crowded oropharynx.

> Adenotonsillectomy—The first-line treatment option for otherwise healthy children who have OSA and hypertrophy of adenoids and tonsils is referral to an otorhinolaryngologist, or ear—nose–throat (ENT) doctor, for adenotonsillectomy [33]. Adenotonsillectomy may also be the initial therapy for children with other contributors to OSA, such as obesity or other comorbidities, if considerable adenotonsillar tissue is present [33].
> Watchful waiting for up to 6 months—According to the study Childhood Adenotonsillectomy Trial (CHAT) [38], in otherwise healthy children with mild to moderate OSA that was diagnosed by PSG, watchful waiting

with supportive care is a reasonable alternative to adenotonsillectomy, with an acceptable outcome.

PAP therapy—For patients with minimal adenotonsillar tissue or a strong preference for a nonsurgical approach, PAP therapy is an alternative to adenotonsillectomy [33]. It may also be appropriate to stabilize children with severe OSA prior to surgical intervention or for children with persistent OSA despite surgery [39].

Medication—In children with mild to moderate OSA and nasal obstruction due to adenoidal hypertrophy/allergic rhinitis, a trial of intranasal corticosteroids and/or leukotriene modifier therapy (monteleukast [Singulair*]) may be prescribed. A trial of 2 to 4 weeks should be initiated prior to determining whether the therapy should be continued long-term as an adjunct or alternative to adenotonsillectomy or PAP therapy [40].

Other treatment options—Upper surgery such as maxillary expansion, lingual tonsillectomy, or glossectomy may be used, depending on the upper airway anatomy and site of obstruction. Weight loss may be used for obese children with OSA, and avoidance of environmental irritants such as tobacco smoke or allergens can be useful in children with allergies that cause upper airway congestion.

CENTRAL SLEEP APNEA DISORDERS

Central sleep apnea (CSA) is characterized by recurrent apneas during sleep with no associated respiratory effort; this occurs due to lack of proper brain signals to the muscles that control breathing. This condition differs from OSA, in which breathing is abnormal due to upper airway obstruction. Although CSA is less common than OSA, it is quite common in patients with heart failure, neurologic disorders such as stroke, and those on high doses of opiates. Symptoms of CSA include nocturnal awakenings, insomnia, and daytime sleepiness; however, most patients are asymptomatic.

CSA Definition

CSA is a cessation in airflow for ≥20 seconds in the absence of any inspiratory effort *or* a cessation of at least two baseline breaths in the absence of any inspiratory effort, which is associated with either arousal or a decrease in oxygen saturation >3%. A frequency of five or more central apneas per hour of sleep is considered abnormal, while the diagnosis is made when 50% or more of the events are central. Diagnosis is based on laboratory PSG, which is the gold standard. Home sleep study is still not validated for the diagnosis of CSA. The overall prevalence of CSA on PSG is almost 1% [41]. The median age of patients with CSA is 69 years, and the prevalence is higher among males. CSA can be either primary (idiopathic, unknown cause), which is a rare condition, or secondary to one of major causes described in the following discussion.

Cheyne–Stokes Breathing

Approximately half of CSA cases are associated with Cheyne–Stokes breathing; hence, this is the most common type of CSA. Generally, Cheyne–Stokes respiration with CSA is a form of periodic breathing (pauses in breathing for no more than 10 seconds at a time, followed by a series of rapid, shallow breaths), commonly observed in patients with heart failure or patients who have a had a stroke. In this type of apnea, central apneas alternate with hypopneas (an increase in depth and rate of breathing) with a crescendo–decrescendo pattern of tidal volume and a recurrence of this pattern throughout the night. Each cycle usually takes 30 seconds to 2 minutes (Figure 17.3) [42]. This type of breathing has profound effects on the cardiopulmonary system, causing oxygen desaturation, cardiac arrhythmias, and changes in mental status. The mechanism for Cheyne–Stokes respiration is ventilatory control system instability characterized by a tendency to hyperventilate followed by central apnea when partial pressure of carbon dioxide ($PaCO_2$) falls below the threshold for apnea [43].

Treatment

Initial treatment of CSA should focus on any condition that may be causing or exacerbating the CSA, such as stabilizing congestive heart failure. If CSA persists,

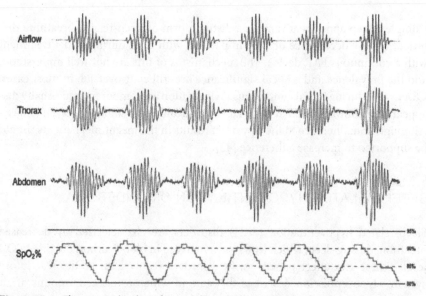

Figure 17.3 Cheyne–Stokes breathing with central apneas. Characterized by crescendo-decrescendo pattern of airflow and effort. SpO2, oxygen saturation.

CSA-specific therapies are indicated for patients with symptoms or significant physiological sequelae attributable to CSA (e.g., daytime sleepiness, prolonged or repetitive oxyhemoglobin desaturation during sleep). Continuous PAP is the preferred first-line therapy for symptomatic patients, although this recommendation is based on a limited number of randomized trials. For severe cases who fail continuous PAP treatment, other modes of advanced noninvasive ventilation are possible.

High Altitude Periodic Breathing

High altitude periodic breathing is characterized by periods of central apnea cycling with periods of hyperpnea during sleep upon ascent to high altitudes. This typically occurs when climbing at least to 2500 meters, although some individuals may exhibit the disorder at altitudes as low as 1500 meters. However, it occurs in virtually everyone at altitudes higher than 4000 meters. The hypoxemia and hypocapnia, universally seen in subjects exposed to high altitude are the main factors leading to instability of the ventilatory system and the development of periodic breathing and central apneas during sleep.

TREATMENT
Treatment options are supplemental oxygen, which stabilizes the ventilatory control; interventions that improve sleep quality, including medication such as acetazolamide; and, obviously, return to a lower altitude [44].

COMPLEX SLEEP APNEA

Complex sleep apnea syndrome is a distinct form of sleep-related breathing disorder. It is the occurrence of CSA in patients with OSA during initial treatment with a continuous PAP device. The mechanisms of this are not well understood, and the prevalence and clinical significance are still controversial. In most cases, CSA events during initial continuous PAP titration are temporary and usually disappear after continued PAP use for 4 to 8 weeks (although sometimes even longer). Although nonadherence to therapy often results in the meantime, patients should be supported to increase adherence [45].

SLEEP-RELATED HYPOVENTILATION DISORDERS

Sleep-related hypoventilation (SRH) disorders are characterized by decreased breathing during sleep, which leads to an increase in blood carbon dioxide (CO_2) levels. These can affect patients with disorders at any level of the respiratory system. Hypoventilation describes the state in which a reduced amount of air enters the alveoli in the lungs, resulting in low blood levels of oxygen (O_2) and increased levels of the body's waste gas, carbon dioxide (CO_2).

Definition

Hypoventilation can be due to breathing that is too shallow, breathing that is too slow, obstructed airways, or restricted or damaged lungs. Conventionally, hypoventilation is defined as arterial blood gas partial pressure of CO_2 (pCO_2) above the normal levels of 35 to 45 mmHg in an awake patient. Hypoventilation is often, but not always, accompanied by hypoxemia. Clinicians may suspect hypoventilation on the basis of capillary or venous blood gas with unexplained elevations of CO_2 (>50 mmHg) and bicarbonate (>25 mEq/L), or pulse oximetry with a baseline oxygen saturation <96% at rest.

Diagnosis

Diagnosis is based on the observed hypercapnia during PSG. In adults, either an increase in the arterial PCO_2 to a value >55 mmHg for ≥10 minutes, or ≥10 mmHg increase in arterial PCO_2 during sleep (in comparison to an awake supine value) to a value >50 mmHg for ≥10 minutes. Diagnosis in children is defined as hypercapnia (>50 mmHg) for more than 25% of total sleep time [4].

Clinical Presentation

Signs and symptoms of SRH are related to the higher levels of carbon dioxide in the blood and to sleep disturbance including morning headaches, restless sleep, daytime tiredness or sleepiness, and difficulty concentrating during the day. Recurrent respiratory problems can also be present, including chest infections and shortness of breath. Although these signs and symptoms are common, they may not be recognized as signs of SRH. The major types of SRH are described next.

Obesity Hypoventilation Syndrome

Obesity hypoventilation syndrome also known as Pickwickian syndrome is defined as the presence of awake alveolar hypoventilation ($PaCO_2$ >45 mmHg) in an obese individual with a body mass index >30 kg/m², which cannot be attributed to other conditions associated with hypoventilation.

CLINICAL MANIFESTATIONS

The clinical manifestations are nonspecific and more reflective of the manifestations of obesity and coexisting OSA, or the related complications such as pulmonary hypertension. Sleep-related desaturation and daytime hypoxemia are common. For those with suspected obesity hypoventilation syndrome in whom a diagnosis of OSA does not already exist, in-laboratory PSG should be performed based upon the rationale that 90% of patients have coexisting OSA and the remainders have SHR. Once diagnosed, all patients with obesity hypoventilation syndrome should be assessed for common complications, including pulmonary hypertension and cardiovascular disorders

TREATMENT
A comprehensive and multidisciplinary approach is used to target the immediate initiation of noninvasive PAP therapy, along with lifestyle modifications for weight loss. Morbidity and mortality in untreated patients are high, with most deaths occurring due to cardiovascular complications, including pulmonary hypertension and right heart failure. The impact of therapy on cardiovascular complications and mortality is uncertain.

CONGENITAL CENTRAL ALVEOLAR HYPOVENTILATION SYNDROME
Congenital central alveolar hypoventilation syndrome (CCHS), also referred to as Ondine's curse, is a life-threatening disorder manifesting as sleep-associated alveolar hypoventilation. The literary misnomer Ondine's curse is based on the German folk epic, in which the nymph Ondine falls in love with a mortal. When the mortal is unfaithful to the nymph, he is cursed by the king of the nymphs. The king's curse makes the mortal responsible for remembering to perform all bodily functions, even those that occur automatically, such as breathing. When the mortal falls asleep, he "forgets" to breathe and dies.

CCHS is a rare syndrome that should be considered in children with episodic or sustained hypoventilation and hypoxemia in the first months of life, in the absence of apparent respiratory distress and no obvious metabolic, cardiopulmonary, or neuromuscular disease. Most patients breathe normally while awake but hypoventilate during sleep. It is a genetic disease caused by mutation in the paired-like homeobox 2B gene *(PHOX2B)* gene located on chromosome 4.

DIAGNOSIS
CCHS requires exclusion of other causes of SRH and demonstration of a mutation in the *PHOX2B* gene. CCHS is associated with a wide variety of abnormalities including neurocognitive deficits, Hirschsprung disease, tumors such as neuroblastoma, ophthalmologic abnormalities, and other autonomic system abnormalities.

TREATMENT
Treatments includes artificial ventilation during sleep and often during wakefulness, most commonly via tracheostomy. Monitoring of oxygen saturation, end-tidal CO_2, and extensive home care support are required, as well as scheduled follow-up with PSG, cardiac testing, cognitive testing, and surveillance for tumors [46,47].

Sleep-Related Hypoventilation Due to Medication or Substance

Medications and other substances that suppress the central nervous system, such as benzodiazepines, opiates, and alcohol, can also cause SRH [42].

Sleep-Related Hypoventilation Due to Medical Disorder

A wide range of medical disorders can affect ventilation and lead to, or present with, SRH: for example, pulmonary parenchymal or vascular pathologies (pulmonary hypertension); lower airway obstructions, such as chronic obstructive pulmonary disease; neuromuscular disease; metabolic disease [48]; and chest wall disorders, particularly scoliosis. Treatment should focus on stabilizing the primary medical disorder and noninvasive ventilation such as bilevel PAP therapy.

REFERENCES

1. Sateia MJ. International classification of sleep disorders-third edition: highlights and modifications. *Chest.* 2014;146:1387–1394.
2. Young T, Palta M, Dempsey J, Peppard PE, Nieto FJ, Hla KM. Burden of sleep apnea: rationale, design, and major findings of the Wisconsin Sleep Cohort study. *WMJ.* 2009;108:246–249.
3. Peppard PE, Young T, Barnet JH, Palta M, Hagen EW, Hla KM. Increased prevalence of sleep-disordered breathing in adults. *Am J Epidemiol.* 2013;177:1006–1014.
4. Berry RB, Brooks R, Gamaldo C, et al. AASM scoring manual updates for 2017 (Version 2.4). *J Clin Sleep Med,* 2017;13:665–666.
5. Jennum P, Riha RL. Epidemiology of sleep apnoea/hypopnoea syndrome and sleep-disordered breathing. *Eur Res J.* 2009;33:907–914.
6. Tufik S, Santos-Silva R, Taddei JA, Bittencourt LR. Obstructive sleep apnea syndrome in the Sao Paulo Epidemiologic Sleep Study. *Sleep Med.* 2010;11:441–446.
7. Quintana-Gallego E, Carmona-Bernal C, Capote F, et al. Gender differences in obstructive sleep apnea syndrome: a clinical study of 1166 patients. *Resp Med,* 2004;98:984–989.
8. Peppard PE, Young T, Palta M, Dempsey J, Skatrud J. Longitudinal study of moderate weight change and sleep-disordered breathing. *JAMA.* 2000;284:3015–3021.
9. Redline S, Tishler PV, Hans MG, Tosteson TD, Strohl KP, Spry K. Racial differences in sleep-disordered breathing in African-Americans and Caucasians. *Am J Resp Crit Care Med.* 1997;155:186–192.
10. Ancoli-Israel S, Klauber MR, Stepnowsky C, Estline E, Chinn A, Fell R. Sleep-disordered breathing in African-American elderly. *Am J Resp Crit Care Med,* 1995;152:1946–1949.
11. Punjabi NM, Shahar E, Redline S, Gottlieb DJ, Givelber R, Resnick HE. Sleep-disordered breathing, glucose intolerance, and insulin resistance: the Sleep Heart Health Study. *Am J Epidemiol.* 2004;160:521–530.
12. Togeiro SM, Carneiro G, Ribeiro Filho FF, et al. Consequences of obstructive sleep apnea on metabolic profile: a population-based survey. *Obesity.* 2013;21:847–851.
13. Kent BD, Grote L, Ryan S, et al. Diabetes mellitus prevalence and control in sleep-disordered breathing: the European Sleep Apnea Cohort (ESADA) study. *Chest.* 2014;146:982–990.
14. Kendzerska T, Gershon AS, Hawker G, Tomlinson G, Leung RS. Obstructive sleep apnea and incident diabetes: a historical cohort study. *Am J Resp Crit Care Med.* 2014;190:218–225.

15. Drager LF, Togeiro SM, Polotsky VY, Lorenzi-Filho G. Obstructive sleep apnea: a cardiometabolic risk in obesity and the metabolic syndrome. *J Am Coll Card.* 2013;62:569–576.

16. Turkay C, Ozol D, Kasapoglu B, Kirbas I, Yildirim Z, Yigitoglu R. Influence of obstructive sleep apnea on fatty liver disease: role of chronic intermittent hypoxia. *Resp Care.* 2012;57:244–249.

17. Minville C, Hilleret MN, Tamisier R, et al. Nonalcoholic fatty liver disease, nocturnal hypoxia, and endothelial function in patients with sleep apnea. *Chest.* 2014;145:525–533.

18. Chen YH, Keller JK, Kang JH, Hsieh HJ, Lin HC. Obstructive sleep apnea and the subsequent risk of depressive disorder: a population-based follow-up study. *J Clin Sleep Med.* 2013;9:417–423.

19. Peppard PE, Szklo-Coxe M, Hla KM, Young T. Longitudinal association of sleep-related breathing disorder and depression. *Arch Internal Med.* 2006;166:1709–1715.

20. Wheaton AG, Perry GS, Chapman DP, Croft JB. Sleep disordered breathing and depression among U.S. adults: National Health and Nutrition Examination Survey, 2005–2008. *Sleep.* 2012;35:461–467.

21. George CF. Sleep apnea, alertness, and motor vehicle crashes. *Am J Resp Crit Care Med.* 2007;176:954–956.

22. Strohl KP, Brown DB, Collop N, et al. An official American Thoracic Society Clinical Practice Guideline: sleep apnea, sleepiness, and driving risk in noncommercial drivers: an update of a 1994 statement. *Am J Resp Crit Care Med.* 2013;187:1259–1266.

23. Punjabi NM, Caffo BS, Goodwin JL, et al. Sleep-disordered breathing and mortality: a prospective cohort study. *PLOS Med.* 2009;6:e1000132.

24. Lavie P, Lavie L, Herer P. All-cause mortality in males with sleep apnoea syndrome: declining mortality rates with age. *Eur Resp J.* 2005;25:514–520.

25. Dixon JB, Schachter LM, O'Brien PE, et al. Surgical vs conventional therapy for weight loss treatment of obstructive sleep apnea: a randomized controlled trial. *JAMA.* 2012;308:1142–1149.

26. Foster GD, Borradaile KE, Sanders MH, et al. A randomized study on the effect of weight loss on obstructive sleep apnea among obese patients with type 2 diabetes: the Sleep AHEAD study. *Arch Int Med.* 2009;169:1619–1626.

27. Araghi MH, Chen YF, Jagielski A, et al. Effectiveness of lifestyle interventions on obstructive sleep apnea (OSA): systematic review and meta-analysis. *Sleep.* 2013;36:1553–1562.

28. Giles TL, Lasserson TJ, Smith BH, White J, Wright J, Cates CJ. Continuous positive airways pressure for obstructive sleep apnoea in adults. *Cochrane Db Sys Rev.* 2006;25:Cd001106.

29. Epstein LJ, Kristo D, Strollo PJ, et al. Clinical guideline for the evaluation, management and long-term care of obstructive sleep apnea in adults. *J Clin Sleep Med.* 2009;5:263–276.

30. Sawyer AM, Gooneratne NS, Marcus CL, Ofer D, Richards KC, Weaver TE. A systematic review of CPAP adherence across age groups: clinical and empiric insights for developing CPAP adherence interventions. *Sleep Med Rev,* 2011;15:343–356.

31. Schwab RJ, Badr SM, Epstein LJ, et al. An official American Thoracic Society statement: continuous positive airway pressure adherence tracking systems: the optimal

monitoring strategies and outcome measures in adults. *Am J Resp Crit Care Med.* 2013;188:613–620.

32. Kryger MH, Malhotra A. Management of obstructive sleep apnea in adults. UpToDate. https://www.uptodate.com/contents/management-of-obstructive-sleep-apnea-in-adults. Published 2019. Accessed May 10, 2019.

33. Marcus CL, Brooks LJ, Draper KA, et al. Diagnosis and management of childhood obstructive sleep apnea syndrome. *Pediatrics.* 2012;130:e714–e755.

34. Marcus CL, Greene MG, Carroll JL. Blood pressure in children with obstructive sleep apnea. *Am J Resp Crit Care Med.* 1998;157:1098–1103.

35. Nieminen P, Lopponen T, Tolonen U, Lanning P, Knip M, Lopponen H. Growth and biochemical markers of growth in children with snoring and obstructive sleep apnea. *Pediatrics.* 2002;109:e55.

36. Beebe DW, Ris MD, Kramer ME, Long E, Amin R. The association between sleep disordered breathing, academic grades, and cognitive and behavioral functioning among overweight subjects during middle to late childhood. *Sleep.* 2010;33:1447–1456.

37. Paruthi S. Evaluation of suspected obstructive sleep apnea in children. UpToDate. https://www.uptodate.com/contents/evaluation-of-suspected-obstructive-sleep-apnea-in-children. Published 2019. Accessed May 10, 2019.

38. Marcus CL, Moore RH, Rosen CL, et al. A randomized trial of adenotonsillectomy for childhood sleep apnea. *N Engl J Med.*2013;368:2366–2376.

39. Guilleminault C, Pelayo R, Clerk A, Leger D, Bocian RC. Home nasal continuous positive airway pressure in infants with sleep-disordered breathing. *J Ped,* 1995;127:905–912.

40. Liming BJ, Ryan M, Mack D, Ahmad I, Camacho M. Montelukast and nasal corticosteroids to treat pediatric obstructive sleep apnea: a systematic review and meta-analysis. *Otolaryngol Head Neck Surg.* 2019;160:594–602.

41. Donovan LM, Kapur VK. Prevalence and characteristics of central compared to obstructive sleep apnea: analyses from the Sleep Heart Health Study Cohort. *Sleep.* 2016;39:1353–1359.

42. Correa D, Farney RJ, Chung F, Prasad A, Lam D, Wong J. Chronic opioid use and central sleep apnea: a review of the prevalence, mechanisms, and perioperative considerations. *Anesth Analg.* 2015;120:1273–1285.

43. Muza RT. Central sleep apnoea: a clinical review. *J Thorac Dis.* 2015;7:930–937.

44. Ainslie PN, Lucas SJ, Burgess KR. Breathing and sleep at high altitude. *Respir Physiol Neurobiol.* 2013;188:233–256.

45. Boing S, Randerath WJ. Chronic hypoventilation syndromes and sleep-related hypoventilation. *J Thorac Dis.* 2015;7:1273–1285.

46. Brouillette RT. Congenital central hypoventilation syndrome and other causes of sleep-related hypoventilation in children. UpToDate. https://www.uptodate.com/contents/congenital-central-hypoventilation-syndrome-and-other-causes-of-sleep-related-hypoventilation-in-children. Published 2019. Accessed May 10, 2019.

47. Chin TW, Chen JJ, Maharaj S. Congenital central hypoventilation syndrome clinical presentation. *Medscape.* https://emedicine.medscape.com/article/1002927-overview. Updated June 2, 2017. Accessed February 26, 2020.

48. Labanowski M, Schmidt-Nowara W, Guilleminault C. Sleep and neuromuscular disease: frequency of sleep-disordered breathing in a neuromuscular disease clinic population. *Neurology.* 1996;47:1173–1180.

18

Insomnia

JASON G. ELLIS ■

INTRODUCTION

In the broadest sense, insomnia is a problem with not getting enough sleep. While this definition is quite sensitive (i.e., it is likely to capture most, if not all, people who have insomnia), it lacks specificity (i.e., the ability to exclude people who do not have insomnia but may not be getting enough sleep for other reasons). To be relevant to clinicians and researchers, however, we need a definition that has a good balance between sensitivity and specificity—so that we can correctly identify all, but only, those people with insomnia. There are currently three diagnostic manuals that attempt this: the *International Classification of Disorders* (ICD-10) [1] by the World Health Organization; the *International Classification of Sleep Disorders* (ICSD-3) [2] by the American Academy of Sleep Medicine; and the *Diagnostic and Statistical Manual of Mental Disorders* (DSM-5) [3] by the American Psychiatric Association. Although these three differ significantly in terms of how they define insomnia, they share some features [4]. Most notably, all three rely on the individual's self-reports.

The manual used most often in research and clinical practice, and the one on which we will focus here, is the DSM-5 [3]. The DSM-5 defines insomnia disorder as a self-reported dissatisfaction with sleep that is characterized as a difficulty in initiating sleep (i.e., getting off to sleep), maintaining sleep (i.e., waking during the night and being unable to get back off to sleep), and/or early morning awakening (i.e., waking up earlier than needed and unable to get back off to sleep). Further, the problem should exist despite adequate opportunity for sleep, occur at least 3 nights in a week, and have been present for at least 3 months; prior to 3 months duration, it is known as acute insomnia. Again, relying of self-report, the individual should also report that the insomnia is causing them distress and/or impairment to their daily functioning. This criterion can include feelings of daytime sleepiness or distress; difficulties with memory, attention or concentration; and/or increased challenge to normal work, caregiving, or school activities. Finally, the insomnia should not be better explained by another sleep disorder, adequately explained by a medical or mental condition, or attributed to use of a substance or medication.

Why are these particular criteria necessary for a diagnosis? The first criterion is clearly very sensitive to those with insomnia, whereas all the others aim to differentiate insomnia from other issues (i.e., specificity). For example, the 3 disrupted nights per week minimum differentiates insomnia from normal sleep—even people who sleep "normally" are likely to have the odd disrupted night [5]. The adequate opportunity criterion accounts for individuals who may be getting insufficient amounts of sleep (usually voluntarily), and the daytime distress/dysfunction criterion differentiates those with insomnia from people who spend more time in bed (TIB) than they actually need (usually termed "short sleepers").

The final criterion is challenging, as it is sometimes difficult to determine whether some other factor or issue "adequately" or even "better" explains the insomnia. For example, there is a large overlap between insomnia and depression, but how can we determine whether the depression adequately explains the insomnia? I tend to ask which came first in an attempt to answer this question. The most significant contribution the DSM-5 makes to our understanding of insomnia, however, is that it was the first diagnostic manual to reject the idea insomnia is only a symptom—as opposed to a disorder in its own right—if it occurs alongside any another illness, disease, disorder (including another sleep disorder), or substance or medication use. When you read the later section on the consequences of insomnia, you will understand why this was such an important step forward.

HOW WE MEASURE INSOMNIA IN RESEARCH

Outside of the diagnostic criteria, for which a clinical interview is generally needed, few psychometric (i.e., valid and reliable) questionnaires measure insomnia. Having a psychometric tool that can do this is very helpful for research, especially if it is short but still has sufficient sensitivity and specificity. The most widely used psychometric for measuring insomnia is the Insomnia Severity Index (ISI) [6]. This questionnaire asks the individual to answer seven questions relating to their symptoms of insomnia over the past month. Each question is rated, by the individual, on a scale of zero (meaning "no problem") to 4 ("very severe"), with a possible range of scores between zero and 28. The individual's scores are then interpreted, with a score of zero to 7 indicating no insomnia, 8 to 14 indicating subthreshold insomnia, 15 to 21 indicating moderate insomnia, and 22 to 28 indicating severe insomnia. Importantly for research and clinical practice, it has recently been shown that a reduction of 8.4 points on the ISI is associated with a moderate treatment response and 9.9 points with a marked treatment response, following cognitive-behavioral therapy for insomnia (CBT-I; see later discussion) [7]. While the ISI does not ask about adequate opportunity, number of nights affected in a given week, or the duration of insomnia (it only addresses the past month), it focuses on both the daytime and night-time symptoms.

The other questionnaire you are likely to see used in the context of insomnia is the Pittsburgh Sleep Quality Index (PSQI) [8]. The PSQI contains 19 questions about how the individual slept over the last month; when scored, the PSQI scale ranges between zero and 21, with higher scores indicating more of a problem with sleep. A score >5 suggests clinically relevant sleep disturbance. The main disadvantage of the PSQI, over the ISI, is that it lacks specificity for insomnia and may actually be measuring the individual's response to another type of sleep disorder.

The other main method of tracking the signs and symptoms of insomnia is through a sleep diary (Figure 18.1). Looking at the questions, you can see where I, as a clinician, might identify the different symptoms of insomnia. For example, question 5 asks how long it took the individual to get to sleep—sleep latency; question 6 asks how many times they awoke in the night—number of awakenings; and question 7 asks how long they were awake in the night after getting to sleep in the first place—wake after sleep onset.

By asking what time the individual gets into and out of bed, we can also determine other variables that will become very helpful when we try to treat insomnia. The first of these is their TIB. For example, if they got into bed at 11 PM and out of bed at 6 AM, their TIB would be 6 hours (360 minutes). Another important variable can be determined by looking at how much sleep the individual actually obtained—total sleep time (TST). Let us say they were in bed for 6 hours, but it took them 30 minutes to fall asleep, they were awake for 15 minutes in the night, and awoke 15 minutes earlier than they needed to. In this case, their TST would be 5 hours (300 minutes). TST and TIB can then be used to work out how efficiently the individual is sleeping, using the following formula (TST/TIB × 100). Known as sleep efficiency (SE) in this individual's SE would be 83.3% (300 minutes/360 minutes × 100). The final questions in the sleep diary ask about sleep quality and two of the main issues reported by people with insomnia: physical tension and/or mental anxiety while in bed.

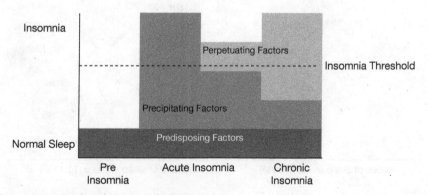

Figure 18.1 Spielman's 3P Model of Insomnia.

HOW INSOMNIA DEVELOPS

The most influential model, which outlines the development of insomnia, comes from Spielman and colleagues—the 3P model of insomnia [9, 10]. Spielman suggested that insomnia develops from a combination of three factors: those that are predisposing, precipitating, and perpetuating. According to Spielman, predisposing factors are individual differences or circumstances that determine our vulnerability to getting insomnia. For example, an anxious or worry-prone personality (aspects of the trait neuroticism) is associated with having insomnia [11]. As you can see in Figure 18.2, predisposing factors are insufficient, on their own, to result in insomnia, but they do determine how close we are to the insomnia threshold (i.e., how likely we are to get insomnia). Precipitating factors, according to Spielman, are stressful events that push us over the insomnia threshold, resulting in acute insomnia. This is a biologically driven "fight or flight" response to the stressor—anyone who has watched a horror movie is likely to have observed this phenomenon. How many times in the horror movie does the heroine (or hero), who is being pursued by a monster or serial killer—usually through a forest or disused factory—in the middle of the night, stop to have a sleep? Not likely! She (or he) seems able to run all night without the need for sleep. This is the flight-or-fight response in action.

Although Spielman suggested that a precipitant should be a stressful life event, such as a bereavement or divorce, this idea has been questioned in light of our understanding of how chronic stressors (e.g., caregiving) and daily hassles affect our

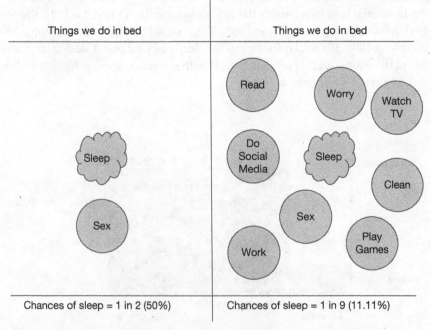

Figure 18.2 The impact of daytime activities in the bedroom.

health and well-being [12, 13]. Irrespective of the source of the stress, this flight or fight response results in initial difficulties with sleep. What happens next, and the final aspect of Spielman's model, is the introduction of perpetuating factors. During this phase, which he termed "early insomnia," the stressor is still the main thing fueling the insomnia, but the individual starts to compensate for their poor sleep. One of the most common things people do to compensate for poor sleep is to spend more TIB—either by going to bed earlier than normal, staying in bed after awaking in the morning, or napping during the daytime [14]. Unfortunately, as explained in Chapter 4 of this volume, each of those strategies are likely to disrupt the sleep homeostat and/or the circadian rhythm, potentially making things worse.

Additionally, what people do while waiting for the sandman to come and whisk them off to sleep can also make the problem worse. In my experiences, talking to patients with insomnia generally sounds like this:

> Well . . . when I go to bed I will take a book to read, or a magazine . . . but then I know I get thirsty when I read, so I take something to drink . . . okay . . . well, I also know that I sometimes get hungry at night so I will take a snack as well, just in case. Then I think I suppose I should take my tablet, phone, laptop, just in case I can't sleep so I can catch up on some work or watch a movie, so I take those as well.

All these strategies seem innocuous enough, but what the individual has done is introduce several daytime activities into their bedtime routine and into their bedroom itself. What this means is the association between the bedroom and sleep has become blurred—in other words, their body becomes confused as to whether it should be awake or sleep in bed [15]. This is likely to decrease the odds of sleeping (see Figure 18.3). Other compensatory strategies include consuming caffeine over the course of the day to stay awake and/or consuming alcohol at night to help get to sleep, both of which are not good for sleep. A final compensation strategy is to "try" to sleep. Otherwise known as sleep effort, an individual with insomnia is likely to lie in bed willing themselves to sleep while also monitoring for physical signs and symptoms of sleepiness, such as sore eyes or yawning, or indeed alertness [16]. Unfortunately, the more we "try" to sleep, the less likely it is to occur, leading to anger, frustration, and/or being miserable in bed pretty quickly, which is also not sleep-compatible.

According to Spielman, by the time insomnia has become chronic (full insomnia disorder) the influence of the precipitating factor is minimal but perpetuating factors fuel the insomnia in a vicious cycle of poor sleep and compensatory behavior. Since Spielman, numerous others have attempted to model why insomnia occurs or how it is maintained [see 17]. These explanations all tend to agree with Spielman's basic premise of the 3Ps, but add new insights or sophistication, based on new research. The newer models have largely focused on the role of cognition in insomnia and/or how insomnia is maintained at a biological/neurological level. Most notably, researchers have started to incorporate issues such as sleep-related

MEASURING THE PATTERN OF YOUR SLEEP	Day 1	Day 2	Day 3	Day 4	Day 5	Day 6	Day 7
1. What time did you wake this morning?							
2. At what time did you get out of bed?							
3. At what time did you go to bed last night?							
4. Lights Out:- At what time did you put the lights out to go to sleep?							
5. How long did it take you to fall asleep (minutes)? (After Lights Out)							
6. How many times did you wake up during the night?							
7. How long were you awake during the night (in total)?							
8. About how long did you sleep altogether (hours/mins)?							
9. Did you use anything to help you sleep (medication, herbal, alcohol)? (Y/N)							

MEASURING OTHER ACTIVITIES

1. How was the quality of your sleep last night?

0	1	2	3	4
very poor		moderately ok		very poor

2. How physically tense were you last night at bedtime?

0	1	2	3	4
not at all		moderately		very

3. How mentally alert were you last night at bedtime?

0	1	2	3	4
not at all		moderately		very

4. Did you nap in the daytime and for how long? (time and duration)

Figure 18.3 Sleep diary example.

dysfunctional attitudes and beliefs, attentional and interpretative biases (i.e., we are more likely to seek out sleep-related stimuli or interpret neutral stimuli as sleep related), and catastrophic thoughts and feelings related to sleep into our understanding of perpetuating factors [e.g. 18–22].

In terms of the research supporting the 3P model, and indeed other, subsequent models, a significant number of studies have examined both the predisposing and precipitating aspects of insomnia. Overall, research has shown that those with insomnia tend to display the personality characteristics of high neuroticism and perfectionism, and low extraversion [23, 24]. Furthermore, stress in any form (life events, chronic stress, and daily hassles) has been shown to result in an increase in insomnia symptoms [25, 26]. Even experimentally induced stress results in poor sleep for people who otherwise sleep "normally" [27, 28]. In terms of perpetuating factors, there is now a great deal of research support for the notion that people with insomnia have both attention and interpretative biases toward sleep and have more dysfunctional attitudes and beliefs about their sleep [29–31]. That said, virtually no studies have assessed whether people with insomnia engage in the more behaviorally based perpetuating factors (i.e., going to be early, lying in, napping, sleep effort or using the bedroom for daytime activities). However, as you will see in the later section on treatment section, strategies to address these behavioral perpetuating factors are the main focus of CBT-I, the primary nonpharmacological approach, which works!

THE SIGNIFICANCE OF INSOMNIA

When we consider whether any condition, illness, or disability is an important issue, we need to ask ourselves two questions: (i) How common is the condition, and (b) what are the costs and consequences of having that condition, compared to not having that condition? To answer the first question, naturally, we need a definition, so we can determine how many people have or will develop the condition. Then, we can perform epidemiological studies to count the number of people with the condition at a certain point in time (prevalence) or who develop the condition over a specific period of time (incidence). Using the DSM-5 diagnosis for identifying those with insomnia, research suggests that acute insomnia (fewer than 3 months) affects around 8% of the population [32]. Chronic insomnia affects somewhere between 9% to 15% of the population (although these studies used earlier versions of our diagnostic tools—the ICSD-2 or DSM-IV) [33]. In terms of incidence, approximately a third of the population will develop an episode of acute insomnia (36.6%) [32], in a given year, whereas only around 3% of the population will develop insomnia disorder in a given year [34]. What this suggests is that every year many people will get acute insomnia, but not many of them will go on to develop insomnia disorder. For those who do develop full insomnia disorder, however, the news is not great, with one study showing that most people with insomnia are likely to still have it 2 years later (74%) and over

half (54%) will still have it 3 years later [35]. In essence, insomnia is a highly in-
cidental and prevalent condition which, without intervention, is likely to persist.

So, what about the costs and consequences of insomnia? To answer these
questions, we look at two types of outcomes—health-related and nonhealth-
related. Both dimensions can be examined based on the impact of insomnia on
the individual and on society. In terms of an individual's health, research has
shown that you are more likely to have a physical (e.g., cancer, cardiovascular
disease, type 2 diabetes) or psychological (e.g., anxiety, posttraumatic stress disorder) illness if you have insomnia, compared to if you do not [36, 37]. However,
the issue of causality should be noted here: Is the illness causing the insomnia or
is insomnia causing the illness? Irrespective, individuals with insomnia do demonstrate overall poorer health-related quality of life than "normal" sleepers [38].
The most conclusive evidence for a causal link between insomnia and health is in
the area of depression research, with numerous studies now demonstrating that
insomnia poses a significant risk for both first and future episodes of depression
[39–41]. Beyond an individual's health, research has also shown that having insomnia is linked to accidents and poor performance in the workplace [42, 43],
marital disharmony at home [44], and increased risk-taking behavior among both
adolescents and adults [45, 46]. Overall, the direct (health-related) and indirect
(nonhealth related) costs of insomnia have been estimated at CAD$6.6 billion (or
approximately US$5.1 billion or £4.03 billion) per year [47].

Once we have determined the prevalence and incidence of a condition, like
insomnia, and its direct and indirect costs, the next thing we do is determine
what increases the chances of developing that condition (i.e., increased risk).
Identifying these risk factors can help prevent the condition. In terms of demographic factors, being female, older, and from a lower socioeconomic status
group have consistently been shown to increase the risk for developing insomnia
[4, 48]. As previously mentioned, having had a previous episode of insomnia also
increases the risk of a future episode [49]. Beyond demographic factors, having
an illness (either physical or psychological), exposure to stress (including bullying
and discrimination), and/or being hospitalized or imprisoned have all been
shown to increase the risk for getting insomnia [50–52]. Together, this picture
gives us a clue as to whom we should target, and where we should aim our prevention strategies.

HOW WE MANAGE INSOMNIA

Insomnia is currently managed using two main approaches: pharmacologically
and nonpharmacologically, both of which have advantages and disadvantages.
Pharmacological approaches generally incorporate benzodiazepines or Z-
hypnotics (both of which work by increasing, albeit in slightly different ways, the
potency and activity of the gamma-aminobutyric acid, a sleep-promoting neurotransmitter). Studies have shown that both types of drugs improve sleep to
differing degrees; however, benzodiazepines have long been associated with side

effects (e.g., insomnia tends to recur after discontinuing use [known as rebound insomnia], daytime hangover effects, nausea) in addition to being addictive and less effective with longer-term use (i.e., increased tolerance). The Z-hypnotics were designed to address these issues and are consequently shorter acting (i.e., their effects do not last as long). That said, Z-hypnotics have still been associated with some side effects [53]. General practitioners in the United Kingdom are now reluctant to prescribe either of these drugs; a recent study showed that 95% were more likely to either offer sleep hygiene advice (detailed in the following discussion) or prescribe a low-dosage antidepressant (e.g., amitriptyline) [54].

The main alternative to hypnotics and/or antidepressants is CBT-I. CBT-I is a talking therapy that usually involves 6 to 8 weekly sessions of about an hour each week. At each of the sessions, new techniques are introduced that aim to reduce or eliminate different perpetuating factors while also increasing the drive to sleep via the sleep homeostat (see Table 18.1 for an overview). In terms of sleep hygiene, lifestyle factors such as caffeine, alcohol, and tobacco use are normally discussed, in addition to whether the bedroom is cool, dark, and quiet; each of these factors (i.e., heat, light, and noise) are well-known for their potential to negatively affect sleep. Clinicians also ask about exercise, food, and liquid intake, especially in terms of when these things occur, as doing them too close to bedtime can interrupt the normal sleep process.

The final aspect of sleep hygiene is to stop an individual from clock-watching, as we all have a tendency to want to know the time when we awaken, even in the middle of the night. This can be stressful, further preventing sleep, especially when we start to calculate how long we have been asleep and how much time we have left before we are due to get up. To avoid clock-watching, we ask the patient to remove visible clock faces from their bedroom. The interesting thing to note about sleep hygiene is that patients usually have reasonable knowledge of sleep hygiene before they begin CBT-I, so that sleep hygiene alone is unlikely to fix an individual's insomnia [55].

Sleep diaries are completed every day throughout the CBT-I treatment, to track the patients' symptoms—sleep onset latency, number of awakenings, and time wake after sleep onset are collected, in addition to working out the level of sleep restriction that is to be prescribed to the patient. To calculate this prescription, the average TST from a pretreatment sleep diary (completed for 1 or 2 weeks beforehand) becomes their TIB for the first week of sleep restriction. Each following week we calculate the average SE for that week to help us determine how much sleep restriction or extension needs to take place. If an individual's SE is between 85% and 90%, then we would continue with the originally prescribed sleep restriction schedule, but if it goes over 90%, then we would give the individual a further 15 minutes in bed each night for the following week. The most important thing to remember is to never restrict the patients' sleep too much; otherwise, it could be harmful, and so we tend to set a limit of 5 hours TIB minimum.

Both the sleep restriction and stimulus control techniques (getting out of bed if you are not asleep, potentially several times a night) are the most challenging to patients, as we are asking them to spend a lot less time in the bedroom, and this, we

Table 18.1 SLEEP DIARY EXAMPLE

MEASURING THE PATTERN OF YOUR SLEEP	Day 1	Day 2	Day 3	Day 4	Day 5	Day 6	Day 7
1. What time did you wake this morning?							
2. At what time did you get out of bed?							
3. At what time did you go to bed last night?							
4. Lights Out: At what time did you put the lights out to go to sleep?							
5. Flow long did it take you to fall asleep (minutes)? (After Lights Out)							
6. Flow many times did you wake up during the night?							
7. Flow long were you awake during the night (in total)?							
8. About how long did you sleep altogether (hours/mins)?							
9. Did you use anything to help you sleep (medication, herbal, alcohol)? (Y/N)							

MEASURING OTHER ACTIVITIES

1. How was the quality of your sleep lagt night?
0   1   2   3   4
very poor   moderately ok   very good

2. How physically tense were you last night at bedtime?
0   1   2   3   4
not at all   moderately   very

3. How mentally alert were you last night at bedtime?
0   1   2   3   4
not at all   moderately   very

4. Did you nap in the daytime and for how long? time and duration)

believe, is the main reason a patient will drop out of therapy [56]. I find it helpful to discuss what the patient will do with all their extra time outside the bedroom and work with them to find things that are not going to seem like a punishment but that will also not make their sleep problem worse (e.g., drinking alcohol). It has recently been determined that CBT-I should be the first treatment used for insomnia [57–59], despite these issues with drop out and the fact that there are very few clinicians who are properly trained in delivering CBT-I. This recommendation was based on several hundred studies which cumulative suggest that CBT-I is (i) equally effective and potentially longer lasting than pharmacotherapy; (ii) effective for between 70% to 80% of those with insomnia; (iii) effective for people with a variety of physical and psychological conditions; and (iv) results in significant reductions in the symptoms of anxiety and depression [60–63].

CONCLUSION

The aim of this chapter was to introduce you to the concept of insomnia. After defining the condition, we moved on to discuss how insomnia develops, and what makes some people more vulnerable to insomnia. We then examined how common insomnia is and how problematic for the individual's health and well-being, as well as how much it costs society in terms of increased healthcare and non-healthcare costs. Insomnia is a remarkably common issue that increases the chances that an individual will develop other physical and/or psychological problems. Moreover, the combined costs of insomnia to society are quite large and not just in terms of the increased burden on the healthcare system. Finally, we examined the various options currently used to treat insomnia. Both the advantages and disadvantages of drugs (pharmacological) and nonpharmacological approaches were outlined. In summary, insomnia is best managed using CBT-I, even for those with other illnesses alongside their insomnia. However, much work remains to be done, including to help those who do not benefit from CBT-I, find CBT-I too challenging, or do not want to undertake CBT-I in the first place.

REFERENCES

1. World Health Organization. *The ICD-10 Classification of Mental and Behavioural Disorders: Clinical Descriptions and Diagnostic Guidelines*. Geneva, Switzerland: World Health Organization; 1992.
2. American Academy of Sleep Medicine. *International Classification of Sleep Disorders*. 3rd ed. Darien, IL: American Academy of Sleep Medicine; 2014.
3. American Psychiatric Association. *Diagnostic and Statistical Manual of Mental Disorders*. 5th ed. Arlington, VA: American Psychiatric Publishing; 2013.
4. Ellis JG. Insomnia: nosological classification, definitions, epidemiology. In: Bassetti C, Dogas Z, Peigneux P, eds. *Sleep medicine textbook*. Regensburg, Germany: European Sleep Research Society; 2014:151–165.

5. Buysse DJ, Cheng Y, Germain A, et al. Night-to-night sleep variability in older adults with and without chronic insomnia. *Sleep Med.* 2010;11:56–64.

6. Bastien CH, Vallières A, Morin CM. Validation of the Insomnia Severity Index as an outcome measure for insomnia research. *Sleep Med.* 2001;2:297–307.

7. Morin CM, Belleville G, Bélanger L, Ivers H. The Insomnia Severity Index: psychometric indicators to detect insomnia cases and evaluate treatment response. *Sleep.* 2011;34:601–608.

8. Buysse DJ, Reynolds CF 3rd, Monk TH, Berman SR, Kupfer DJ. The Pittsburgh Sleep Quality Index: a new instrument for psychiatric practice and research. *Psychiatr Res.* 1989;28:193–213.

9. Spielman AJ. Assessment of insomnia. *Clin Psychol Rev.* 1986;6:11–25.

10. Spielman AJ, Caruso LS, Glovinsky PB. A behavioral perspective on insomnia treatment. *Psychiatr Clin.* 1987:10:541–553.

11. Watts FN, Coyle K, East MP. The contribution of worry to insomnia. *Brit J Clin Psychol.* 1994;33:211–220.

12. Ellis JG, Gehrman P, Espie CA, Riemann D, Perlis ML. Acute insomnia: current conceptualizations and future directions. *Sleep Med Rev.* 2012;16:5–14.

13. McCurry SM, Gibbons LE, Logsdon RG, Vitiello MV, Teri L. Insomnia in caregivers of persons with dementia: who is at risk and what can be done about it?. *Sleep Med. Clin.* 2009;4:519–526.

14. Spielman AJ, Saskin P, Thorpy MJ. Treatment of chronic insomnia by restriction of time in bed. *Sleep.* 1987;10:45–56.

15. Bootzin RR, Epstein D, Wood JM. Stimulus control instructions. In: Hauri PJ, ed. *Case studies in insomnia.* Boston, MA: Springer; 1991:12–28.

16. Broomfield NM, Espie CA. Towards a valid, reliable measure of sleep effort. *J Sleep Res.* 2005;14:401–407.

17. Perlis M, Ellis J, Kloss J, Riemann D. Insomnia: Etiology and pathophysiology of insomnia. In: Kryger MH, Roth T, Demen WC, eds. *Principles and Practice of Sleep Medicine.* 6th ed. Philadelphia, PA: Elsevier Saunders; 2016:769–784.

18. Morin CM. *Insomnia: Psychological Assessment and Management.* New York, NY: Guilford Press; 1993.

19. Harvey AG. A cognitive model of insomnia. *Behav Res Thera.*2002;40:869–893.

20. Espie CA, Broomfield NM, MacMahon KM, Macphee LM, Taylor LM. The attention–intention–effort pathway in the development of psychophysiologic insomnia: a theoretical review. *Sleep Med Rev.* 2006;10:215–245.

21. Perlis ML, Giles DE, Mendelson WB, Bootzin RR, Wyatt JK. Psychophysiological insomnia: the behavioural model and a neurocognitive perspective. *J Sleep Res.* 1997;6:179–188.

22. Buysse DJ, Germain A, Hall M, Monk TH, Nofzinger EA. A neurobiological model of insomnia. *Drug Disc Today Dis Mod.* 2011;8:129–137.

23. van de Laar M, Verbeek I, Pevernagie D, Aldenkamp A, Overeem S. The role of personality traits in insomnia. *Sleep Med Rev.* 2010;14:61–68.

24. LeBlanc M, Beaulieu-Bonneau S, Mérette C, Savard J, Ivers H, Morin CM. Psychological and health-related quality of life factors associated with insomnia in a population-based sample. *J Psychosom Res.*2007;63:157–166.

25. Bastien CH, Vallieres A, Morin CM. Precipitating factors of insomnia. *Behav Sleep Med.* 2004;2:50–62.

26. Morin CM, Rodrigue S, Ivers H. Role of stress, arousal, and coping skills in primary insomnia. *Psychosom Med.* 2003;65:259–267.
27. Hall M, Vasko R, Buysse D, et al. Acute stress affects heart rate variability during sleep. *Psychosom Med.* 2004;66:56–62.
28. Germain A, Buysse DJ, Ombao H, Kupfer DJ, Hall M. Psychophysiological reactivity and coping styles influence the effects of acute stress exposure on rapid eye movement sleep. *Psychosom Med.* 2003;65:857–864.
29. Ree MJ, Pollitt A, Harvey AG. An investigation of interpretive bias in insomnia: an analog study comparing normal and poor sleepers. *Sleep.* 2006;29:1359–1362.
30. Akram U, Ellis JG, Myachykov A, Barclay NL. Misperception of tiredness in young adults with insomnia. *J Sleep Res* 2016;25:466–474.
31. Barclay NL, Ellis JG. Sleep-related attentional bias in poor versus good sleepers is independent of affective valence. *J Sleep Res.* 2013;22:414–421.
32. Ellis JG, Perlis ML, Neale LF, Espie CA, Bastien CH. The natural history of insomnia: focus on prevalence and incidence of acute insomnia. *J Psychiatr Res.* 2012;46:1278–1285.
33. Ohayon MM. Epidemiology of insomnia: what we know and what we still need to learn. *Sleep Med Rev.* 2002;6:97–111.
34. Jansson-Fröjmark M, Linton SJ. The course of insomnia over one year: a longitudinal study in the general population in Sweden. *Sleep.* 2008;31:881–886.
35. Morin CM, Bélanger L, LeBlanc M, et al. The natural history of insomnia: a population-based 3-year longitudinal study. *Arch Intern Med.* 2009;169:447–453.
36. Taylor DJ, Lichstein KL, Durrence HH. Insomnia as a health risk factor. *Behav Sleep Med.* 2003;1:227–247.
37. Roth T. Insomnia: definition, prevalence, etiology, and consequences. *J Clin Sleep Med.* 2007;3:S7.
38. Kyle SD, Morgan K, Espie CA. Insomnia and health-related quality of life. *Sleep Med Rev.* 2010;14:69–82.
39. Baglioni C, Battagliese G, Feige B, et al. Insomnia as a predictor of depression: a meta-analytic evaluation of longitudinal epidemiological studies. *J Affect Dis* 2011;135:10–19.
40. Chang PP, Ford DE, Mead LA, Cooper-Patrick L, Klag MJ. Insomnia in young men and subsequent depression: the Johns Hopkins Precursors Study. *Am J Epidemiol.* 1997;146:105–114.
41. Ellis JG, Perlis ML, Bastien CH, Gardani M, Espie CA. The natural history of insomnia: acute insomnia and first-onset depression. *Sleep.* 2014; 37:97–106.
42. Leger D, Guilleminault C, Bader G, Levy E, Paillard M. Medical and socioprofessional impact of insomnia. *Sleep.* 2002;25:625–629.
43. Kuppermann M, Lubeck DP, Mazonson PD, et al. Sleep problems and their correlates in a working population. *J Gen Intern Med.* 1995;10:25–32.
44. Troxel WM, Robles TF, Hall M, Buysse DJ. Marital quality and the marital bed: Examining the covariation between relationship quality and sleep. *Sleep Med Rev.* 2007;11:389–404.
45. Catrett CD, Gaultney JF. Possible insomnia predicts some risky behaviors among adolescents when controlling for depressive symptoms. *J Gen Psychol* 2009;170:287–309.

46. Roehrs T, Greenwald M, Roth T. Risk-taking behavior: effects of ethanol, caffeine, and basal sleepiness. *Sleep.* 2004;27:887–893.

47. Daley M, Morin CM, LeBlanc M, Gregoire JP, Savard J. The economic burden of insomnia: direct and indirect costs for individuals with insomnia syndrome, insomnia symptoms, and good sleepers. *Sleep.* 2009;32:55–64.

48. Hall MH, Matthews KA, Kravitz HM, et al. Race and financial strain are independent correlates of sleep in midlife women: the SWAN sleep study. *Sleep.* 2009;32:73–82.

49. Klink ME, Quan SF, Kaltenborn WT, Lebowitz MD. Risk factors associated with complaints of insomnia in a general adult population: influence of previous complaints of insomnia. *Arch Intern Med.* 1992;152:1634–1637.

50. Slopen N, Lewis TT, Williams DR. Discrimination and sleep: a systematic review. *Sleep Med.* 2016;18:88–95.

51. Griffiths MF, Peerson A. Risk factors for chronic insomnia following hospitalization. *J Advanc Nurs.* 2005;49:245–253.

52. Dewa LH, Kyle SD, Hassan L, Shaw J, Senior J. Prevalence, associated factors and management of insomnia in prison populations: an integrative review. *Sleep Med Rev.* 2015;24:13–27.

53. Wilson SJ, Nutt DJ, Alford C, et al. British Association for Psychopharmacology consensus statement on evidence-based treatment of insomnia, parasomnias and circadian rhythm disorders. *J Psychopharmacol* 2010;24:1577–15601.

54. Everitt H, McDermott L, Leydon G, Yules H, Baldwin D, Little P. GPs' management strategies for patients with insomnia: a survey and qualitative interview study. *Brit J Gen Pract.* 2014;64:e112–e119.

55. Ellis JG, Allen SF. Sleep hygiene and the prevention of chronic insomnia. In: Grandner MA, ed. *Sleep and Health.* London, UK: Academic Press; 2019:137–145.

56. Ong JC, Kuo TF, Manber R. Who is at risk for dropout from group cognitive-behavior therapy for insomnia? *J Psychosom Res.* 2008;64:419–425.

57. Wilson SJ, Nutt DJ, Alford C, et al. British Association for Psychopharmacology consensus statement on evidence-based treatment of insomnia, parasomnias and circadian rhythm disorders. *J Psychopharmacol.* 2010;24:1577–1601.

58. Qaseem A, Kansagara D, Forciea MA, Cooke M, Denberg TD. Management of chronic insomnia disorder in adults: a clinical practice guideline from the American College of Physicians. *Ann Intern Med.* 2016;165:125–133.

59. Riemann D, Baglioni C, Bassetti C, et al. European guideline for the diagnosis and treatment of insomnia. *J Sleep Res.* 2017;26:675–700.

60. Mitchell MD, Gehrman P, Perlis M, Umscheid CA. Comparative effectiveness of cognitive behavioral therapy for insomnia: a systematic review. *BMC Fam Pract.* 2012;13:40.

61. Trauer JM, Qian MY, Doyle JS, Rajaratnam SM, Cunnington D. Cognitive behavioral therapy for chronic insomnia: a systematic review and meta-analysis. *Ann Intern Med.* 2015;163:191–204.

62. Smith MT, Huang MI, Manber R. Cognitive behavior therapy for chronic insomnia occurring within the context of medical and psychiatric disorders. *Clin Psychol Rev.* 2005;25:559–592.

63. Manber R, Bernert RA, Suh S, Nowakowski S, Siebern AT, Ong JC. CBT for insomnia in patients with high and low depressive symptom severity: adherence and clinical outcomes. *J Clin Sleep Med.* 2011;7:645–652.

Parasomnias, Narcolepsy, and Restless Legs Syndrome

**OLIVIERO BRUNI, MARCO ANGRIMAN,
MARIA GRAZIA MELEGARI, AND RAFFAELE FERRI ■**

INTRODUCTION

The term *parasomnia* derives from the Greek "para" meaning "around" and the Latin "somnus" meaning "sleep." The most recent *International Classification of Sleep Disorder* (ICSD-3) [1] defines parasomnias as "undesirable physical events or experiences that occur during entry into sleep, within sleep, or during arousal from sleep."

All parasomnias events appear episodically (i.e., at regular intervals) during sleep, without disrupting the architecture of sleep. They also have specific features: they are each associated with specific sleep phases; they might be associated with partial awakenings; and they commonly have a benign evolution, with spontaneous resolution during puberty.

Parasomnias include several specific disorders that share clinical and physiological characteristics: (i) clear and dramatic symptoms associated with autonomic nervous system changes and skeletal muscle activity; (ii) correlation with age; (iii) unassociated medical problems; (iv) absence of specific polysomnographic anomalies; (v) spontaneous resolution; and (vi) unknown etiology. The classification of parasomnias is related to the sleep stage during which they occur: nonrapid eye movement (NREM)-related parasomnias, including disorders of arousal (DoA; confusional arousals, sleepwalking, sleep terrors, and sleep-related eating disorder [SRED]), rapid eye movement (REM)-related parasomnias (REM sleep behavior disorder [RBD], recurrent isolated sleep paralysis, and nightmare disorder), and other parasomnias (exploding head syndrome, sleep-related hallucinations, and sleep enuresis [SE]). Table 19.1 describes the classification we

Table 19.1 Classification of Parasomnias Based on ICSD-3

NREM-related parasomnias	REM-related parasomnias	Other parasomnias
Confusional arousals	REM sleep behavior disorder	Exploding head syndrome
Sleepwalking	Recurrent isolated sleep paralysis	Sleep-related hallucinations
Sleep terrors	Nightmare disorder	Sleep enuresis
Sleep-related eating disorder		

use for each of these disorders—and the details of each are described in the following discussion, after a general introduction to this class of disorders.

Physicians base their diagnosis of the majority of parasomnias on clinical manifestations and history; therefore, it is extremely important for them to have an accurate description of the features of the patient's episode and, ultimately, a video recording of the event. Questions they use to evaluate the patient include:

- Timing of appearance of the symptom.
- Exact behavior: manifested movements and symptoms.
- Possible movement of the child from the bed.
- Moment of nocturnal/daytime sleep in which symptoms occur.
- Reaction to external interventions (if the symptom worsens).
- Recall of the episode.
- Presence of stereotypies (rhythmic, repetitive movements) during the episode.

If the physician has clinical doubts, polysomnographic recordings (also see Chapter 22 of this volume) are essential to differentiate their diagnosis from other, potentially comorbid (simultaneously co-occurring), sleep disorders like sleep-disordered breathing or narcolepsy or with nocturnal seizures.

The current pathophysiological theories consider parasomnias to be state dissociation, characterized by the coexistence of both wake- and sleep-like activities within cortical and subcortical areas of the brain. Although parasomnias are not usually associated with a primary complaint of insomnia or excessive sleepiness, they are considered clinical disorders because they may result in injuries, adverse health, and psychosocial effects.

The main treatment for parasomnias is based on patient education and behavioral management, but pharmacological treatment (also see Chapter 21 of this volume) may be needed when episodes are frequent and persist despite resolution of possible inducing factors, are associated with a high risk of injury, or cause secondary consequences [2].

NREM-RELATED PARASOMNIA

NREM-related parasomnia or DoA are defined in the ICSD-3 as recurrent episodes of incomplete awakening from sleep, characterized by inappropriate or absent responsiveness to efforts of others to intervene or redirect the person during the episode and with limited or no associated cognition or dream imagery. Subjects have partial or complete amnesia for the episode [1].

DoA includes confusional arousals, sleep terrors, sleepwalking (also called somnambulism), and SRED. There is usually only one event per night, which typically occurs during the first third of the major (usually nocturnal) sleep episode and the individual may continue to appear confused and disoriented for several minutes, or even longer, following the episode. They are usually benign events, habitually occurring in childhood and ceasing by adolescence; in rare cases they may begin in, or persist into, adulthood. Sometimes, however, they involve complex behavior with potentially violent or injurious features.

In some cases, differential diagnosis (the process of differentiating between two or more conditions sharing similar signs or symptoms) is not simple. This is because DoA may mimic nocturnal seizures or RBD (described in detail later in the chapter) and the parents' descriptions of events may be inaccurate, especially when the events make them anxious or even terrified. Thus, a video of the episode can be extremely important to correctly define the event, and if there are still doubts, polysomnographic recordings with video help in the clinical diagnosis. Some individual may even experience more than one type of arousal parasomnia [2].

At the end of each NREM period, we experience a state transition leading to one of three possible manifestations: transition to a lighter sleep stage, complete awakening, and partial arousal (a state in which the individual, most often a child, is unable to awaken completely, to get out of deep sleep, or to transition to the next sleep cycle).

Pathophysiology

NREM parasomnias occur when there is an incomplete dissociation of NREM sleep into wakefulness. There are several potential causes for this. First, phenomena that deepen sleep and enhance sleep inertia promote NREM parasomnias by impairing normal arousal mechanisms. Second, conditions that cause repeated cortical arousals lead to NREM parasomnias through sleep fragmentation. Third, an impaired arousal mechanism and the persistence of sleep drive result in a failure of the brain to fully transition into wakefulness [3].

The DoA is considered a phenotypical (i.e., physical, or somatic) expression of simultaneous states of sleep and wakefulness. For example, investigators captured a sleepwalking event in a 16-year-old boy using cranial single photon emission computed tomography, a functional neuroimaging technique; the event was characterized by activation (increased regional cerebral blood flow) of thalamocingulate (motor coordination) pathways, with simultaneous deactivation in the frontal lobe [4]. Two studies with depth electroencephalogram (EEG) electrodes have shown frequent, short-lasting, local activations of the motor cortex, paralleled by a concomitant increase in slow waves in the dorsolateral prefrontal cortex—suggesting the coexistence of sleep and wakefulness in different brain regions [5, 6]. This group also found an EEG pattern of wakefulness in the motor and central cingulate cortices and concomitant increased delta bursts (indicative of sleep) in the frontal and parietal dorsolateral associative cortices [5]. When a short, local activation appears in the motor cortex, a burst of slow waves characterizes the other two EEG derivations [6].

Apart from the phenomenon of state dissociation, other mechanisms seem to contribute to the appearance of these sleep disorders:

1 *Activations of innate behaviors and locomotor centers.* It has been hypothesized that clinical features of parasomnias could result from a release of inhibition of central pattern generators that are functional neural organizations regulating innate behavioral automatisms and survival behaviors, which are located in the spinal cord, mesencephalon, pons, and bulb [7].
2. *Arousal instability.* Subjects with NREM parasomnia show increased arousals and cyclic alternating pattern rate during slow-wave sleep, even on nights without episodes, reflecting an alteration of NREM sleep continuity and different dynamics of slow wave activity throughout the night [8].
3. *Genetic influences.* About 80% of sleepwalkers have at least one family member affected by this parasomnia and the prevalence of somnambulism is higher in children of parents with a history of sleepwalking [9].
4. *Psychopathology.* Not all research studies agree that psychological factors contribute to arousal parasomnias; there is a lack of a definitive association between a history of major psychological trauma, severe psychopathology, and sleepwalking/night terrors [10].

Epidemiology

NREM parasomnias are a common pediatric sleep disorder that tends to decrease across development. Almost all children occasionally have confusional arousals; in particular, during the preschool years, they frequently experience minor episodes of partial awakening from sleep, which their parents may not even notice. Laberge et al. [11] found that about 17% of children between 3 and 13 years old experience occasional or frequent episodes of confusional arousals. In another study, Ohayon et al. observed that confusional arousal affect 4.2% of the general population, decreasing from 6.1% among those 15 to 24 years old to 3.3% among those ages 25 to 34, and stabilizing around 2% after age 35 years [12]. The prevalence of sleepwalking in children ranges from 3% to 14.5%, and most episodes resolve after age 10 years. Sleep terrors have the greatest incidence in preschool children, with a reported overall prevalence of 17.3% in children between 3 to 13 years. Another longitudinal study reported the frequency of this sleep disorder to be 39.8% among children ages 2½ to 6 years, with a peak incidence at ages 2½, 3½, and 4 years [13]. NREM parasomnias in adults mostly represent a continuation of episodes after adolescence.

Clinical Features

NREM parasomnias occur along a continuum, ranging from confusional arousals with low motor and autonomic activation at the lower end of the spectrum, up to sleepwalking characterized by intense motor activity and mild autonomic activation at the high end of the spectrum. For example, a child might present a sequence of confusional arousals in early childhood and sleepwalking when they are slightly older, followed by sleep terrors in their late childhood and adolescence. These three disorders show common features (see Table 19.2).

Any factor that deepens sleep (e.g., sleep deprivation, stress, febrile [fever-inducing] illness, medications, alcohol) or is associated with arousals (external or internal stimuli) may increase the occurrence of NREM parasomnias.

Table 19.2 CLINICAL FEATURES OF DISORDERS OF AROUSAL

	Confusional Arousal	Sleepwalking	Night terrors
Age	2–10 years	4–12 years	18 months–10 years
Onset	First third of night	First third of night	First third of might
Agitation	Mild	No/poor	Marked
Autonomic activity	Medium	Mild	Marked
Motor activity	Low	Complex	Rarely complex
Ictal behavior	Whimpering, some articulation, sitting up in bed, inconsolable	Screaming, agitation, flushed face, sweating, inconsolable	Walking around, quiet or agitated, unresponsive to verbal commands
Amnesia	Yes	Yes	Yes
Threshold of arousal	High	High	High
Familiarity	High	High	High

CONFUSIONAL AROUSAL

Confusional arousals are episodes characterized by mental confusion or confused behavior that occurs while the patient is in bed, in the absence of terror or ambulation outside of the bed [1]. The child looks awake but is confused, disoriented, sometimes aggressive, does not respond adequately to orders, and can speak but in an inconsistent way. Episodes usually start with a moan and some movements and then progresses toward crying; the expression of terror typical of the *pavor nocturnus* is missing. The duration varies from a few minutes to 40 to 60 minutes.

The exact prevalence is unknown due to the difficulty of classification (i.e., distressed parents' descriptions are usually highly inaccurate). The debut is before the child turns 5 years old.

SLEEPWALKING

Sleepwalking is a series of complex behaviors that are usually initiated during arousals from slow-wave sleep and culminate in leaving the bed in an altered state of consciousness. The subject acts out more or less complex, automatic movements that vary from simply sitting on the bed to walking around the house in an agitated manner associated with semipurposeful behaviors such as eating, drinking, leaving home, etc. These episodes can be concomitant with vocalization, often in an incomprehensible language and sometimes aggressive acts can occur, usually in relation to attempts to block the child or to awaken him. The average duration of the episodes is around 10 minutes. Typically, parents report that the episode ends after the child has gone to the bathroom to urinate; this has led to the supposition that bladder repletion may contribute to these episodes.

The age of onset is generally between 4 and 8 years, with a peak at 12 years and then episodes disappear during adolescence. The prevalence is between 15% and 30% for sporadic episodes and 3% for frequent episodes. There is no difference between males and females.

A high level of familiarity is characteristic: around 80% have other family members with sleepwalking or other arousal disorders, with a chance of recurrence of 45% if one parent is affected and 60% if two parents are affected.

Some precipitating factors have been identified, including fever, sleep deprivation, obstructive apnea, bladder distension, external noises, and drugs (neuroleptics, chloral, some tricyclic antidepressants). The concomitance and association with a psychopathological profile has only been highlighted in adulthood [8].

SLEEP TERRORS

During a sleep terror episode, the child presents with a sudden onset of partial awakening, a loud cry, intense agitation, autonomic symptoms (pallor, sweating, tachycardia, tachypnea, increased arterial pressure, mydriasis) and increased muscle tone. In this state, the child is not very responsive to environmental stimulation and will not recognizing those close to them; they may seem to "look beyond," appear terrified, and be inconsolable. Less often, they may also get out of bed and walk around the house. These episodes are short (typically a few minutes) in duration but can range from 30 seconds to 30 minutes. If awakened, the child will be confused and disoriented, although will usually return to sleep quickly and in the morning will not remember the episode (unlike nightmares, with which memories are often vivid). Some of these characteristics overlap with those of somnambulism, although sleep terrors differ in their autonomic activation and distinct expression of terror. They can occur more than once a night and up to several times per week.

The prevalence of sleep terrors varies between 1% to 6% and is slightly higher among males; the typical age of onset is from 2 to 4 years, with a peak between 5 and 7 years old. There is a high overlap between sleep terrors and other parasomnias. The precipitating factors are stress, fever, bladder distension, and sleep deprivation. As with sleepwalking, there is no apparent relationship with psychopathology [14].

The diagnosis of sleep terrors is mainly based on clinical descriptors: a general and hypnic anamnesis, questionnaire, and sleep diaries; a video recording of a typical episode in the home by the parents is also extremely important. A clear clinical history can be sufficient to diagnose the presence of NREM parasomnia in the majority of cases, but in others only video polysomnographic (PSG) recording can clarify the nature of the disorder. Typical polysomnographic features of sleep architecture of patients with NREM parasomnia include hypersynchronous delta waves, irregular buildup of slow-wave activity, and NREM sleep instability. NREM parasomnia needs to be distinguished from other parasomnias, nocturnal panic attacks, and sleep-related seizures [16].

Nightmares can sometimes resemble sleep terrors, although nightmares occur during REM sleep and are therefore more prominent in the second half of the night; children who arouse after a nightmare usually become fully alert quickly, respond positively to comforting, may report the dream content after awakening, and show lower levels of autonomic activation (e.g., palpitations or dyspnea), vocalization, and mobility.

NOCTURNAL PANIC ATTACKS

Nocturnal panic attacks consist in waking from sleep in a state of panic, with intense fear or discomfort. They are more frequent in adults and are sometimes appear indistinguishable from sleep terrors. However, patients with sleep panic attacks do not become physically agitated or aggressive during the attack; immediately after the episodes, they also appear oriented, can vividly recall their attack, and usually have difficulty returning to sleep [15].

NOCTURNAL FRONTAL LOBE EPILEPSY OR SLEEP HYPERMOTOR EPILEPSY

Initially recognized as nocturnal paroxysmal dystonia and included in the parasomnias group, nocturnal frontal lobe epilepsy (NFLE) or sleep hypermotor epilepsy is actually acknowledged as an epileptic syndrome with seizures occurring almost exclusively during sleep. These seizures usually begin before 20 years of age and peak during childhood. NFLE or sleep hypermotor epilepsy patients may show a variety of different sleep-related motor attacks of increasing complexity and duration, varying from short-lasting stereotyped movements to paroxysmal arousals, major attacks, and epileptic nocturnal wandering. Taking into account the similarities and possible coexistence of parasomnias in those with NFLE, the differential diagnosis between these disorders can be complicated [17].

NREM Parasomnia Treatment

Parasomnia attacks in healthy children and adolescents are often benign and normally require no treatment. Reassuring the patient and caregivers about the generally benign nature of the episodes is sometimes sufficient. Sleep medicine specialists also work with parents on adopting the principles of sleep hygiene, such as maintaining a regular sleep–wake rhythm, avoiding sleep deprivation and medications that may contribute to the episodes, discouraging parental interventions, and not trying to awaken the child. The latter are because the child can react and get hurt; interventions can even prolong the episode. Relaxation techniques prior to sleep and hypnosis have also been recommended. Identifying coexisting sleep disorders is another important step.

So-called anticipatory or scheduled awakenings consist of awakening the child about 15 minutes before the presumed time when the episode will occur (they usually occur at very regular times and always within 2 hours of falling asleep). This may shift the child into a lighter state of sleep, thereby aborting the event.

A psychotherapeutic approach can be feasible if there is a suspicion that there may be a psychological problem. Especially in the case of sleepwalking, environmental safety issues should be discussed with the parents and represent a first-line approach.

Pharmacotherapy should be considered only when the episodes are frequent or dangerous to the patient or others or when they cause undesirable secondary consequences, such as excessive daytime sleepiness (EDS) or distress to the patient or their family. Patients should therefore be advised that prescribed drugs are considered "off-label" [18, 19]. L-5-hydroxytryptophan, a precursor of serotonin that may modify central serotoninergic system dysfunction or enhance production of sleep-promoting factors [20], can be effective in the treatment of sleep terrors. Melatonin has also proven helpful for patients with sleepwalking and sleep terrors [21]. For more detailed information, also see Chapter 21 of this volume.

SLEEP-RELATED EATING DISORDER

SRED consists of "recurrent episodes of involuntary eating and drinking during arousals from sleep, associated with diminished levels of consciousness and subsequent recall, with problematic consequences" (p. 240) [1]. Episodes typically occur during partial arousals from sleep during the first third of the night, with impaired subsequent recall [22]. SRED occurs predominantly in adult women, and the average age of onset is approximately 22 to 27 years, with a typical 12 to 16 years before patients present their symptoms to their healthcare provider.

REM-RELATED PARASOMNIA

The main differences between NREM parasomnias and REM-related parasomnias are the latter's occurrence during the second half of the night, when REM is more prevalent in the sleep cycle. REM-related parasomnias also feature dream enactment behaviors and the absence of mental confusion upon awakening. Some patients may meet the diagnostic criteria for both NREM and REM parasomnias; these patients are diagnosed with parasomnia overlap disorder.

REM Sleep Behavior Disorder

RBD is characterized by complex and violent behaviors. sometimes associated with dream-like thoughts and images. These usually occur in the first REM episode. The pathogenesis is linked to the absence of the REM-typical elimination of muscle tone (atonia). In the absence of normal atonia, and patients present recurrent episodes of enacting their dreams—behaviors that can vary from small hand movements to violent activities, such as punching, kicking, or leaping out of bed [23]. RBD in childhood and adolescence is rare and is usually associated with narcolepsy or idiopathic hypersomnia, neurodevelopmental–neurodegenerative disorders, or structural brainstem abnormalities; it can also represent a side effect of pharmacological agents, such as selective serotonin reuptake inhibitors agents [24, 25].

Nightmare Disorder

Nightmare disorder is characterized by "recurrent, highly dysphoric dreams, which are disturbing mental experiences that generally occur during REM sleep and that often result in awakening" (p. 257) [1].

Occasional nightmares are very common in children, ranging from 60% to 75%, but the prevalence of nightmare disorder is estimated to be 1.8% to 6% and is more frequent in children with posttraumatic stress disorder [26]. A child with nightmare disorder may be scared, but usually manages to report the dream and is well oriented, with an intact sensory (distinct from parasomnias). In this case, parental intervention is well accepted, and the child recognizes them immediately. Unlike night terrors, nightmares occur during REM and are rarely associated with vegetative symptoms; it is difficult for the child to move out of bed, there is little motor activity (due to the atony typical of REM).

Emotional contents of nightmares are characteristically negative, with significant anxiety and fear but also anger, rage, embarrassment, and disgust. Monsters or other fantastical images often characterize the dreams of young children, whereas adolescent and adults may experience more realistic images, often derived from daytime stressors or traumatic events.

Recurrent Isolated Sleep Paralysis

Recurrent isolated sleep paralysis is defined as a period of inability to perform voluntary movements, which occurs at the beginning of sleep of a sleep period (hypnagogic) and/or after waking up (hypnopompic). This can occur in the absence of narcolepsy, which is described in detail in the following discussion [1].

The individual experiencing sleep paralysis is conscious and alert but feel paralyzed; all of their muscle groups are involved, with the exception of their diaphragm and the extrinsic muscles of the eye. The attacks usually last a few minutes and end spontaneously, although they may occasionally be stopped intentionally if they individual moves their eyes rapidly or are administered tactile stimuli. These episodes commonly begin in adolescence but can also appear in childhood. Hallucinations can also occur during paralysis and commonly include sensing the presence of others nearby, pressure on the chest, or hearing footsteps.

The pathogenesis of this disorder is linked to the persistence of REM sleep into wakefulness; thus, normal mental activity occurs in the presence of body paralysis. Prevalence estimates vary widely, between 6% and 40%. Isolated episodes are exacerbated by sleep deprivation, stress, and sleep–wake rhythm irregularities [27].

The first-line treatments are reassuring the patient that the episodes are benign and to avoid sleep deprivation and other triggering factors. Pharmacologic treatment is based on REM-suppressing agents such as low doses of tricyclics, clonidine, or clonazepam.

Sleep-Related Hallucinations

Sleep-related hallucinations are "hallucinatory experiences that occur at sleep onset (hypnagogic) or on awakening from sleep (hypnopompic)" (p. 267) [1]. These can be visual, auditory, tactile, or kinetic phenomena. Complex nocturnal visual hallucinations may represent a distinct form of sleep-related hallucinations, with vivid images of people or animals, sometimes distorted in shape or size.

These hallucinations may remain present for many minutes but usually disappear if the room light is turned on. Within the general population, there is a reported prevalence of 25% to 37% for hypnagogic hallucinations and 7% to 13% for hypnopompic hallucinations. Reassurance may be sufficient for many patients but in severe cases, tricyclic antidepressants can be useful.

SLEEP ENURESIS

SE is characterized by

> recurrent involuntary voiding that occurs during sleep. In primary SE, recurrent involuntary voiding occurs at least twice a week during sleep after 5 years of age in a patient who has never been consistently dry during sleep for six consecutive months. SE is considered secondary in a child or adult who had previously been dry for six consecutive months and then began wetting at least twice a week. Both primary and secondary enuresis must be present for a period of at least three months. [1] (p. 270)

SE is defined as monosymptomatic when the subject has no associated daytime symptoms of bladder dysfunction (such as wetting, increased voiding frequency, urgency, jiggling, squatting, and holding maneuvers). However, when a meticulous history is obtained, the majority of children have at least some light daytime void symptoms, and their SE is classifiable as non-monosymptomatic [28].

Sleep enuresis is one of the most common problems in pediatrics, with a general prevalence of 3% to 15%. SE is more frequent in boys under 11 years of age, though after age 11 no sex differences are reported. Spontaneous remission during childhood occurs in around 15% of patients with this disorder.

From a developmental point of view, complete control of the bladder at night is usually achieved by age 5 years; thus, bed-wetting in toddlers is considered physiologic.

The most accepted hypothesis for the pathogenesis of sleep enuresis is that it involves three systems: excessive nocturnal urine production, nocturnal bladder overactivity, and failure to awaken in response to bladder sensations [29]. Other pathophysiological mechanisms are mostly related to sleep fragmentation, which can be secondary to sleep-disordered breathing [30] or periodic limb movements (PLM) during sleep (PLMS) [31].

Children with enuresis are often described as "deep sleepers," who have arousal thresholds that seem to be higher during all sleep stages compared to children without enuresis [28]. Enuretic events happen mainly during the first part of the night and can occur in all sleep stages; however, sleep structure is similar regardless of enuresis occurring or not on a given night [32]. One recent study reported that patients with enuresis are subjectively sleepier than normal control patients and more difficult to awaken; this was attributed to sleep fragmentation, which might be responsible for the higher arousal threshold and is consistent with a large body of research [33, 34]. There is a strong genetic predisposition for primary SE. The reported prevalence is 77% when both parents were enuretic as children and 44% when only one parent had a history of enuresis.

Secondary SE is more commonly associated with organic factors (e.g., urinary tract infections, malformations of the genitourinary tract), medical conditions that result in an inability to concentrate urine (diabetes mellitus or insipidus, sickle cell disease), increased urine production secondary to excessive evening fluid intake (caffeine ingestion, diuretics, or other agents), neurologic diseases (spinal cord abnormalities with neurogenic bladder or seizures), and psychosocial stressors (parental divorce, neglect, physical or sexual abuse, institutionalization).

Enuresis can reduce a child's self-esteem and lead to development of personality problems, although treatment should only be carried out in children over the age of 5 years. Behavioral therapy is considered the front-line approach and is based on general hygiene measures (moderate restriction of evening drinks), elimination of negative family habits (e.g. repeated intimate care, excessively careful attitudes toward sphincter control), sphincter conditioning exercises and "bladder gymnastics" training, behavioral and conditioning measures (keeping a diary, scheduled awakenings), and motivational techniques with positive reinforcement. The established drug therapy of SE is desmopressin, imipramine, and oxybutynin [35].

The most effective treatment for enuresis is an alarm. This is a system consisting of a small sensor clipped to the underwear, which is connected to a small battery-powered speaker that is activated when the sensor becomes wet. The resulting alarm awakens the wearer, alerting them that enuresis has begun. Controlled studies have shown that this approach is superior to all other approaches, including pharmacological or psychotherapeutic treatment, and that it leads to very low recurrence.

NARCOLEPSY

The ICSD-3 [1] defines narcolepsy, based on clinical features and cerebrospinal hypocretin 1 (CSF hcrt-1) levels in two forms: narcolepsy type 1 (NT1) with cataplexy and CSF hcrt-1 deficiency and narcolepsy type 2 (NT2) without cataplexy and normal CSF hcrt-1 levels.

The pathogenesis of NT1 a loss of hypothalamic hypocretin (orexin) producing neurons that lead to undetectable CSF hcrt-1 levels [36]. The etiological mechanism is linked to an autoimmune reaction, supported by an association with a specific human leukocyte antigen (HLA-DQB1 0602) and by the connection with streptococcal infections and anti-H1N1 vaccination in several European countries and the H1N1 pandemic in China [37]. Narcolepsy onset usually occurs in adolescence or young adulthood, although the first symptoms often appear during childhood.

Clinical Features

The clinical features of narcolepsy are historically represented by four symptoms: EDS, cataplexy, hypnagogic hallucinations, and sleep paralysis. Recently, sleep fragmentation has been added to the classic presentation of narcolepsy.

EDS is often the first symptom, isolated or concomitant to other key features and characterized by a prolongation of the nocturnal sleep period, an increase of daytime napping behavior, and great difficulty awakening in the morning [38]. Sleep attacks occur several times a day as uncontrollable episodes of sleep during monotonous activities (e.g., watching TV or performing tasks that do not require attention).

Those with NT1 may show aggressive behavior, irritability, and hyperactivity that are coping strategies used to fight against drowsiness. They may feel constant drowsiness with episodes of microsleep lasting 1 to 10 seconds, which may go unnoticed because the patient's eyes are open (although with an absent look) and they can speak (although their words are out of context and they respond to questions slowly or inappropriately); they may also show hesitation during automatic behaviors and loss of memory.

Cataplexy attacks can cause "ground loss" (i.e. falling) due to a sudden loss of muscle tone, or they can appear as just a slight tremor of the legs (without falling to the ground) or even brief speech pauses. These episodes are typically triggered by intense emotion (most often laughter, anger, surprise). In some patients, all voluntary muscles (except the ocular muscles and the diaphragm) are affected, while in others only muscles of the head and neck may be affected. The duration of cataplectic attacks can vary anywhere from 1 to 2 seconds to 20 to 30 seconds. Consciousness is preserved during the initial stage, but if the episode continues, then hallucinations may occur, and the patient may fall directly into REM sleep.

Recently, the motor phenomenon of the childhood cataplexy has been accurately described as consisting of both "negative" and "active" motor features [39]. Negative motor phenomena constitute intermittent or subcontinuous hypotonia with wide-based gait, spontaneous falls to the ground, and a characteristic "cataleptic facies" with ptosis and tongue protrusion. Active motor phenomena include perioral/tongue movements, body sways together with eyebrow raising, stereotyped motor behaviors, facial grimacing and dyskinetic and/or dystonic movements of the arms and tongue.

Hypnagogic hallucinations are reported less frequently, which may be partly due to the self-perception of the phenomena and the ability to distinguish oneiric mentation from reality. It is sometimes difficult to differentiate these from the individual's fears of falling asleep. Because of the vivid visual and auditory hallucinations, nocturnal or diurnal sleep can be a very unpleasant, or even a terrifying experience. Teenagers may doubt their sanity and avoid sharing such experiences.

Sleep paralysis appears predominantly upon awakening, is temporary, and is completely reversible. It can be blocked by tactile stimuli or being shaken by another person, by rapid eye movements or by rapid compressions of the eyeballs. The patient cannot speak or move and may have a sensation of suffocating. Sleep paralyses are difficult to investigate in young children, who often have difficulties with both properly reporting the experience of being unable to move and distinguishing the transitional condition between rapid REM sleep and wakefulness.

The nocturnal sleep of patients with narcolepsy is fragmented, with frequent awakenings and dreamlike states associated with terrifying dreams. Other sleep disorders are frequent in patient with narcolepsy, mainly non-REM and REM sleep-related parasomnias, including RBD [37].

Diagnosis

The diagnostic criteria for narcolepsy, according to the ICSD-3, are in Table 19.3.

Polysomnography, including the associated multiple sleep latency test (MSLT—a daytime nap assessment to determine how quickly and into what stage the sleeper falls asleep), is essential for a correct diagnostic procedure. The differential diagnosis should be addressed with other diseases such as obstructive sleep apnea syndrome, epilepsy, trauma and central nervous system tumors, drug abuse, night-time sleep deprivation, psychological disorders, metabolic diseases, essential hypersomnia, and Kleine–Levin syndrome.

Treatment

Especially in the initial phases, a behavioral approach is preferred. The patient's life must be well-organized, accommodate their EDS, and provide an adequate amount of nocturnal sleep, by advancing bedtime when necessary. The so-called nap schedule should be used (scheduled 20- to 30-minute naps at midday and during the late afternoon can increase vigilance for the next 3 hours). Adequate sleep hygiene can also help prevent the onset of behavioral disturbances. Physical activity can ameliorate fatigue, maintaining arousability. Reminding patients about the dangers of driving while sleepy is particularly important. Narcolepsy symptoms can affect the patient's emotions and self-esteem, which may worsen their response to any treatment [40].

Since no U.S. Food and Drug Administration/European Medicines Agency–approved pharmacotherapy is available for narcoleptic patients younger than 16 years, medication used to treat pediatric narcolepsy are off-label. The most appropriate drug is chosen based on symptom prevalence. Treatment typically starts with stimulating drugs, although because pharmacological therapy alone does not lead to a constant remission of the symptoms, it is prescribed along with one or two daily scheduled naps (20–30 minutes each, in the morning at school and in the afternoon).

Table 19.3 ICSD-3 DIAGNOSTIC CRITERIA FOR NARCOLEPSY

Diagnostic criteria of narcolepsy type 1

Criteria A and B must be met

A. The patient has daily periods of irrepressible need to sleep or daytime lapses into sleep occurring for at least 3 months.

B. The presence of one or both of the following:

1. Cataplexy (as defined under essential features) and a mean sleep latency of 8 minutes and 2 or more sleep onset rapid eye moment periods (SOREMPs) on an multiple sleep latency test (MSLT) performed according to standard techniques. A SOREMP (within 15 minutes of sleep onset) on the preceding nocturnal polysomnogram may replace one of the SOREMPs on the MSLT 2.

2. Cerebrospinal fluid (CSF) hypocretin-1 concentration, measured by immunoreactivity, is either 110 pg/mL or <1/3 of mean values obtained in normal subjects with the same standardized assay.

Diagnostic criteria of narcolepsy type 2

Criteria A–E must be met

A. The patient has daily periods of irrepressible need to sleep or daytime lapses into sleep occurring for at least 3 months.

B. A mean sleep latency of 8 minutes and 2 or SOREMPs are found on a MSLT performed according to standard techniques. A SOREMP (within 15 minutes of sleep onset) on the preceding nocturnal polysomnogram may replace one of the SOREMPs on the MSLT

C. Cataplexy is absent.

D. Either CSF hypocretin-1 concentration has not been measured or CSF hypocretin-1 concentration measured by immunoreactivity is either >110 pg/mL or >1/3 of mean values obtained in normal subjects with the same standardized assay 2.

E. The hypersomnolence and/or MSLT findings are not better explained by other causes such as insufficient sleep, obstructive sleep apnea, delayed sleep phase disorder, or the effect of medication or substances or their withdrawal.

Modafinil is a wake-promoting drug with unknown mechanism of action; it is highly effective for treating sleepiness yet has only minimal benefits on cataplexy and other REM sleep-related symptoms. Methylphenidate is a dopamine and catecholamine reuptake inhibitor that reduces EDS, increases sleep onset and REM sleep latency, and reduces the percentage of REM sleep. Like modafinil, its common side effects include irritability, headaches, and anorexia. Sodium oxybate is highly effective for the treatment of cataplexy, EDS, disrupted sleep, hypnagogic hallucinations, and sleep paralysis. This medication is usually split into two doses during the night. Tricyclic antidepressants, selective serotonin reuptake inhibitors, venlafaxine, and reboxetine are commonly used for cataplexy. Pitolisant is an inverse agonist of the histamine H3 receptor that increases the secretion of histamine and is effective on EDS; it is also well tolerated [41].

RESTLESS LEGS SYNDROME

Restless legs syndrome (RLS), or Willis–Ekbom disease, is a neurological disorder initially described by Sir Thomas Willis in 1685 and further defined by Dr. Ekbom in 1944; however, pediatric RLS was not described in the literature until 1994. Diagnostic criteria for pediatric-onset RLS were introduced in 2003 and updated in 2013 [42] to allow the use of age-related descriptive terms and words outlining specific considerations for diagnosis in children. Herein we will refer to this disorder simply as RLS.

Clinical Features

The primary feature of RLS is the urge to move one's legs, with or without accompanying leg sensations. If sensations are present, they invariably involve the legs, although the arms and other body parts are sometimes affected.

RLS is relatively common in pediatrics with an estimated prevalence of 2% to 4% in school-aged children and adolescents [43]. It is often misdiagnosed and is generally ignored by most pediatricians and general practitioners because of the mild and intermittent nature of the symptoms at younger ages. However, RLS is usually progressive and thus it is likely that these children will become more symptomatic in the future. Pediatricians need to be aware of RLS because it is relatively common and, when left untreated, can cause significant functional impairment.

Since RLS symptoms occur during bedtime, they are most likely to interfere with sleep onset, and, in children, these symptoms may be confused with bedtime resistance and limit-setting–type behaviors. The typical increase in symptoms during the evening or at night that adults experience may not be reported by children. The majority of children with RLS (66%) report daytime leg discomfort. One explanation for this is the number of hours children spend sitting during the school day [44].

Diagnosis

The current ICSD-3 criteria for RLS are in Table 19.4.

The ICSD-3 states that "for children, the description of these symptoms should be in the child's own words" (p. 282) [1]. The interview questions should be phrased using words developmentally appropriate for the child. Language and cognitive development determine the applicability of the RLS diagnostic criteria, rather than age. The clinical course criteria do not apply for pediatric cases; it is not certain that at least twice weekly can be considered the best determinant of chronicity in pediatric cases.

Differentiating pediatric RLS from other conditions, or mimics, can be complicated [45]. Some of the common mimics of pediatric RLS are positional

Table 19.4 ICSD-3 CRITERIA FOR RESTLESS LEGS SYNDROME

A. An urge to move the legs, usually accompanied by uncomfortable and unpleasant sensations in the legs:
   - Begin or worsen during periods of rest or inactivity such as lying down or sitting.
   - Be partially or totally relieved by movement, such as walking or stretching, as least as long as the activity continues.
   - Occur exclusively or predominantly in the evening or night rather than during the day.
B. The previous features are not solely condition (e.g., leg cramps, positional discomfort, myalgia, venous stasis, leg oedema, arthritis, accounted for as symptoms of another medical or a behavioural habitual foot-tapping). For pediatric condition, there is the need to exclude mimics of restless legs syndrome, which are disorders.
C. The symptoms of restless legs syndrome cause concern, distress, sleep disturbance or impairment in mental, physical, social, occupational, educational, behavioural or other important areas of functioning and cannot be better explained by other disorders, medication use, or substance use disorder.

discomfort, sore leg muscles, ligament sprain/tendon strain, positional ischemia (numbness), dermatitis, bruises, growing pains, leg cramps, arthritis, peripheral neuropathy, radiculopathy, myelopathy, myopathy, fibromyalgia, and sickle cell disease.

RLS is also difficult to diagnose in children because they may be unable to provide a precise description of the symptoms. Sensory symptoms are difficult for children to explain, so simple descriptions such as a funny feeling, pain, hurting, tickling, bugs, spiders, ants, and goose bumps in the legs can be accepted. Sometimes children may draw pins, needles, tiny sand particles, bugs, or a saw over their legs when asked to depict their symptoms. It is very important for the healthcare provider to establish a good rapport with the child to facilitate expression of the sensation in the child's own words. RLS-related pain in children typically occurs from both knees down and especially involves the calves, although thigh pain may also appear. These pains can be symmetric or asymmetric.

RLS symptoms can be confused with growing pains, which are characterized by intermittent bilateral leg pain that occur in the late afternoon or evening [46]. Leg rubbing to obtain relief from leg discomfort is common to both disorders, although walking to obtain relief seems unique to RLS. However, growing pains are always described as painful, while childhood RLS is considered painful in only 45% of cases. It has been hypothesized that the two conditions could represent different phenotypic expressions of the same disorder. Furthermore, growing pains commonly do not affect the arms, and there is no relief from growing pains, as there is with RLS, by engaging activity. Symptoms of growing pains resolve during adolescence [47]. In both conditions, massage, ice packs, warm compresses, and acetaminophen or ibuprofen may alleviate symptoms.

There are no specific tests for RLS and the diagnosis is made through a complete medical history and physical examination. An overnight sleep study may be helpful to evaluate the presence of other sleep disorders, especially PLM disorder (PLMD) [48].

It is also extremely important to evaluate family history of RLS. It is not uncommon, when taking the history of the child, to discover that another family member has been affected by RLS without being aware of it. Early onset RLS has a familial pattern and about 40% to 92% of children with RLS have affected family members [49].

Causes of secondary RLS include peripheral neuropathy and uremia. Medications, such as antidepressants, sedating antihistamines, and dopamine receptor antagonists, may worsen or precipitate RLS. In patients who are thought to have secondary RLS, screening for renal disease, thyroid dysfunction, and vitamin B12 and folic acid deficiency (peripheral neuropathy) should be considered [50].

Comorbidities

An association between RLS and PLMS has been reported in children. Most individuals with RLS have PLMS, and PLMS is considered to be supportive of an RLS diagnosis in children. Often a diagnosis of PLMD precedes the diagnosis of RLS in children under 6 years of age who do not yet have sufficiently well-developed language skills to describe the sensory component of RLS [51].

Attention-deficit/hyperactivity (ADHD) symptoms have also been frequently described, in both clinical and community samples of children with RLS. Sleep disruption associated with RLS may lead to ADHD symptoms, RLS may mimic the symptomatology of ADHD, or it may be comorbid with idiopathic ADHD [52]. About 25% of adults and school-aged children with RLS meet the criteria for ADHD, whereas 12% to 35% of children with ADHD met the criteria for RLS. Several studies have shown that diurnal manifestations of RLS mimic ADHD and that RLS and PLM are more prevalent in children with ADHD [53].

The exact relationship among ADHD, RLS, and PLMD is unclear, but we can hypothesize that RLS may lead to symptoms of ADHD via sleep disruption or that RLS and ADHD may coexist as comorbid disorders that share a common dopamine dysfunction.

Both ADHD and RLS have been associated with iron deficiency (ID), which may affect dopaminergic hypoactivity, since iron is a cofactor for tyrosine hydroxylase, the rate-limiting enzyme for dopamine synthesis. Children with ADHD are more likely to have ID and treatment with supplemental iron has been reported to help reduce their PLMD symptoms, improve sleep quality, and subsequently decrease ADHD symptoms [54]. ADHD symptom severity is also higher in children with ADHD when RLS is present as a comorbid disorder [29], and low doses of dopaminergic agents (levodopa, pergolide, and ropinirole) and/or iron supplementation have been effective [55].

Treatment

Successful pediatric RLS therapy is especially important, since the associated sleep disturbances can lead to determine significant developmental, behavioral and cardiovascular morbidities, as well as impact family well-being.

Nonpharmacologic interventions mainly consist of establishing healthy sleep habits and sleep hygiene rules, with adequate sleep duration and regular bed timings. For leg symptom relief, the individual or in the children, their parents, may try applying a heating pad or cold compress; rubbing the legs as well as massage, acupressure, walking, stretching, or other relaxation techniques can also be effective. Avoiding medications or other factors that could aggravate RLS and PLMD and examining ways of discontinuing these medications (such as selective serotonin reuptake inhibitors, tricyclic antidepressants, metoclopramide, diphenhydramine, nicotine, caffeine, and alcohol [56] may also help.

Since the most common cause of RLS in children appears to be ID, serum ferritin is the best indicator of early ID. Saturation of peripheral iron stores typically occurs at ferritin levels of 80 to 100 ng/mL. Current evidence suggests that achieving and maintaining serum ferritin above 50 ng/mL can be beneficial for RLS, PLMS, and ADHD [57]. A recent study found that 10-year-old children who experienced ID anemia in infancy showed a mild but significant increase of tibialis anterior electromyographic activity during sleep when compared to age-matched normal controls, pointing to the possibility of long-term consequences of ID in infancy, despite iron therapy [58]. The dopaminergic theory of RLS further support the ID hypothesis, since iron is fundamental for the biosynthesis of dopamine and is necessary for tyrosine hydroxylation, which is a rate-limiting step for dopamine production.

Iron supplementation in children with RLS should be started when ferritin level is <50 lg/L with 3 mg elemental iron/kg/day or ferrous sulfate at a dose of 50 to 65 mg of elemental iron for 3 months and then recheck ferritin level. To enhance absorption, iron should ideally be taken in the morning on an empty stomach with a source of vitamin C such as orange juice. Some foods (e.g., milk, cereals, fiber, eggs) may decrease iron absorption for 2 hours. However, it may take weeks or even months of treatment with iron supplementation to detect improvements in RLS symptoms.

Currently, neither the U.S. Food and Drug Administration nor the European Medicines Agency have approved medications for RLS in children. The initial form of treatment is to reduce factors or conditions that may worsen or precipitate RLS and evaluate for the presence of ID. Careful monitoring for adverse events and periodic reassessment of treatment are recommended and family understanding of the pathology is crucial. When starting a drug for RLS in children, it is prudent to begin with the lowest possible dose and slowly titrate upward with close monitoring for adverse effects.

Dopaminergic medications (i.e. L-dopa, ropinirole, pramipexole) have proven successful in case reports and small open-label studies of children with RLS with and without ADHD but very few double-blind, placebo-controlled trials have been carried out. Anticonvulsants (e.g., gabapentin), levetiracetam, or benzodiazepines (e.g., clonazepam) have shown some efficacy in small series of patients. Other options are clonidine or melatonin, although little evidence supports their use in children with RLS [56].

CONCLUSIONS

The clinician and the psychologist have multidisciplinary tasks when managing these disorders in children like education of regular lifestyle, adequate sleep hygiene, avoiding sleep deprivation, and providing quiet sleeping conditions. It is important to create a personalized sleep ritual with a regular bedtime even on the weekends. For narcolepsy, allowing multiple naps might be a successful therapy in mild cases.

Psychotherapies/hypnosis, cognitive behavioral therapy, or relaxation may be helpful and possibly lead to a long-term benefit to the patient if they learns how to recognize the signs of their disease and how to cope with it. Finally, this can have a repercussion on the patient's awareness and, ultimately, on the quality of life.

REFERENCES

1. American Academy of Sleep Medicine. *International Classification of Sleep Disorders*. 3rd ed. Darien, IL: American Academy of Sleep Medicine; 2014.
2. Proserpio P, Nobili L. Parasomnias in children. In: Nevsimalova S, Bruni O, eds. *Sleep Disorders in Children*. Cham, Switzerland: Springer International; 2017:305–335.
3. Mahowald MW, Cramer Bornemann MA, Schenck CH. State dissociation, human behavior, and consciousness. *Curr Top Med Chem*. 2011;11:2392–2402.
4. Bassetti C, Vella S, Donati F, Wielepp P, Weder B. SPECT during sleepwalking. *Lancet*. 2000;356:484–485.
5. Terzaghi M, Sartori I, Tassi L, et al. Evidence of dissociated arousal states during NREM parasomnia from an intracerebral neurophysiological study. *Sleep*. 2009;32:409–412.
6. Terzaghi M, Sartori I, Tassi L, et al. Dissociated local arousal states underlying essential clinical features of non-rapid eye movement arousal parasomnia: an intracerebral stereo-electroencephalographic study: local sleep and NREM parasomnia. *J Sleep Res*. 2012;21:502–506.
7. Tassinari CA, Cantalupo G, Högl B, et al. Neuroethological approach to frontolimbic epileptic seizures and parasomnias: the same central pattern generators for the same behaviours. *Rev Neurol*. 2009;165:762–768.
8. Zadra A, Desautels A, Petit D, Montplaisir J. Somnambulism: clinical aspects and pathophysiological hypotheses. *Lancet Neurol*. 2013;12:285–294.
9. Hublin C, Kaprio J. Genetic aspects and genetic epidemiology of parasomnias. *Sleep Med Rev*. 2003;7:413–421.

10. Nevsimalova S, Prihodova I, Kemlink D, Skibova J. Childhood parasomnia—a disorder of sleep maturation? *Eur J Paediatr Neurol.* 2013;17:615–619.

11. Laberge L, Tremblay RE, Vitaro F, Montplaisir J. Development of parasomnias from childhood to early adolescence. *Pediatrics.* 2000;106:67–74.

12. Ohayon MM, Priest RG, Zulley J, Smirne S. The place of confusional arousals in sleep and mental disorders: findings in a general population sample of 13,057 subjects. *J Nerv Ment Dis.* 2000;188:340–348.

13. Petit D, Touchette E, Tremblay RE, Boivin M, Montplaisir J. Dyssomnias and parasomnias in early childhood. *Pediatrics.* 2007;119:e1016–e1025.

14. Mason TBA, Pack AI. Sleep terrors in childhood. *J Pediatr.* 2005;147:388–392.

15. Craske MG, Tsao JCI. Assessment and treatment of nocturnal panic attacks. *Sleep Med Rev.* 2005;9:173–184.

16. Derry CP, Davey M, Johns M, et al. Distinguishing sleep disorders from seizures: diagnosing bumps in the night. *Arch Neurol.* 2006;63:705–709.

17. Derry C. Nocturnal frontal lobe epilepsy vs parasomnias. *Curr Treat Options Neurol.* 2012;14:451–463.

18. Kotagal S. Treatment of dyssomnias and parasomnias in childhood. *Curr Treat Options Neurol.* 2012;14:630–649.

19. Howell MJ. Parasomnias: an updated review. *Neurotherapeutics.* 2012;9:753–775.

20. Bruni O, Ferri R, Miano S, Verrillo E. L-5-Hydroxytryptophan treatment of sleep terrors in children. *Eur J Pediatr.* 2004;163:402–407.

21. Jan JE, Freeman RD, Wasdell MB, Bomben MM. A child with severe night terrors and sleepwalking responds to melatonin therapy. *Dev Med Child Neurol.* 2004;46:789.

22. Schenck CH, Mahowald MW. Review of nocturnal sleep-related eating disorders. *Int J Eat Disord.* 1994;15:343–356.

23. Arnulf I. REM sleep behavior disorder: motor manifestations and pathophysiology. *Mov Disord.* 2012;27:677–689.

24. Kotagal S. Rapid eye movement sleep behavior disorder during childhood. *Sleep Med Clin.* 2015;10:163–167.

25. Lloyd R, Tippmann-Peikert M, Slocumb N, Kotagal S. Characteristics of REM sleep behavior disorder in childhood. *J Clin Sleep Med.* 2012;8:127–131.

26. Zadra A, Donderi DC. Nightmares and bad dreams: their prevalence and relationship to wellbeing. *J Abnorm Psychol.* 2000;109:273–281.

27. Sharpless BA, Barber JP. Lifetime prevalence rates of sleep paralysis: a systematic review. *Sleep Med Rev.* 2011;15:311–315.

28. Harari MD. Nocturnal enuresis. *J Paediatr Child Health.* 2013;49:264–271.

29. Butler RJ, Holland P. The three systems: a conceptual way of understanding nocturnal enuresis. *Scand J Urol Nephrol.* 2000;34:270–277.

30. Alexopoulos EI, Malakasioti G, Varlami V, Miligkos M, Gourgoulianis K, Kaditis AG. Nocturnal enuresis is associated with moderate-to-severe obstructive sleep apnea in children with snoring. *Pediatr Res.* 2014;76:555–559.

31. Dhondt K, Baert E, Van Herzeele C, et al. Sleep fragmentation and increased periodic limb movements are more common in children with nocturnal enuresis. *Acta Paediatrica.* 2014;103:e268–e272.

32. Nevéus T, Stenberg A, Läckgren G, Tuvemo T, Hetta J. Sleep of children with enuresis: a polysomnographic study. *Pediatrics.* 1999;103:1193–1197.

33. Wolfish N, Pivik R, Busby K. Elevated sleep arousal thresholds in enuretic boys: clinical implications. *Acta Paediatr.* 1997;86:381–384.

34. Soster LA, Alves RC, Fagundes SN, et al. Non-REM sleep instability in children with primary monosymptomatic sleep enuresis. *J Clin Sleep Med.* 2017;13:1163–1170.

35. Caldwell PHY, Deshpande AV, Gontard AV. Management of nocturnal enuresis. *Brit Med J.* 2013;347:f6259.

36. Nishino S, Ripley B, Overeem S, Lammers GJ, Mignot E. Hypocretin (orexin) deficiency in human narcolepsy. *Lancet.* 2000;355:39–40.

37. Rocca FL, Pizza F, Ricci E, Plazzi G. Narcolepsy during childhood: an update. *Neuropediatrics.* 2015;46:181–197.

38. Aran A, Einen M, Lin L, Plazzi G, Nishino S, Mignot E. Clinical and therapeutic aspects of childhood narcolepsy-cataplexy: a retrospective study of 51 children. *Sleep.* 2010;33:1457–1464.

39. Plazzi G, Pizza F, Palaia V, et al. Complex movement disorders at disease onset in childhood narcolepsy with cataplexy. *Brain.* 2011;134:3480–3492.

40. Nevsimalova S. The diagnosis and treatment of pediatric narcolepsy. *Curr Neurol Neurosci Rep.* 2014;14:469.

41. Franceschini C, Pizza F, Antelmi E, Folli MC, Plazzi G. Narcolepsy treatment: pharmacological and behavioral strategies in adults and children. *Sleep Breath.* 2019 doi:10.1007/s11325-019-01894-4. [Epub ahead of print]

42. Picchietti DL, Bruni O, de Weerd A, et al. Pediatric restless legs syndrome diagnostic criteria: an update by the International Restless Legs Syndrome Study Group. *Sleep Med* 2013;14:1253–1259.

43. Picchietti D, Allen RP, Walters AS, Davidson JE, Myers A, Ferini-Strambi L. Restless legs syndrome: prevalence and impact in children and adolescents: the Peds REST study. *Pediatrics.* 2007;120:253–266.

44. Picchietti MA, Picchietti DL. Advances in pediatric restless legs syndrome: iron, genetics, diagnosis and treatment. *Sleep Med.* 2010;11:643–651.

45. Benes H, Walters AS, Allen RP, Hening WA, Kohnen R. Definition of restless legs syndrome, how to diagnose it, and how to differentiate it from RLS mimics. *Mov Disord.* 2007;22:S401–S408.

46. Walters AS, Gabelia D, Frauscher B. Restless legs syndrome (Willis–Ekbom disease) and growing pains: are they the same thing? A side-by side comparison of the diagnostic criteria for both and recommendations for future research. *Sleep Med.* 2013;14:1247–1252.

47. Evans AM. Growing pains: contemporary knowledge and recommended practice. *J Foot Ankle Res.* 2008;1:4.

48. Hamilton-Stubbs PE, Walters AS. Sleep disorders in children: simple sleep-related movement disorders. In: Nevšímalová S., Bruni O, eds. *Sleep Disorders in Children.* Cham, Switzerland: Springer; 2017:227–251.

49. Picchietti MA, Picchietti DL. Advances in pediatric restless legs syndrome: iron, genetics, diagnosis and treatment. *Sleep Med.* 2010;11:643–651.

50. Bruni O, Angriman M. Management of RLS in children (unique features). In: Manconi M, Garcia-Borreguero D, eds. *Restless Legs Syndrome/Willis Ekbom Disease. Long-Term Consequences and Management.* New York, NY: Springer:261–278.

51. Picchietti MA, Picchietti DL. Restless legs syndrome and periodic limb movement disorder in children and adolescents. *Semin Pediatr Neurol.* 2008;15:91–99.

52. Picchietti DL, England SJ, Walters AS, Willis K, Verrico T. Periodic limb movement disorder and restless legs syndrome in children with attention-deficit hyperactivity disorder. *J Child Neurol.* 1998;13:588–594.

53. Lewin DS, Di Pinto M. Sleep disorders and ADHD: shared and common phenotypes. *Sleep.* 2004;27:267–273.

54. Cortese S, Konofal E, Lecendreux M, et al. Restless legs syndrome and attention-deficit/hyperactivity disorder: a review of the literature. *Sleep.* 2005;28(8):1007–1013.

55. Konofal E, Lecendreux M, Deron J, et al. Effects of iron supplementation on attention deficit hyperactivity disorder in children. *Pediatr Neurol.* 2008;38:20–26.

56. DelRosso L, Bruni O. Treatment of pediatric restless legs syndrome. In: Clemens S, Ghorayeb I, eds. *Advances in Pharmacology.* Vol. 84. New York, NY: Academic Press, 2019:237–253.

57. Simakajornboon N, Gozal D, Vlasic V, Mack C, Sharon D, McGinley BM. Periodic limb movements in sleep and iron status in children. *Sleep.* 2003;26:735–738.

58. Peirano P, Algarin C, Chamorro R, Manconi M, Lozoff B, Ferri R. Iron deficiency anemia in infancy exerts long-term effects on the tibialis anterior motor activity during sleep in childhood. *Sleep Med.* 2012;13:1006–1012.

20

Sleep and Psychiatric Disorders

ARGELINDA BARONI, SHILPA M. AGRAHARKAR,
AND MARC P. HALPERIN ■

INTRODUCTION

The relationship between sleep and psychiatric disorders is simultaneously obvious and elusive. It is obvious insofar as most psychiatric disorders present with sleep complaints, and sleep disruptions affect both psychological well-being and cognition. It is elusive as the causality of these relationships, as well the underlying mechanisms, remain objects of debate and investigation. However, the importance of sleep for mental health is finally being recognized, and in recent years, we have witnessed a major change in the paradigms related to sleep and mental health. Historically, most clinicians would consider sleep complaints, such as insomnia or nightmares, which co-occurred with a psychiatric disorder, simply a symptom of the disorder. Today, sleep problems are also seen as key risk factors for psychiatric disorders, as multiple longitudinal studies (i.e., studies that observe individuals over long periods of time) have shown that sleep symptoms often precede the development of full psychiatric syndromes, especially mood and anxiety disorders, and possibly schizophrenia. This new appreciation of sleep's role has been conveyed by the American Psychiatric Association; the fifth edition of the *Diagnostic and Statistical Manual of Mental Disorders* (DSM-5) [1] allows clinicians to diagnose sleep and psychiatric disorders independently when they are indicated, which is a major change from prior editions. Additionally, interest in sleep and circadian rhythm manipulations as treatment tools—including sleep phase advance, scheduled sleep deprivation, and bright light—is growing, as these appear to improve depressive syndromes.

However, we are still far from understanding the biological mechanisms behind the relationship between sleep and psychiatric disorders. Sleep–wake phases, sleep cycles, and, to some extent, circadian rhythms are influenced and regulated by the same neurotransmitters implicated in most psychiatric disorders. For example, depressive disorders are characterized by dopamine, noradrenaline, and serotonin imbalances, among other major players in wake–sleep balance. Given these commonalities, the frequent co-occurrence of insomnia or hypersomnia in depressive syndromes, and that insomnia often precedes depressive episodes, make sense. In this chapter, we will review the most common sleep disorders or complaints associated with specific psychiatric disorders, their current treatments, and clinical examples—topics about which we hope you will share our enthusiasm.

ATTENTION-DEFICIT/HYPERACTIVITY DISORDER

Attention-deficit/hyperactivity disorder (ADHD) is a common psychiatric disorder, characterized by inattention, impulsivity, and hyperactivity. In the United States, at least 5% of school age children and 2.5% of adults are estimated to have ADHD [1]. Symptoms of inattention include carelessness mistakes, difficulty sustaining attention and following instructions, distractibility, and frequent daydreaming. Those who are primarily hyperactive/impulsive have pronounced difficulty staying still and often act impulsively or recklessly. Other symptoms include frequent fidgetiness, feeling restless, and constantly moving about, along with difficulty waiting their turn, both in actions and when speaking, leading them to interrupt others often. ADHD can lead to lifelong consequences, including lower academic and professional attainment, more car accidents, and increased rate of incarcerations [2, 3]. While the specific mechanisms behind ADHD remain unknown, the dopaminergic and noradrenergic systems, major wake-promoting neurotransmitters, appear to be implicated in ADHD symptoms [4].

Sleep in ADHD

> Charlie is a 19-year-old college student who has ADHD. His symptoms were present since elementary school. When he does not take his medications for ADHD, he can't focus in class, feels restless, dreads long assignments, and often procrastinates. When he finally mobilizes himself, he tries to complete multiple assignments at once, ending up staying up late and waking up quite late.

Sleep disturbances have long been understood to be associated with ADHD, and in earlier editions of the DSM, sleep disturbances were a diagnostic criterion of the disorder. Approximately 25% to 50% children with ADHD suffer from sleep disturbances, and up to 75% of adults have sleep onset insomnia or delayed sleep disorder [5, 6]. While it is well-established that sleep complaints are common in those with ADHD, researchers currently debate whether sleep issues are inherent in ADHD, due to a comorbid sleep disorder, or share causes [5]. Clinically, it is important to exclude a sleep disorder, such as obstructive sleep apnea (OSA), or chronic sleep loss, prior to diagnosing ADHD, as chronic sleep disruptions can lead to inattention and hyperactivity, mimicking ADHD, especially in children and adolescents.

Clinicians who work with children are well aware that sleep disturbances often accompany ADHD. Parents report that children with ADHD often struggle to fall asleep at night, exhibit resistance to bedtime, have more difficulty waking in the morning, and show increased daytime drowsiness, all of which can be symptoms of insomnia and delayed sleep phase disorder [5]. Insomnia and delayed sleep phase disorder are common in adults with ADHD as well, and delayed melatonin secretion has been observed in adults with ADHD [6]. Melatonin is a hormone produced by a small gland in the brain, the pineal gland, and it is essential for regulation of circadian rhythms and sleep–wake cycles; delayed secretion of melatonin determines later sleep times and later wake-up times [6]. ADHD is also associated with increased likelihood of having restless legs syndrome (RLS) and periodic limb movement disorder (PLMD), two common sleep disorders [5, 7]. RLS is characterized by uncomfortable sensations in one's legs and uncontrollable urges to move them, which occur predominantly at night when trying to sleep. PLMD is characterized by small twitches of the limbs while sleeping, which can affect how deeply one sleeps. RLS affects approximately 3% to 5% of children and 5% to 10% of adults; among those with ADHD, it appears to be much more common [7]. Similarly, between 25% to 75% of children with ADHD are estimated to suffer from PLMD [8]. RLS is caused by, among other factors, iron deficiency, which may, in turn, be connected to dopamine metabolism. Abnormalities in dopamine metabolism may link ADHD and RLS, as both conditions are ameliorated by medications, which act on dopamine [7].

While the prevalence of sleep disordered breathing in ADHD is unclear, increased rates of snoring and obstructive apneas have been reported in those with ADHD [5]. For this reason, if a child or an adult presents with symptoms of ADHD in concomitance with chronic snoring and enuresis or increased urination overnight, OSA should be suspected and a sleep study performed to assess for this. In positive cases, the sleep disruption associated with OSA likely drives the ADHD-like symptoms, as sleep deprived individuals tend to be forgetful, distracted, unable to focus, and possibly physically hyperactive. In fact, it is important to remember that any chronic sleep loss can mimic ADHD. For example, neurotypical children who reduce their sleep time by 1 hour per night for five consecutive nights score within the ADHD range on standardized scales [9].

In addition to primary sleep disorders co-occurring with ADHD, the first-line medications to treat ADHD (stimulants such as methylphenidate or amphetamines) have the common side effect of making it difficult to sleep. Therefore, when a patient with ADHD and sleep difficulties is evaluated, their current and prior medications must be examined to determine whether these may be a factor in the sleep disturbances. Clinicians managing sleep symptoms that are exacerbated or caused by medication can usually decrease the medication dose or change to an alternate medication class with fewer sleep-related side effects [10].

Objective Findings

In ADHD, objective studies (polysomnography [PSG] and actigraphy) have not detected a clear pattern of abnormalities, although some have found lower sleep efficiency, delayed sleep onset, higher apnea–hypopnea index, more phase shifts, and more irregular sleep-wake phases [11].

Treatment

Treating sleep disturbances both with melatonin and sleep hygiene changes has been shown to ameliorate sleep symptoms but without significantly improving core ADHD symptoms (i.e., inattention and hyperactivity). The first step is to assess and evaluate the child or adult's sleep symptoms and sleep hygiene. A person with difficulty sleeping should have consistent behaviors and routines surrounding their bedtime, with a stable bedtime and wake time. Screens and bright lights should be turned off 2 hours prior to bedtime. Caffeine, nicotine, and alcohol should be avoided. Additionally, cognitive behavioral therapy (CBT) approaches can be used to manage difficulty sleeping, in those with or without ADHD, including relaxation training. In addition to, or if behavioral approaches are not completely effective, use of melatonin can be helpful [12]. While mela-tonin is produced naturally by our bodies, it can also be taken by mouth as an over-the-counter sleep aid. Unfortunately, as melatonin is not a regulated drug but a natural product in the United States, melatonin supplements can vary in purity and integrity, and this is associated with significant variations in effective doses and blood concentrations.

AUTISM SPECTRUM DISORDER

Autism spectrum disorder (ASD) is a complex neurodevelopmental syndrome characterized by impairments of interpersonal connectedness, social communica-tion, and cognitive flexibility. As the name implies, the spectrum of presentations within ASD is wide, ranging from mild social difficulties to severe impairment that can be accompanied by intellectual disability and may necessitate contin-uous care. Hallmarks of the syndrome include: poor eye contact and difficulties appreciating interpersonal nuances and social conventions such as greetings or turn-taking in conversations; restricted interests such as unusual interest in trains, astronomy, or specific TV shows; repetitive behaviors such as flapping, spinning, lining up objects; and hyper- or hyposensitivity to noise or physical sensations [1]. ASD is a relatively common condition, with prevalence ranging between 1% and 1.5% in children, with boys diagnosed three to five times more frequently than girls [1]. The condition is diagnosed via interviews and structured activities with the child or adolescent to assess communicative ability, social interaction, and interactive play. While the diagnosis is typically made in early childhood, milder forms of ASD can be diagnosed at any age.

Sleep in ASD

> Danny is an 18-year-old college student with a diagnosis of mild ASD. He is a physics major and does well academically but struggles socially. He is passionate about physics but has difficulties asking a girl out or engaging in small talk with peers in between classes. He has never been a good sleeper and has chronic difficulties sleeping, worsened by late night on-line socialization and videogames. He sleeps slightly better when he takes over-the-counter melatonin.

Poor sleep is extremely common in individuals with ASD [13]. Sleep disturbances are present in 60% to 86% of children with ASD and include difficulties falling asleep, night awakenings, and early morning awakenings [13]. Studies on sleep in adults with ASD are few but suggest that, at least for some, sleep disturbances persist into adulthood. Poor sleep appears to exacerbate some of the behavioral difficulties that individuals with ASD experience and can worsen reciprocal social interactions and mood disorders and increase anxiety, irritability, and aggression [14]. Moreover, there is often a ripple effect on the family unit: parents of children with ASD who are poor sleepers themselves experience significantly higher levels of stress and poor sleep, compared to parents of children with ASD who are good sleepers [14].

There is no clear explanation for sleep problems in ASD, and they are most likely multifactorial (i.e., due to a combination of poor sleep hygiene, comorbid disorders, and biological reasons). Among the biological reasons, abnormalities of melatonin have been noted, though this is a controversial topic [15]. Children with ASD, particularly prepubertal children, have been reported to have a relative deficiency of melatonin or an abnormal timing of secretion of melatonin, either of which may drive sleep disturbances and disrupt circadian rhythms [16–18]. At night, children with ASD may not register that it is time to go to sleep; similarly, in the morning, their bodies may not be aware that it is time to rise. Low iron is another biological factor implicated in sleep difficulties in ASD. Low iron has been associated with the development of RLS and subsequent poor sleep. Iron is ingested mainly via foods that are often not preferred by children, including legumes, leafy vegetables, and red meat. Picky eating, common in children with ASD, might lead to low iron stores and RLS. Some studies have shown an association between low iron stores and poor sleep in ASD, but results are mixed [19]. Nevertheless, assessment for RLS is advisable in all individuals with ASD with sleep disturbances, especially if poor iron intake is suspected.

Objective Findings

Objectively, compared with neurotypical children, those with ASD have approximately 30 minutes less total sleep time per day, longer sleep onset latency (i.e., it takes them longer to fall asleep), and decreased sleep efficiency (i.e., they spend more time awake in bed) [20].

Regarding sleep architecture, there is evidence for increase in N1, decrease in N2 and N3, fewer sleep spindles, and lower number of REMs during REM sleep [21].

Of note, people with ASD who have normal intelligence may have fewer objective differences in sleep physiology compared to their peers than do individuals with ASD and intellectual disabilities, suggesting that other brain factors are responsible for sleep abnormalities.

Treatment

Good sleep hygiene is considered the mainstay for children and adults with ASD, but this is often difficult to implement [13], given that people with ASD can struggle with transitions and rigidity. However, they usually appreciate routines and the use of visual bedtime routines (e.g., pictures of a child/person changing into pajamas, brushing teeth, going to bed) can be extremely helpful. Additionally, while the presence of electronic devices in the bedroom is associated with shorter sleep in children and adolescents in general, it seems that the presence of a TV or computer can cause more sleep loss in boys with ASD compared with their neurotypical peers and that, specifically among boys with ASD, playing video games is associated with less sleep [22]. Low doses of melatonin are also often used in people with ASD to facilitate sleep, with good results [23].

ANXIETY DISORDERS AND POSTTRAUMATIC STRESS DISORDER

Anxiety is a normal cognitive, physical, and emotional reaction in many situations and mild levels of anxiety can help us perform better. For example, if one were to be confronted by a lion, a robust anxiety response would be beneficial for survival, and, similarly, mild anxiety might help us to study harder for a test. However, when the anxiety is excessive in relation to the stimulus or is persistent, we might be facing an anxiety disorder. Anxiety disorders are characterized by pathological fear responses to neutral or mild stimuli, like an insect or talking in front of class, that the brain mischaracterizes as dangerous. These include separation anxiety disorder, generalized anxiety disorder (GAD), social anxiety disorder, and panic disorder, each of which is described in the DSM-5 [1]. Anxiety disorders are the most commonly diagnosed mental health disorders; their estimated prevalence is around 25% to 30% in children and adolescents and around 18% in adults [24, 25]. In separation anxiety disorder, patients experience excessive anxiety when separated from close caregivers or attachment figures; approximately 1% to 2% of adults and adolescents are affected [1]. For example, a child might refuse to go to school because she does not want to separate from her mother as she worries that her mother might not return. Patients with GAD have excessive worries and ruminations about everyday experiences and events. Such worries can include school or job performance, health of family members, or everyday chores. Poor sleep is a criterion for GAD in the DSM-5, and some researchers think that GAD and insomnia share many features, including chronic hyperarousal (i.e., abnormal alertness and responsiveness to stimuli). GAD affects approximately 3% of adults and 1% of adolescents [1]. In social anxiety disorder, worries are focused in the social realm, with patients experiencing significant difficulty in social situations; approximately 6% of adults and 8% of adolescents are affected [1]. Panic disorder is characterized by brief, repeated periods of intense fear, often without a clear trigger, accompanied by physical and emotional symptoms of fear. Panic disorder is present in 2% to 3% of the general population [1].

While posttraumatic stress disorder (PTSD) is no longer classified as an anxiety disorder in the DSM-5, its symptoms stem from abnormal fear responses that arise after trauma. PTSD is seen frequently in military veterans exposed to war trauma, but it is also seen in children and adults with histories of physical or sexual abuse. PTSD affects approximately 4% of adults and adolescents, and up 9% of the US population has met criteria for PTSD at some time during their lives [1]. Symptoms of PTSD include intrusive thoughts or images related to trauma, avoidance of stimuli that remind the person of the trauma, negative feelings and thoughts in relation to the trauma, and disruptions in arousal and reactivity that begin after the trauma. Nightmares related to the trauma and insomnia are specific criteria for PTSD, related to intrusive trauma memories and hyperarousal, respectively. Neurochemically, anxiety disorders and PTSD have been associated with alterations in serotonin, noradrenaline, and gamma-aminobutyric acid (GABA) which are likely also related to the sleep disturbances [4].

Sleep in Anxiety Disorders and PTSD

Maggie is a 21-year-old college student with a diagnosis of GAD. She worries about everything, and her worries are often overwhelming. For example, she worries that if she does not pass her next biology test, she will fail the class and won't find a job and will end up homeless. Paradoxically, her anxiety about school ends up interfering with her ability to focus on studying. When she goes to sleep, she ruminates about school, bills, relationships, and her inability to sleep. It usually takes her a long time to fall asleep and she wakes up multiple times during the night. She wakes up feeling tired.

Annie is a 19-year-old college student who was mugged at gunpoint while walking alone to her dorm after a party. She started sleeping poorly after the episode and three months later has symptoms of PTSD. She has intrusive images of the person who mugged her during the day, is afraid to walk around the campus alone even during the day, startles at any loud sounds (known as "hyperarousal") and feels anxious and depressed. She struggles to fall asleep at night, wakes up tired, and dreams of the incident at least twice a week.

Sleep disturbances are extremely common in anxiety disorders. In children and adolescents, up to 90% of patients report sleep subjective complaints and between 50% to 70% of adults with GAD report sleep complaints [26]. In children with GAD and separation anxiety, parents note resistance to bedtime, problems initiating or maintaining sleep, and not feeling rested upon waking as some of the more common complaints, in addition to sleep terrors, sleep walking, nightmares, and refusal to sleep alone or away from home. Among youth, subjective sleep complaints are most common in GAD and subjective sleep complaints have been linked to the future development of GAD in both adults and children in several studies.

In panic disorder, approximately 50% of patients have at least one experience with a panic episode which arises during sleep, usually during the transition between stages N2 to N3 and thus not related to nightmares [27]. The mechanism behind these panic episodes originating in sleep is still unclear.

In PTSD, sleep complaints are even more common. Approximately 70% to 90% of adults and 80% of children report insomnia and nightmares related to the trauma [28]. Sleep disturbances are usually among the first symptoms of PTSD to occur after the traumatic experience and some researchers think that initial sleep disruption might play a role in the pathogenesis of PTSD [29]. It is likely that sleep disturbances actually mediate and predict PTSD and mood symptoms after the trauma occurs. Other studies have found that sleep disturbances may also exacerbate other PTSD symptoms, worsening the disorder's severity. Children with PTSD, along with nightmares and insomnia, often present with bedtime fearfulness and avoidance, in an attempt to avoid nightmares. Additionally, for those who were sexually abused in their bedroom, there is often a negative association with the bedroom as a reminder of the abuse, which triggers fear responses at bedtime and thus poor sleep.

Objective Findings

Objective measures, including PSG or actigraphy, have mostly failed to demonstrate clear sleep abnormalities in the majority of youth with anxiety disorders [30]. However, in both children and adults with GAD, PSG studies show increased sleep onset latency and decreased REM onset latency [31].

Among adults with anxiety, PSG studies show more consistent abnormalities. In GAD, in addition to the increased sleep onset latency also seen in children, decreased total sleep time, increased N2 percentage and time, and increased wake after sleep onset are all seen [31]. Studies in panic disorder are few and have only been done in adults, with decreased sleep efficiency and total sleep time, along with increased sleep onset latency. Research on PTSD and sleep in adults is more robust than any other anxiety disorder, and generally finds decreased sleep efficiency, decreased total sleep time, increased sleep onset latency, increased wake after sleep onset, and increased sleep fragmentation [31].

Treatment

Treatment of sleep disturbances in anxiety disorders should include the sleep hygiene steps recommended for treating ADHD (previously discussed) but should also involve treating the underlying disorder itself. CBT is the first-line psychotherapy for most anxiety disorders, with trauma-focused CBT specifically used for PTSD. Medications (e.g., sedating antidepressants) may also be used, particularly when therapy has not been completely successful.

Chronic nightmares related to PTSD can be treated with imagery rehearsal therapy, which is now considered the standard of care for this symptom in adults and has shown some positive results in children as well. In imagery rehearsal therapy, the patient rehearses alternative positive variants of their nightmares during the day and prior to sleep. For example, a woman who has recurrent nightmares of being attacked might rehearse becoming incredibly powerful or being able to fly and overcome her aggressor [32]. While there is some controversy over their use, medications that decrease noradrenergic tone, such as prazosin, are also indicated for nightmares in patients with PTSD [32].

MOOD DISORDERS

Mood disorders, including depressive and bipolar disorders, affect one's mood, thoughts, level of activity, and ability to perform. During a major depressive episode, a person experiences feelings of sadness, emptiness, and/or irritability, along with several other symptoms. Depressive symptoms can include decreased interest or pleasure in usual activities and hobbies, constant boredom, self-doubt, low self-esteem and guilt, poor concentration, changes in appetite (decrease or increase, often with weight variations), fatigue, decreased or increased psychomotor activity (e.g., excessive slowness in talking or thinking or agitation, such as pacing or restlessness), suicidal thoughts, and sleep symptoms. Specifically, both insomnia and hypersomnia (increased total sleep time, often accompanied by residual fatigue, or perception of unrestful sleep) represent possible symptoms for the diagnosis. The symptoms should last at least two weeks to meet DSM-5 criteria for major depressive episode. Depression is very common and is the leading cause of disability worldwide due to decreased productivity and need for hospitalizations [33]. Epidemiological data show that, in the United States, approximately 13% of adults, experience at least one depressive episode in their lifetime [34]. Persistent depressive disorder (previously known as dysthymic disorder or dysthymia) is a milder but more persistent form of depressive disorder, the symptoms of which include chronic low mood for at least two years; insomnia or hypersomnia are one of the possible criteria [1].

Those with bipolar disorders often experience depressive episodes; however, diagnostically, they must also experience manic or hypomanic episodes to meet the criteria of this diagnosis. Mania and hypomania can be grossly described as opposites of depression. Mania is characterized by elated or expansive mood, or irritability, increased energy or activities, inflated self-esteem or full-blown grandiosity, distractibility, and impulsivity lasting at least 1 week. During these episodes, patients feel more confident, attractive, social, and energetic than usual and often engage in dangerous or inappropriate behaviors, both sexually and socially. They can dress more provocatively or spend money excessively. During manic episodes, these individuals often experience delusions (i.e., fixed and false beliefs that are unwavering at times despite evidence to the contrary) or hallucinations (i.e., false perceptions, such as voices in one's head). Often the delusions are grandiose in theme, with patients believing they have special powers, wealth, or knowledge. Hypomania includes similar symptoms, although less intense, and, by definition, the person's functioning is not impaired by them. Actually, during hypomania, people often feel or function better than at baseline. The presence of a manic episode determines the diagnosis of bipolar disorder type I; the presence of hypomanic and depressive episodes determines the diagnosis of bipolar disorder type II. Sleep-wise, mania and hypomania present with decreased need for sleep, which is a sleep symptom unique (or pathognomonic, in medical terminology) to these syndromes. Classically, during manic and hypomanic episodes, patients sleep significantly less (less than 2 hours below their baseline, as a rule of thumb) and wake up energized. In severe cases of mania, patients do not feel the need for sleep for up to several days.

Sleep in Mood Disorders

Mary is a 23-year-old college senior. During the last 2 months she has been feeling progressively more depressed. She feels sad, tired and bored. Even theater, which was one of her passions, seems less interesting. She has been eating less and has lost some weight. At times she thinks she would rather not wake up in the morning. Her sleep is poor; she has difficulties falling asleep and often wakes up too early, without being able to fall back to sleep.

Steve is an 18-year-old college freshman. He was depressed last semester but since last week he has been having some hypomanic symptoms. He is elated and optimistic. He feels more attractive, more confident, and smarter than usual. His friends have noted that he talks more and faster than usual and is more social. He is thinking about setting up a new business and investing his money in it. He usually sleeps 8 hours, but since his mood symptoms started, he noted that he sleeps only 5 to 6 hours per night and still wakes up energized and ready to go.

Sleep symptoms are very common in both depressive and bipolar patients. In some studies, up to 90% of depressive patients report sleep disturbances, with the vast majority (~80%) reporting insomnia, and roughly half reporting hypersomnia (alone or with insomnia) [35]. Studies of patients with bipolar disorder show that an overwhelming 78% to 100% of people in the active manic or hypomanic phase of their bipolar illness report a decreased need for sleep [36]. Additionally, and possibly more interestingly, there is growing evidence that sleep disturbances often precede the development of mood disorders. For example, in longitudinal studies in which young adults have been followed for prolonged periods of time, insomnia appears to increase the risk of developing depression up to fourfold and hypersomnia up to threefold [37]. Similarly, the presence of sleep disturbances (usually difficulties falling asleep and early awakenings) have been associated with an increased risk of bipolar disorder and sleep disturbances often precede a relapse [36]. It is not known whether treating sleep disturbances decreases the risk of developing depression or mania, but it is recognized that regular sleep–wake cycles are essential to maintain mood stability.

Objective Findings

Despite the symptoms experienced by patients with depressive and manic episodes appearing antithetical, objectively, sleep appears affected is similar ways. Although few studies have been conducted in manic patients, both manic and depressive episodes appear to disrupt sleep architecture, shorten REM latency (i.e., the period between sleep-onset and initiation of REM sleep), increase REM density (i.e., the number of eye movements during REM), prolong first REM episode, and decrease slow wave sleep [36].

Treatment

Sleep and mood are deeply biologically intertwined. Treatments that address sleep–wake cycles represent both clinical resources and useful tools for researching the causes of mood disorders. Some of these treatments are also surprising. Sleep deprivation (skipping a whole night of sleep) has a rapid antidepressant effect (i.e., effects are evident in 1–2 days) in the majority of patients with major depressive disorder. However, its results are usually not sustained, and 80% of patients relapse when they resume sleeping. For this reason, some researchers are looking into sustainable ways to "administer sleep deprivation" long-term (e.g., with partial sleep deprivation once a week) [38]. Similarly, a profound phase advance (e.g., going to sleep and falling asleep 4–6 hours earlier than usual) reduces depressive symptoms in 75% of depressed patients in 2 to 3 weeks. However, the mismatch between sleep–wake periods and social activities makes this regimen difficult to sustain for most people [38]. Bright light is also used to address depressive symptoms and it is administered in ways resembling the treatment of delayed sleep phase disorder, with high intensity (2,5000–10,000 lux) around wake-up time. Conversely, extended periods of darkness are being explored as adjunctive treatment for manic symptoms, with initial promising results [38]. Stabilizing circadian rhythms and sleep is also a mainstay of evidence-based treatments for bipolar disorder, including social rhythm therapy. Finally, addition of medications for insomnia has shown to hasten recovery and reduce relapse in both depressive and bipolar disorders.

SCHIZOPHRENIA

Schizophrenia is a disorder involving recurrent bouts of psychosis, which can be roughly defined as symptoms that mark a break from reality. Symptoms of schizophrenia include hallucinations, delusions, disorganized thinking and/or impoverished thinking and speech, cognitive decline, and emotional blunting [1]. Depression and anxiety are also often present. As described in relation to mania, hallucinations are false perceptions such as "hearing voices" in the absence of real stimuli (i.e., auditory hallucinations). Hallucinations can be also visual, physical, olfactory, or gustatory, but these are less common in schizophrenia. Delusions are false beliefs, characteristically firm despite being bizarre or with evidence of contrary, such as believing that others can read their mind or are after them (i.e., paranoid delusion). Disorganized thoughts and behaviors are also seen in schizophrenia; these can include thought patterns that are difficult to follow, such as a person jumping from topic to topic without ever answering the question.

Patients with schizophrenia often have also diminished emotional expression and a decrease in volitional behavior. The prevalence of schizophrenia worldwide is approximately 0.3% to 0.7%, with the majority of cases diagnosed in adolescence and early adulthood [1]. Prior to puberty, schizophrenia is extremely rare.

Sleep in Schizophrenia

Mike is a 19-year-old college freshman who was recently been diagnosed with schizophrenia. He is now taking antipsychotic medication and feels better but previously had multiple symptoms. He became suspicious that his roommates were spying on him and, along with other students, plotting against him. He was hearing voices denigrating him and commenting on his actions. He felt disinterested and stopped caring for himself and couldn't study anymore. He had difficulty falling asleep, was waking frequently, and did not feel rested on waking.

In schizophrenia, sleep disturbances are a common complaint throughout the illness, including the prodromal period, which precedes the full expression of the disorder and during which patients do not have all the symptoms but show some signs. Depending on the study, approximately 30% to 80% of patients with schizophrenia report sleep disturbances, although it is very rarely the presenting complaint [39]. Sleep disturbances in schizophrenia can vary depending on whether a person is acutely psychotic, in which case complaints include difficulty falling asleep, decrease in total sleep time, multiple awakenings, and worsening quality of sleep. In general, treatment with antipsychotics improves insomnia and withdrawal of antipsychotics significantly worsens sleep disruptions [39, 40]. However, even among those with schizophrenia who are clinically stable, circadian rhythm disruption is common, with a higher likelihood of sleeping during the day and waking at night [41, 42]. This is seen in both patients who have never received medications and patients on medications. In addition, acute and severe changes in the sleep of patients with schizophrenia is a warning sign that an acute psychotic decompensation may be forthcoming [40].

Objective Findings

Objective tests have confirmed the subjective complaints in sleep. While there have been some divergent data, patients with schizophrenia are most consistently found to have a prolonged sleep onset latency, increased wake time after sleep onset, poor sleep efficiency, decreased overall total sleep time (due to initial, middle, and late insomnia), shortening of REM latency, slow-wave sleep reduction, and spindle abnormalities [39, 43]. Of note, not only is insomnia frequently seen in schizophrenic patients, but patients who suffer from insomnia commit suicide at higher rates compared with patients with schizophrenia who did not complain of sleep disturbances [44]. Given that the rate of suicide in patients with schizophrenia is alarmingly high (nearly 5%) overall, this is cause for concern [45]. Quality of life among those with schizophrenia who suffer from sleep disturbances has been found to be lower [46, 47]. Several studies have also found correlations between poor sleep and neurocognitive deficits, seen in both medicated and nonmedicated patients with schizophrenia [48, 49].

Treatment

As previously discussed, treatment for sleep in schizophrenia should begin with treating schizophrenia itself. In patients treated with antipsychotics, total sleep time is increased and sleep efficiency improves [39]. Primary treatments for schizophrenia include first- and second-generation antipsychotics, which work by targeting dopamine receptors, and frequently have the side effect of sedation [4]. However, some sleep disorders can also present as side effects of antipsychotics, including PLMD, RLS, and OSA (likely as a result of weight gain secondary to antipsychotics). A few promising studies using CBT for insomnia have showed positive results, albeit in small groups of patients, with improvements in insomnia, persecutory delusions, anxiety, and depression [50].

CONCLUSION

These are exciting days for researchers and clinicians interested in sleep and mental health. Sleep and circadian rhythms are now regarded as key fields to study in basic science and medicine, as shown, for example, by the award of the 2017 Nobel Prize for Medicine to circadian rhythms researchers. Additionally, the involvement of researchers with diverse expertise (e.g., genetics, neuroscience, cognitive psychology) in sleep science will lead to a greater understanding of mechanisms underlying associations between mental disorders and sleep. Sleep is a robust biological phenomenon that provides multiple insights into the mechanisms related to mental illness—and likely valuable tools for prevention and treatment of mental disorders. For example, understanding spindle abnormalities present in schizophrenia might shed light on the pathogenesis and brain changes associated with this disorder. Similarly, altering sleep phase and light–dark exposure patterns in patients with mood disorders might represent alternative or adjunctive treatment modality for mood episodes and help clarify how circadian rhythms affect these disorders. The value of sleep for good mental health has been discussed since the days of Hippocrates; finally, both scientists and the public have a greater appreciation of this.

REFERENCES

1. American Psychiatric Association. *Diagnostic and Statistical Manual of Mental Disorders.* Arlington, VA: American Psychiatric Association; 2013.
2. Caye A, Rocha TB, Anselmi L, et al. Attention-deficit/hyperactivity disorder trajectories from childhood to young adulthood: evidence from a birth cohort supporting a late-onset syndrome. *JAMA Psychiatr.* 2016;73:705–712.
3. Erskine HE, Norman RE, Ferrari AJ, et al. Long-term outcomes of attention-deficit/hyperactivity disorder and conduct disorder: a systematic review and meta-analysis. *J Am Acad Child Adolesc Psychiatr.* 2016;55:841–850.
4. Sadock BJ, Sadock VA, Ruiz P, Kaplan HI. *Kaplan & Sadock's Comprehensive Textbook of Psychiatry.* Philadelphia, PA: Wolters Kluwer Health/Lippincott Williams & Wilkins; 2009.
5. Yoon SY, Jain U, Shapiro C. Sleep in attention-deficit/hyperactivity disorder in children and adults: past, present, and future. *Sleep Med Rev.* 2012;16:371–388.
6. Van Veen MM, Kooij JJ, Boonstra AM, Gordijn MC, Van Someren EJ. Delayed circadian rhythm in adults with attention-deficit/hyperactivity disorder and chronic sleep-onset insomnia. *Biol Psychiatr.* 2010;67:1091–1096.
7. Cortese S, Konofal E, Lecendreux M, et al. Restless legs syndrome and attention-deficit/hyperactivity disorder: a review of the literature. *Sleep.* 2005;28:1007–1013.

8. Walters AS, Silvestri R, Zucconi M, Chandrashekariah R, Konofal E. Review of the possible relationship and hypothetical links between attention deficit hyperactivity disorder (ADHD) and the simple sleep related movement disorders, parasomnias, hypersomnias, and circadian rhythm disorders. *J Clin Sleep Med*. 2008;4:591–600.

9. Gruber R, Cassoff J, Frenette S, Wiebe S, Carrier J. Impact of sleep extension and restriction on children's emotional lability and impulsivity. *Pediatrics*. 2012;130:e1155–e1161.

10. Ganelin-Cohen E, Ashkenasi A. Disordered sleep in pediatric patients with attention deficit hyperactivity disorder: an overview. *Isr Med Assoc J*. 2013;15:705–709.

11. Cortese S, Faraone SV, Konofal E, Lecendreux M. Sleep in children with attention-deficit/hyperactivity disorder: meta-analysis of subjective and objective studies. *J Am Acad Child Adolesc Psychiatr*. 2009;48:894–908.

12. Hvolby A. Associations of sleep disturbance with ADHD: implications for treatment. *Atten Defic Hyperact Disord*. 2015;7:1–18.

13. Souders MC, Zavodny S, Eriksen W,] et al. Sleep in children with autism spectrum disorder. *Curr Psychiatry Rep*. 2017;19:34.

14. Johnson CR, Smith T, DeMand A, et al. Exploring sleep quality of young children with autism spectrum disorder and disruptive behaviors. *Sleep Med*. 2018;44:61–66.

15. Veatch OJ, Goldman SE, Adkins KW, Malow BA. Melatonin in children with autism spectrum disorders: how does the evidence fit together? *J Nat Sci*. 2015;1:e125.

16. Kulman G, Lissoni P, Rovelli F, Roselli MG, Brivio F, Sequeri P. Evidence of pineal endocrine hypofunction in autistic children. *Neuro Endocrinol Lett*. 2000;21:31–34.

17. Tordjman S, Najjar I, Bellissant E, et al. Advances in the research of melatonin in autism spectrum disorders: Literature review and new perspectives. *Int J Mol Sci*. 2013;14:20508–20542.

18. Melke J, Goubran Botros H, Chaste P, et al. Abnormal melatonin synthesis in autism spectrum disorders. *Mol Psychiatr*. 2008,13:90–98.

19. Lane R, Kessler R, Buckley AW, et al. Evaluation of periodic limb movements in sleep and iron status in children with autism. *Pediatr Neurol*. 2015;53:343–309.

20. Elrod MG, Hood BS. Sleep differences among children with autism spectrum disorders and typically developing peers: a meta-analysis. *J Dev Behav Pediatr*. 2015;36:166–177.

21. Limoges E, Mottron L, Bolduc C, Berthiaume C, Godbout R. Atypical sleep architecture and the autism phenotype. *Brain*. 2005;128:1049–1061.

22. Engelhardt CR, Mazurek MO, Sohl K. Media use and sleep among boys with autism spectrum disorder, ADHD, or typical development. *Pediatrics*. 2013;132:1081–1089.

23. Rossignol DA, Frye RE. Melatonin in autism spectrum disorders: a systematic review and meta-analysis. *Dev Med Child Neurol*. 2011;53:783–792.

24. Kessler RC, Avenevoli S, Costello EJ, et al. Prevalence, persistence, and sociodemographic correlates of DSM-IV disorders in the National Comorbidity Survey Replication Adolescent Supplement. *Arch Gen Psychiatr*. 2012;69:372–380.

25. Kessler RC, Chiu WT, Demler O, Merikangas KR, Walters EE. Prevalence, severity, and comorbidity of 12-month DSM-IV disorders in the National Comorbidity Survey Replication. *Arch Gen Psychiatr*. 2005;62:617–627.

26. Alfano CA, Reynolds K, Scott N, Dahl RE, Mellman TA. Polysomnographic sleep patterns of non-depressed, non-medicated children with generalized anxiety disorder. *J Affect Disord*. 2013;147:379–384.

27. Craske MG, Tsao JC. Assessment and treatment of nocturnal panic attacks. *Sleep Med Rev.* 2005;9:173–184.

28. Kovachy B, O'Hara R, Hawkins N, et al. Sleep disturbance in pediatric PTSD: current findings and future directions. *J Clin Sleep Med.* 2013;9:501–510.

29. Spoormaker VI, Montgomery P. Disturbed sleep in post-traumatic stress disorder: secondary symptom or core feature? *Sleep Med Rev.* 2008;12:169–184.

30. McMakin DL, Alfano CA. Sleep and anxiety in late childhood and early adolescence. *Curr Opin Psychiatr.* 2015;28:483–489.

31. Cox RC, Olatunji BO. A systematic review of sleep disturbance in anxiety and related disorders. *J Anxiety Disord.* 2016;37:104–129.

32. Aurora RN, Zak RS, Auerbach SH, et al. Best practice guide for the treatment of nightmare disorder in adults. *J Clin Sleep Med.* 2010; 6:389–401.

33. World Health Organization. *World Health Statistics 2018.* Geneva, Switzerland: World Health Organization; 2018.

34. Hasin DS, Goodwin RD, Stinson FS, Grant BF. Epidemiology of major depressive disorder: results from the National Epidemiologic Survey on Alcoholism and Related Conditions. *Arch Gen Psychiatr.* 2005;62(10):1097–1106.

35. Geoffroy PA, Hoertel N, Etain B, et al. Insomnia and hypersomnia in major depressive episode: Prevalence, sociodemographic characteristics and psychiatric comorbidity in a population-based study. *J Affect Disord.* 2018;226:132–141.

36. Harvey AG, Talbot LS, Gershon A. Sleep disturbance in bipolar disorder across the lifespan. *Clin Psychol.* 2009;16:256–277.

37. Breslau N, Roth T, Rosenthal L, Andreski P. Sleep disturbance and psychiatric disorders: a longitudinal epidemiological study of young adults. *Biol Psychiatr.* 1996;39:411–418.

38. Dallaspezia S, Suzuki M, Benedetti F. Chronobiological therapy for mood disorders. *Curr Psychiatry Rep.* 2015;17:95.

39. Cohrs S. Sleep disturbances in patients with schizophrenia: Impact and effect of antipsychotics. *CNS Drugs.* 2008;22:939–962.

40. Chemerinski E, Ho BC, Flaum M, Arndt S, Fleming F, Andreasen NC. Insomnia as a predictor for symptom worsening following antipsychotic withdrawal in schizophrenia. *Compr Psychiatr.* 2002;43:393–396.

41. Benson KL. Sleep in schizophrenia: impairments, correlates, and treatment. *Psychiatr Clin North Am.* 2006;29:1033–1045.

42. Pritchett D, Wulff K, Oliver PL, et al. Evaluating the links between schizophrenia and sleep and circadian rhythm disruption. *J Neural Transm.* 2012;119:1061–1075.

43. Kamath J, Virdi S, Winokur A. Sleep disturbances in schizophrenia. *Psychiatr Clin North Am.* 2015;38:777–792.

44. Pompili M, Lester D, Grispini A, et al. Completed suicide in schizophrenia: evidence from a case-control study. *Psychiatry Res.* 2009; 167:251–257.

45. Palmer BA, Pankratz VS, Bostwick JM. The lifetime risk of suicide in schizophrenia: a reexamination. *Arch Gen Psychiatr.* 2005;62:247–253.

46. Hofstetter JR, Lysaker PH, Mayeda AR. Quality of sleep in patients with schizophrenia is associated with quality of life and coping. *BMC Psychiatr.* 2005;5:13.

47. Ritsner M, Kurs R, Ponizovsky A, Hadjez J. Perceived quality of life in schizophrenia: relationships to sleep quality. *Qual Life Res.* 2004;13:783–791.

48. Wulff K, Joyce E. Circadian rhythms and cognition in schizophrenia. *Br J Psychiatr.* 2011;198:250–252.
49. Yang C, Winkelman JW. Clinical significance of sleep EEG abnormalities in chronic schizophrenia. *Schizophr Res.* 2006;82:251–260.
50. Myers E, Startup H, Freeman D. Cognitive behavioural treatment of insomnia in individuals with persistent persecutory delusions: a pilot trial. *J Behav Ther Exp Psychiatr.* 2011;42:330–336.

21

Pharmacology of Sleep

JENNIFER L. MARSELLA AND CAROLINA Z. MARCUS ■

INTRODUCTION: HISTORY OF PHARMACOLOGY OF SLEEP

Never under any circumstances take a sleeping pill and laxative on the same night.

—Dave Barry, 19 Things That Took Me 50 Years to Learn

Although behavioral interventions are often used first in treating sleep disorders, one in six adults diagnosed with a sleep disorder use prescription sleep aids [1]. Use of sleep aids dates back to ancient times, when herbs were used to make "sleeping potions." In those times, opium and alcohol were the only drugs available to help oneself drift off to sleep.

During the 19th century came anesthetic drugs to "knock you out." Diethyl ether was widely abused, although not prescribed by physicians for sleep disorders. However, a derivative of this, chloral hydrate, was developed and prescribed as a sedative in 1869. Also used in the 19th century were bromide salts, paraldehyde, and sulfonmenthane. Morphine use increased during the second half of the 19th, century with the introduction of syringes. Morphine was named after Morpheus, the Greek god of dreams, due to its sleep-inducing properties. The term *hypnotic* also has its roots in Greek mythology, coming from Hypnos, the Greek god of sleep.

In the early 1900s, barbiturates were used to treat sleep disturbances [2]. Barbital was introduced in 1903 and phenobarbital in 1912, followed by a slew of others in that class. However, barbiturates were highly addictive and lad to overdoses and suicides. Amphetamines were first introduced in 1927 and then used to treat narcolepsy in 1935 [3]. However, this was not the first use of a stimulant. Rather, stimulants, most commonly cocaine from the coca plant, have been used to alleviate drowsiness for hundreds of years [4]. The effects of these drugs were demonstrated in Jacqueline Susann's 1966 novel *Valley of Dolls*, which told the story of aspiring actresses, termed "dolls," who took barbiturates and amphetamines [3].

Due to the adverse side effects of—and overdoses caused by—barbiturates, researchers began looking for a safer treatment option. In 1957, Leo Sternbach, an organic chemist who worked for Roche, achieved this by testing leftover compounds from earlier projects. He found that one of these compounds, chlordi-azepoxide, had sedative, muscle-relaxant, and anticonvulsive effects. This was the first benzodiazepine (BZD) and demonstrated a safer side effect profile compared to barbiturates. It was first marketed as Librium in 1960. By the 1970s, BZDs were the most commonly prescribed drug in the world [3]. In 1970, the first US Food and Drug Administration (FDA)-approved hypnotic, specifically for sleep, was flurazepam [2].

Antihistamines have been taken over the counter for sleep since the 1940s, but it was not until the late 1970s that the FDA approved them for sleep. In 1988, the first BZD receptor agonist, zolpidem (Ambien™), was introduced in Europe, and became FDA-approved in December of 1992, followed by several other Z-drugs in the 1990s to early 2000s. In the rest of this chapter, we will discuss these and some of the newer medications used to treat disorders of sleep.

MEDICATIONS USED TO TREAT SLEEP DISORDERS

Treatment of Insomnia

Insomnia affects at least 30% of the population and sleeping pills for its treatment are one of the most frequently prescribed medications [5]. Although the gold standard treatment for insomnia is a nonpharmacological therapy, specifically cognitive behavioral therapy for insomnia (also see Chapter 18 of this volume), pharmacological treatment of insomnia is a billion-dollar industry. About 1 in 20 people have used prescription sleep aids in the previous month [1]. If you add over-the-counter drugs, this increases the number to about one in three people who have used some type of sleep aid within the past year. Think about what you, your friends, or your family members have taken to help with sleep—do alcohol, Benadryl™ (diphenhydramine), or melatonin come to mind? When we think about the mechanisms of how these work—and the neurotransmitters and hormones involved—it makes sense that these drugs cause sleepiness (see Table 21.1).

Why does alcohol lead to sleepiness? Alcohol acts on the gamma-aminobutyric acid (GABA) system. GABA in the ventrolateral preoptic area in the hypothal-amus is the main neurotransmitter that causes you to flip the switch to sleep. Drinking alcohol or taking medications that affect GABA receptors will cause you to sleep. This is why muscle relaxants, like baclofen, which act on GABA, are sedating. Which medications for insomnia act on GABA receptors? The BZD agonists and non-BZD receptor agonists (see Table 21.1).

Table 21.1 PHARMACOLOGIC TREATMENT OF INSOMNIA

Benzodiazepine Agonists	Benzodiazepines (BZD): estazolam,* flurazepam,* temazepam,* triazolam,* quazepam,*
	Non-BZD, Z-drugs: eszopiclone,* zaleplon,* zolpidem*
Melatonin/Melatonin Agonists	melatonin, ramelteon,* tasimelteon*
Antidepressants	Tricyclic Antidepressant (TCA): doxepin*
	Histamine antagonists: trazodone, mirtazapine
Barbiturates	butabarbital,* secobarbital*
Hypocretin/orexin Receptor Antagonists	suvorexant*
Atypical Antipsychotics	Serotonin and histamine antagonists: olanzapine, quetiapine, risperidone
Over-the-Counter Medications	Antihistamines: diphenhydramine, doxylamine

*U.S. Food and Drug approved for insomnia.

BZDs, as previously described, were developed as a safer alternative to barbiturates, which decrease latency to sleep and nocturnal awakenings due to their central nervous system (CNS) depressing effects. Remember, barbiturates were heavily abused and could lead to overdoses. Although this class is FDA-approved for insomnia, the side effect profile often outweighs the benefits, which led to the development of BZDs. All of the FDA-approved BZDs, except for temazepam, are effective for difficulties with falling asleep (sleep onset) and staying asleep (sleep maintenance). Temazepam is only effective for sleep onset difficulties in adults ages 18 to 65 and for sleep maintenance in adults ages 65 and older. The most common side effects of this class include sedation, memory difficulties, abnormal sleep behaviors, and difficulty walking, which can lead to falls, especially in the elderly. BZDs can still lead to dependence and tolerance, and they are prone to abuse, especially in those with a history of alcohol and substance abuse. Given that BZDs can be very addicting, it is recommended that they only be used as needed and to avoid using them long-term for sleep [6].

The non-BZD receptor agonists were introduced as a safer option to BZDs. We call these so-called sleeping pills the Z-drugs—zolpidem (Ambien™), (es)zopiclone, and zaleplon. These bind selectively to GABA$_A$ receptors, which may be why they are less likely to lead to dependence and tolerance, are less often abused, and have a more favorable side effect profiles. Despite this, patients can still present with unusual behaviors after taking non-BZDs, such as driving to a fast food restaurant *while asleep* or appearing confused and intoxicated. These are typically worsened when compounded by other sedating medications, alcohol, or illicit substances [7]. Of the non-BZD receptor agonists, all are effective at helping patients fall asleep. Long-acting zolpidem CR and eszopiclone are also effective at helping patients stay asleep [6].

Melatonin is a sleep-promoting hormone that your body naturally produces, by the pineal gland, and is released in response to darkness. Taking exogenous melatonin decreased latency to sleep onset in those with insomnia [8]. However, in the United States, where it is not FDA-regulated, there is wide variability in the actual content of melatonin supplements, making dosing inconsistent [9, 10]. Melatonin agonists act in the same way, but the effectiveness of this class of drug may be minimal [9].

Doxepin is a tricyclic antidepressant with a high affinity for histamine receptors, causing histamine antagonism, which helps with sleep maintenance but not initiation. Trazodone, a serotonin reuptake inhibitor and histamine antagonist, is FDA-approved to treat depression and is sometimes used off-label for insomnia due to its hypnotic effect. Other antidepressants and atypical antipsychotic medications also work to antagonize histamine, leading to sedation [11].

One of the main wake-promoting hormones is hypocretin (also known as orexin), a neuropeptide present in the lateral hypothalamic area. Hypocretin/ orexin-blocking medications, like suvorexant, prevent wakefulness and can initiate and/or maintain sleep [6]. Orexin receptor antagonists improve total sleep time and can be a well-tolerated option for those with insomnia [11].

Diphenhydramine and doxepin, like allergy medications, are in the family of medications that block histamine—remember this neurotransmitter in the tuberomammilary nucleus that promotes wakefulness? Well, when you block it, it does the opposite and causes sleepiness. However, these medications can also reduce the quality of sleep and can cause grogginess the next day. Additionally, tolerance is achieved within 3 days of use, after which they may have minimal effects [11].

Why do we feel sleepy after eating turkey on Thanksgiving? Is it really because of the tryptophan? Studies have shown that increased L-tryptophan reduces latency to sleep and increases subjective sleepiness [12]. This is because L-tryptophan is a precursor to serotonin, which is a precursor to melatonin. However, turkey does not have any more tryptophan than other poultry. This postdinner slump, or "postprandial drowsiness," may actually be mediated by the interaction of orexin/ hypocretin with rising levels of glucose after meals [13].

Treatment of Hypersomnias

Now let us switch to the opposite problem of insomnia: hypersomnia or excessive daytime sleepiness. Are you drinking caffeine right now to stay awake to read this chapter? Stimulants are typically used to combat sleepiness, among which caffeine is the most commonly used. Caffeine acts as an adenosine antagonist. Adenosine increases while you are awake, especially in the basal forebrain, and contributes to sleep pressure, with levels decreasing with sleep. Adenosine causes sleepiness through inhibition of histamine transmission and decreased hypocretin/orexin neuronal activity [14]. However, by antagonizing adenosine receptors, these are increased, and wakefulness is maintained. Have you ever heard people say that they are very sensitive to caffeine or that it does not affect them at all? Well, caffeine responsiveness may vary due to variations in the adenosine system [15].

Another commonly used stimulant is nicotine, which increases acetylcholine signaling within the basal forebrain, leading to increased release of dopamine, resulting in wakefulness. In heavy smokers, the hypothalamic–pituitary–adrenal axis can be activated, leading to increased adrenocorticotropic hormone and cortisone, which are wake-promoting [4]. Nicotine has been shown to decrease total sleep time and efficiency, as well as to prolong sleep latency and reduce rapid eye movement (REM) sleep [4].

Since caffeine, nicotine, and other stimulants may mask underlying sleep disorders, it is important to first identify what is causing this excessive sleepiness and to treat these underlying causes. However, in those who have central disorders of hypersomnolence, like narcolepsy, stimulants can be very helpful. Medications that lead to wakefulness typically work through activation of the ascending arousal pathway (see Table 21.2).

The main class of stimulants is amphetamines and its derivatives, which are similar in structure to amphetamines but with substituents for at least one hydrogen atom. This drug class acts by blocking reuptake of dopamine in the ventral periaqueductal grey area, norepinephrine in the locus coeruleus, and serotonin in the dorsal raphe nucleus, which increases monoamine transmission and promotes wakefulness through its excitatory effects on the ascending arousal pathway and inhibitory effects on sleep-promoting neurons of the ventral lateral preoptic area. Amphetamines increase sleep latency and improve symptoms of sleepiness. These effects have made medications, such as Adderall™ and Ritalin™, popular among college students, both recreationally and to pull an "all-nighter" to finish a paper or study for a test. However, tolerance to these effects increases

Table 21.2 PHARMACOLOGIC TREATMENT OF HYPERSOMNIAS

Drug	Mechanism of Action
Modafinil,* Armodafinil*	Unknown: possibly inhibits dopamine reuptake, norepinephrine reuptake
Amphetamines (amphetamine,* methamphetamine, dextroamphetamine, methylphenidate*)	Inhibits dopamine, norepinephrine, and serotonin reuptake
Sodium oxybate*	Unknown: possibly GABA$_B$ agonism
Solriamfetol	Inhibits selective dopamine and norepinephrine reuptake
Pitolisant	Increases histamine release by histamine 3 auto-receptor antagonism and inverse agonism
Caffeine	Adenosine antagonist
Nicotine	Acetylcholine agonist, increases dopamine

*U.S. Food and Drug approved for pathologic sleepiness in narcolepsy.

over time [14]. Their most common side effects include increased heart rate, elevated blood pressure, appetite suppression, stomach upset, and headaches due to the catecholaminergic effects.

Within the amphetamine class is pseudoephedrine. Often used as a decongestant, this medication has stimulant properties due to its adrenergic receptor activity. The International Olympic Committee has even prohibited its use (of greater that 150 micrograms per milliliter in urine), since athletes have used this as a stimulant [16]. Cocaine acts similarly to amphetamine stimulants, inhibiting monoamine reuptake and increasing dopamine, norepinephrine, and serotonin release. It also decreases sleepiness, increases latency to sleep and REM sleep, and decreases duration of REM sleep [4]. Amphetamines and cocaine have high potentials for abuse and dependence.

Nonamphetamine stimulants, which include modafinil and armodafinil, are better tolerated than amphetamines. Their mechanism of action is unclear, but they appear to increase wakefulness via dopamine, and possibly norepinephrine, reuptake inhibition leading to increased catecholamine transmission, which is involved in the ascending arousal pathway [14]. Given increased catecholamines, these medications can still cause the side effects seen with amphetamines. They can also lower hormonal contraception levels and decrease their effectiveness and carry a rare risk of a serious skin reaction.

In those with narcolepsy (also see Chapter 19 of this volume), a medication called sodium oxybate, or gamma-hydroxybutyric acid, is thought to consolidate night-time sleep, thereby reducing sleep pressure and daytime sleepiness [17]. This medication also can improve cataplectic symptoms. Despite its efficacy and favorable side effect profile, this drug is controlled since it has been abused as a date-rape drug and by athletes to increase release of growth hormone via its increase of slow wave sleep [17, 18].

A recently FDA-approved medication used to treat excessive daytime sleepiness is solriamfetol, which works through selective dopamine and norepinephrine reuptake inhibition, leading to wakefulness through the ascending arousal pathway [19, 20]. Pitolisant is another new medication that improves wakefulness, through a different mechanism. Pitolisant is a histamine 3 receptor antagonist and inverse agonist that increases histamine transmission in the brain and promotes wakefulness [21]. It would seem like an orexin/hypocretin agonist would be a clear target for a medication to decrease sleepiness. However, this peptide is too large to cross the blood–brain barrier to exert its effect on orexin/hypocretin neurons in the lateral hypothalamus.

Parasomnias

When treating parasomnias, you must first identify its type. Is it a NREM parasomnia, like sleepwalking or confusional arousals, or a REM parasomnia, like nightmare disorder or REM sleep behavior disorder? Many of these can improve or resolve with behavioral modifications and various forms of therapy (also see

Chapter 19 of this volume). It is also important to consider removing medications that may be exacerbating parasomnias. If, despite these interventions, disruptive or injurious parasomnias continue, then pharmacologic management may be helpful.

When pharmacologic therapy is used, NREM parasomnias are most commonly treated with BZDs, such as clonazepam. It is possible that this works by decreasing transitions from stage N3 to N2 and stabilizing sleep [22]. However, the mechanism of this is unclear, especially since BZD receptor agonists that also work at the $GABA_A$ receptors can worsen parasomnias, like the bizarre night-time behaviors of those who have taken Ambien™, as previously described [23]. Although the pathophysiology of NREM parasomnias is unclear, serotonin signaling may be involved [23]. Antidepressants, especially those with prominent serotonergic effects, can be helpful in NREM parasomnias. However, it seems that this class of medications, like paroxetine, may improve sleep-talking, but may worsen sleepwalking. Imipramine is a norepinephrine and serotonin reuptake inhibitor; again, it is unclear how this improves parasomnias. There is no evidence that pharmacologic management helps those with confusional arousals. Sleep-related eating disorder, which can lead to significant weight gain, may be treated by pramipexole, a dopamine agonist, or topiramate, an antiseizure medication that also works for appetite suppression [23].

REM sleep behavior disorder is best treated by clonazepam or melatonin [24]. Clonazepam, a BZD, is highly effective initially in low dosages. It works by decreasing phasic motor activity during REM sleep [23]. Since this can be sedating and worsen cognition and gait disturbance in those with neurodegenerative disease, high-dose melatonin is a better tolerated alternative. Melatonin decreases both phasic and tonic motor activity during REM sleep. Clonazepam and melatonin can also be used together.

In nightmare disorder, BZDs (nitrazepam, triazolam) or prazosin can be effective. Atypical antipsychotics (olanzapine, aripiprazole, risperidone), antidepressants (imipramine and other tricyclic antidepressants, fluvoxamine, phenelzine, trazodone), antiepileptics (gabapentin, topiramate), prazosin, clonidine, cyproheptadine, and nabilone can be used to treat PTSD-related nightmares. Prazosin is an alpha-1 adrenergic receptor antagonist and clonidine is an alpha-2 adrenergic receptor agonists. These both work by decreasing sympathetic flow in the brain, which affects REM sleep and decreases PTSD-related nightmares. Olanzapine, an atypical antipsychotic, increases slow-wave sleep and decreases REMs through serotonin receptor antagonism, leading to reduced nightmares and PTSD symptoms. Cyproheptadine and antidepressants also increase serotonin outflow to decrease nightmares. Some people use marijuana to treat their nightmares; a study of a synthetic cannabinoid receptor agonist, nabilone, showed that this reduces nightmares, but its mechanism is unknown [25].

Sleep-Related Movement Disorders

If you have ever experienced an overwhelming and unpleasant urge to move your legs while sitting on an airplane or long car ride, you may have experienced symptoms of restless legs syndrome (RLS), also known as Willis–Ekbom Disease (WED). English physician Sir Thomas Willis first described this condition in 1672 as a phenomenon of chronic sleep disruption triggered by frequent limb movements [26]. While other descriptions of the disorder were published in the interim, it was not until 1945 that Swedish neurologist Dr. Karl-Axel Ekbom detailed a comprehensive report of this condition in his doctoral thesis and coined the term "restless legs." Although Dr. Ekbom devoted much of his career to understanding and better characterizing this syndrome, his work was largely overlooked for decades [26]. Formerly known as RLS, the disorder is now also referred to as WED. Going forward, we will refer to this medical condition with the abbreviations, RLS/WED.

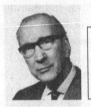

Swedish neurologist, Dr. Karl-Axel Ekbom

Chaudhuri KR. The restless legs syndrome. *Practical Neurology* 2003;3:204-13.

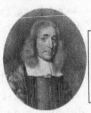

British physician, Sir Thomas Willis

http://www.oxforddnb.com/view/article/29587, Public Domain, https://commons.wikimedia.org/w/index.php?curid=20313755

RLS/WED often involves parts of the body other than the legs. The arms can be involved as well and, in some cases, the torso [27]. RLS/WED is a common disorder, with an estimated 5% to 15% of the general population experiencing symptoms [28]. It is a disorder of the CNS, and the diagnosis is made clinically. There are no specific laboratory tests for RLS/WED, and a sleep study is not routinely indicated in the workup of RLS/WED. Four symptoms are used to describe and confirm the diagnosis [29]:

1. A strong and annoying need or urge to move the limbs (typically legs, but may include arms as well), usually associated with unpleasant or uncomfortable sensations (often aching, tingling, pulling, or crawling in nature).
2. The sensations and urge to move typically worsen during inactivity or rest.
3. The sensations improve (or disappear) with activity.
4. Symptoms are typically worse in the evening or night.

Because the sensations of RLS/WED often happen in the evening hours and while at rest, the disorder can make it difficult for people to fall asleep at night. Over time, the accumulated loss of sleep from this disorder can make a person feel sleepy or fatigued during the daytime and may lead to irritability and impaired concentration or attention. Not surprisingly, people with RLS/WED are more likely to suffer from depression or anxiety as well [30]. Most people with RLS/WED experience symptoms intermittently, but some individuals experience significant discomfort on a regular basis, which can negatively impact their quality of life. I have worked with several patients over the years who could not drive short distances, from their home to the grocery store for example, without pulling over to stretch or move their legs. I also recall a patient who was not able to visit her grandchildren due to severe symptoms while traveling by car or airplane. We should also note that there is a similar, but separate, nocturnal limb movement disorder called periodic limb movement disorder (PLMD). Whereas RLS typically occurs while a person is awake, by definition, PLMD occurs strictly during sleep. A person with PLMD moves their limbs involuntarily and periodically during sleep, which can lead to brief yet repeated arousals from sleep during the night. Generally, a person with PLMD is unaware of the limb movements during the night but may awaken from sleep feeling unrefreshed and will often experience daytime sleepiness and/or fatigue [31].

Various factors may underlie the development of symptoms of RLS/WED—a deficiency of iron stores in the body, genetic predisposition, unintended effects of medications, pregnancy, and renal disease are the most common associations. Up to 19% of women experience symptoms of RLS/WED during pregnancy and symptoms often subside relatively quickly postpartum [27, 29]. RLS/WED also occurs in up to 50% of patients with end-stage renal failure, which can be particularly bothersome during dialysis, as a patient is typically confined to a resting position for a prolonged period during this treatment [32]. Antidepressant medications such as tricyclic antidepressants, selective serotonin reuptake inhibitors (SSRIs), serotonin and norepinephrine reuptake inhibitors, lithium, and dopamine antagonists (used to treat schizophrenia and other psychiatric conditions), may worsen or trigger RLS/WED symptoms. Often, discontinuation of these medications leads to improvement and/or resolution of RLS/WED symptoms [30–32].

Iron is a co-factor in the rate-limiting step of dopamine production inside the brain. In several research studies, low iron levels have been found in the blood and spinal fluid of individuals suffering from RLS/WED, and specifically a low serum ferritin concentration has been associated with an increased severity of RLS/WED symptoms. Ferritin is a protein that our bodies use to store iron and release it where needed. It is an indirect marker of the amount of iron stored in the body's CNS [33]. It is important to note that a person's iron stores can be deficient in the absence of significant anemia; thus, an individual may have normal serum iron levels yet demonstrate a deficiency of serum ferritin. If the serum ferritin level is low (below 75 ng/mL), repletion of iron with a daily oral iron supplement can often lead to a significant improvement in the frequency and intensity of RLS/WED symptoms [34].

In most cases, pharmacologic treatment for RLS/WED is not necessary, given that symptoms are sporadic for most individuals. For many, lifestyle modifications such as regular exercise, avoidance of caffeine, and stopping smoking reduce the frequency of symptoms. For those with more persistent symptoms and whose serum ferritin level is not low, pharmacologic treatment may be indicated. The selection of pharmacologic agents to treat RLS/WED is influenced by a number of factors, including the age of the patient, severity and frequency of symptoms, presence of pregnancy or comorbid medical conditions, and renal failure [31-32].

PHARMACOLOGIC TREATMENT FOR RLS/WED

Recognized treatments for RLS/WED include alpha-2-delta calcium channel ligands, dopamine agonists, opioids, and BZDs. Interestingly, these medications were largely developed for other medical problems, and incidentally found to be beneficial for RLS/WED.

Alpha-2-Delta Calcium Channel Ligands

Alpha-2-delta calcium channel ligands have a broad application in medicine. They are used for management of chronic pain, anxiety, hot flashes, fibromyalgia, and some forms of epilepsy. Alpha-2-delta calcium channel ligands are currently recommended as first line treatment for moderate-to-severe RLS/WED. Gabapentin and pregabalin are alpha-2-delta ligand medications. Both medications have a molecular structure similar to that of the neurotransmitter GABA and act by inhibiting certain calcium channels. Both gabapentin and pregabalin are able to cross the blood-brain barrier and enter the CNS. Gabapentin and pregabalin are taken by mouth. The most common side effects include dizziness, fatigue, drowsiness, ataxia, and peripheral edema (swelling of extremities). The latter side effect of lower extremity swelling is rare but can be quite painful. Alpha-2-delta ligand medications are processed by the kidneys and eliminated in the urine. These medications should be used carefully in people with compromised kidney function, due to possible accumulation and toxicity. It is unclear if the use of these medications is safe during pregnancy or breastfeeding [31].

Dopamine Agonists

The medications pramipexole and ropinirole were initially developed for the treatment of Parkinson's disease. However, they have also been shown to improve RLS/WED symptoms that, as we know, are also thought to derive from impaired dopaminergic signaling in the brain. Dopamine receptor agonists are recommended, with caution, as a first-line treatment for moderate to severe RLS. They are known to cause orthostatic hypotension or sudden drops in blood pressure when shifting from a recumbent to a standing, or sitting, position. This is, of particular, concern with elderly patients who may get up frequently during the night to urinate and could experience dizziness or lightheadedness from orthostatic hypotension. Excessive daytime sleepiness can occur at higher doses and occasionally may manifest as sudden and unexpected sleep attacks. Although rare, compulsive and impulsive behaviors, such as gambling or hypersexuality, may occur with dopaminergic agents.

I worked with one older patient who was treated with high doses of ropinirole for RLS/WED and who was really bothered by daytime sleepiness. In reviewing his history, he casually mentioned that about an hour or two after going to sleep at night, he would wake up to urinate and, upon awakening, would feel compelled to work on his craft projects. This became an ongoing impulse, to the extent that he began to spend hours at night working on his crafts, rather than sleeping. Not surprisingly, this patient struggled to stay awake during the day. As we gradually reduced the dose of the ropinirole, his nocturnal crafting compulsion subsided.

It is important to note that pramipexole is cleared by the kidneys, while ropinirole undergoes metabolism in the liver. Pramipexole should be avoided in individuals with renal disease, and ropinirole should be avoided in those with compromised liver function. Augmentation, which refers to a worsening of RLS/WED symptoms with increasing doses of the medication, including earlier onset and increased intensity of symptoms, is an unfortunate yet common complication of long-term dopaminergic therapy [31].

Benzodiazepines

BZDs are a class of drugs used to treat anxiety, insomnia, seizures, and muscle spasms, among other conditions. All members of the BZD class bind with high affinity to neuronal $GABA_A$ receptors, which mediate synaptic and extrasynaptic forms of neuronal inhibition. GABA is the primary inhibitory CNS neurotransmitter. BZDs can be useful for mild cases of RLS/WED, particularly in younger adult patients. The best-studied BZD for RLS/WED is clonazepam. It is typically effective at a fairly low dose, although its long duration of action may cause more adverse effects, such as unsteadiness, drowsiness, or impaired cognitive function. Older adult patients may have a higher rate of experiencing these adverse effects. Clonazepam may also exacerbate obstructive sleep apnea (OSA). Tolerance to BZDs may develop; thus, clonazepam is best used for patients who require only intermittent therapy [31].

Opioids

Opioid medications, such as codeine, oxycodone, morphine, and methadone, are primarily used for pain management. Interestingly, the benefit of opioids for RLS/WED was first reported by Sir Thomas Willis, in 1685. Specifically, methadone can be highly effective in patients with severe or refractory RLS/WED symptoms that have not responded to other therapeutic agents. It can be used as a monotherapy, or in combination with other medications. It has long-term efficacy and tolerability, and augmentation is not described with methadone. We recognize that the goal of therapy with opioids is to reduce the unpleasant sensations of RLS/

WED, not to manage or alleviate pain [35]. Opioids should be used cautiously for patients who snore and are at-risk for sleep apnea, due to the risk for exacerbation of breathing disturbances during sleep. Long-term opiate therapy may also lead to the development of central sleep apnea. Prior to initiation of opiate therapy, patients should be assessed for the risk of opioid use disorder, and state prescription drug monitoring programs should be queried. A urine drug screen should be performed as well [31].

CIRCADIAN RHYTHM DISORDERS

For an individual with delayed sleep phase syndrome (also see Chapter 15), morning light therapy, along with strategic avoidance of light in the evenings, can be an effective way to help advance the sleep phase [36]. Exposure to bright light directly inhibits melatonin release, while darkness encourages melatonin production by the pineal gland, situated deep in the center of the brain. As such, some have taken to calling melatonin the "hormone of darkness." Melatonin is involved in maintenance of the body's circadian rhythms. Levels of melatonin begin to rise in the evening, promoting sleep, and drop before the sun rises, promoting wakefulness. The American Academy of Sleep Medicine Clinical Practice Guidelines endorses the use of strategically timed melatonin to help regulate the sleep–wake cycle in individuals with delayed sleep–wake phase disorder, for children and adolescents with irregular sleep–wake rhythm disorder, and for blind adults with non-24-hour sleep–wake rhythm disorder [37]. For night owls, low-dose melatonin taken earlier in the evening can help advance the sleep phase [38]. It can also be used to align the endogenous circadian rhythm with the environment in blind individuals who are not able to perceive light. Tasimelteon, a melatonin receptor agonist, is the only FDA-approved treatment for non-24-hour sleep–wake rhythm disorder [39].

For a sustained beneficial effect, it is important that melatonin therapy be given consistently, at a fixed time each night, and maintained on a strict 24-hour cycle. Research suggests that synthetic melatonin is relatively safe. Melatonin is considered a dietary supplement and is therefore not subject to regulation by the FDA. Concerns have been raised about the purity of available preparations, as well as reliability of stated doses [37, 38, 40]. In 2017, a group of Canadian researchers published data on 31 commercially available, over-the-counter melatonin supplements [41]. They found that the actual melatonin content ranged between –83% to +478% of the labeled content on the packaging.

SLEEP-DISORDERED BREATHING

Pharmacologic therapy is generally not a part of the primary treatment recommendations for sleep-disordered breathing or OSA (also see Chapter 17 of this volume). A number of mechanisms have been proposed by which drugs could theoretically reduce the severity of OSA, including increasing in the upper airway dilator muscle tone, enhancing ventilatory drive, reducing the proportion of REM sleep, and reducing upper airway resistance. Although numerous medications have been studied in randomized trials as primary treatment agents for OSA, there is insufficient evidence to recommend the use of drug therapy in the treatment of sleep-disordered breathing. Continuous positive air pressure, a medical device, remains the mainstay of treatment for OSA. However, modafinil, armodafinil, and solriamfetol have been approved by the FDA for use by patients with residual daytime sleepiness, despite adherence to continuous positive air pressure therapy [42, 43].

MEDICATIONS THAT CAUSE SLEEP AND WAKE DISTURBANCES

Many prescription and over-the-counter drugs can adversely impact sleep. Some cause insomnia, while others disrupt sleep continuity, compromise sleep quality, or lead to drowsiness during the daytime. Beta-blockers and clonidine, drugs commonly used to treat elevated blood pressure, can exacerbate insomnia and are associated with nightmares. Interestingly, beta-blockers have been shown to suppress endogenous melatonin production [44]. Diuretics can disrupt sleep continuity by causing frequent night-time urination and can trigger painful muscle cramps during sleep. Corticosteroids, certain antidepressants, thyroid hormone replacement medications, decongestants, caffeine, and some herbal medications can contribute to insomnia. CNS stimulant medications, used for the treatment of attention-deficit/hyperactivity disorder as well as hypersomnia, can make it difficult to fall asleep. Asthma medications, nicotine replacement therapy, and over-the-counter painkillers that contain caffeine can have this effect as well.

Other medications may not interfere with falling asleep but can still disrupt sleep quality. For example, some cholesterol-lowering agents may cause nightmares and trigger frequent night-time awakenings. Certain medications used for anxiety and depression, particularly selective serotonin reuptake inhibitors and serotonin and norepinephrine reuptake inhibitors, as well as BZDs, can lower sleep quality by suppressing REM sleep.

While some medications can keep you awake and make it difficult to sleep, others may lead to daytime drowsiness. For instance, many allergy medicines contain antihistamines, which can cause daytime sleepiness. Some antidepressants and medications used for managing psychosis or anxiety can have sedating effects. Other drugs are known to cause drowsiness, including opioids, muscle relaxants, beta-blockers, and antiseizure medications [45].

CONCLUSIONS

Although pharmacologic treatment of sleep disorders is rarely first line, it is important to understand the underlying mechanisms of these medications in treating sleep disorders and how other drugs can interfere with sleep in various ways.

REFERENCES

1. Chong Y, Fryer CD, Gu Q. Prescription sleep aid use among adults: United States, 2005–2010. *NCHS Data Brief*. 2013;127:1–8.

2. Sateia MJ, Buysse DJ, Krystal AD, Neubauer DN, Heald JL. Clinical practice guideline for the pharmacologic treatment of chronic insomnia in adults: an American Academy of Sleep Medicine clinical practice guideline. *J Clin Sleep Med*. 2017;13:307–349.

3. Mendelson W. *Understanding Sleeping Pills*. n.p.: W Mendelson; 2018.

4. Boutrel B, Koob GF. What keeps up awake: the neuropharmacology of stimulants and wakefulness-promoting medications. *Sleep*. 2004;27:1181–1194.

5. Roth T. Insomnia: definition, prevalence, etiology, and consequences. *J Clin Sleep Med*. 2007;3:S7–S10.

6. Asnis GM, Thomas M, Henderson MA. Pharmacotherapy treatment options for insomnia: a primer for clinicians. *Int J Mol Sci*. 2016;17:50.

7. Poceta JS. Zolpidem ingestion, automatisms, and sleep driving: a clinical and legal case series. *J Clin Sleep Med*. 2011;7:632–638.

8. Auld F, Maschauer EL, Morrison I, Skene DJ, Riha RL. Evidence for the efficacy of melatonin in the treatment of primary adult sleep disorders. *Sleep Med Rev*. 2017;34:10–22.

9. Sullivan SS. Insomnia pharmacology. *Med Clin N Am*. 2010;94:563–580.

10. Erland LA, Saxena PK. Melatonin natural health products and supplements: presence of serotonin and significant variability of melatonin content. *J Clin Sleep Med*. 2017;13:275–281.

11. Lie JD, Tu KN, Shen DD, Wong BM. Pharmacological treatment of insomnia. *Pharm Therapeut*. 2015;40:759–771.

12. George CF, Millar TW, Hanly PJ, Kryger MH. The effect of L-tryptophan on day-time sleep latency in normal: correlation with blood levels. *Sleep*. 1989;12:345–353.

13. Bazar KA, Yun AJ, Lee PY. Debunking a myth: Neurohormonal and vagal modulation of sleep centers, not redistribution of blood flow, may account for postprandial somnolence. *Med Hypotheses*. 2004;63:778–782.

14. Mitchell HA, Weinshenker D. Good night and good luck: norepinephrine in sleep pharmacology. *Biochem Pharmacol*. 2010;79:801–809.

15. Proctor A, Bianchi MT. Clinical pharmacology in sleep medicine. *ISRN Pharmacol*. 2012;2012.914168.

16. World Anti-Doping Agency. What is prohibited. https://www.wada-ama.org/en/content/what-is-prohibited/prohibited-in-competition/stimulants. Accessed July 16, 2019.

17. Mignot EJ. A practical guide to the therapy of narcolepsy and hypersomnia syndromes. *Neurotherapeutics*. 2012;9:739–752.

18. Takenoshita S, Nishino S. Pharmacologic management of excessive daytime sleepiness. *Sleep Med Clin*. 2017;12:461–478.

19. Thorpy MJ, Shapiro C, Mayer G, et al. A randomized study of solriamfetol for excessive sleepiness in narcolepsy. *Ann Neurol*. 2019;85:359–370.

20. Schweitzer PK, Rosenberg R, Zammit GK, et al.; TONES 3 Study Investigators. Solriamfetol for excessive sleepiness in obstructive sleep apnea (TONES 3). a randomized controlled trial. *Am J Respir Crit Care Med*. 2019;199:1421–1431.

21. Dauvilliers Y, Arnulf I, Szakács Z, et al. Long-term evaluation of safety and efficacy of pitolisant in narcolepsy: HARMONY 3 Study. *Neurology.* 2019;92:S46.009.

22. Kotagal S. Treatment of dyssomnias and parasomnias in childhood. *Curr Treat Opt Neurol.* 2012;14:630–649.

23. Howell MJ. Parasomnias: An updated review. *Neurotherapeutics.* 2012;9:753–775.

24. Aurora RN, Zak RS, Maganti RK, et al. Best practice guide for the treatment of REM sleep behavior disorder (RBD). *J Clin Sleep Med.* 2010;6:85–95.

25. Morgenthaler TI, Auerbach S, Casey KR, et al. Position paper for the treatment of nightmare disorder in adults: an American Academy of Sleep Medicine position paper. *J Clin Sleep Med.* 2018;14:1041–1055.

26. Coccagna, G; Vetrugno, R; Lombardi, C; Provini, F. Restless legs syndrome: an historical note. *Sleep Med.* 2004;5:279–283.

27. National Institute of Neurological Disorders and Stroke. Restless legs syndrome information page. www.ninds.nih.gov. Accessed August 13, 2019.

28. Oyayon MM, O'Hara R, Vitiello MV. Epidemiology of restless legs syndrome: a synthesis of the literatura. *Sleep Med Rev.* 2012;16:283–295.

29. Allen RP, Picchietti DL, Garcia-Borreguero D, et al. Restless legs syndrome/Willis–Ekbom disease diagnostic criteria: updated: International Restless Legs Syndrome Study Group (IRLSSG) consensus criteria—history, rationale, description, and significance. *Sleep Med.* 2014;15:860.

30. Hornyak M. Depressive disorders in restless legs syndrome: epidemiology, pathophysiology and management. *CNS Drugs.* 2010;24:89–98.

31. Aurora RN, Kristo DA, Bista SR, et al. The treatment of restless legs syndrome and periodic limb movement disorder in adults—an update for 2012: practice parameters with an evidence-based systematic review and meta-analyses. *Sleep.* 2012;35:1039–1062.

32. National Institute of Health, National Institute of Neurological Disorders and Stroke. Restless legs syndrome fact sheet. https://www.ninds.nih.gov/. Accessed August 13, 2019.

33. Torti FM, Torgi SV. Regulation of ferritin genes and protein. *Blood.* 2002;99:3505–3516.

34. Early CJ, Connor JR, Beard JL, Malecki EA, Epstein DK, Allen RP. Abnormalities in CSF concentrations of ferritin and transferrin in restless legs syndrome. *Neurology.* 2000;54:1698.

35. Silber MH, Becker PM, Buchfuhrer MJ, et al. The appropriate use of opioids in the treatment of refractory restless legs syndrome. *Mayo Clin Proc.* 2018;93:59–67.

36. Gradisar M, Dohnt H, Gardner G, et al. A randomized controlled trial of cognitive-behavior therapy plus bright light therapy for adolescent delayed sleep phase disorder. *Sleep.* 2011;34:1671–1680.

37. Auger RR, Burgess HJ, Emens JS, Deriy LV, Thomas SM, Sharkey KM. Clinical practice guideline for the treatment of intrinsic circadian rhythm sleep–wake disorders: advanced sleep-wake phase disorder (ASWPD), delayed sleep–wake phase disorder (DSWPD), non-24-hour sleep wake rhythm disorder (N24SWD), and irregular sleep-wake rhythm disorder (ISWRD). *J Clin Sleep Med.* 2015;11:1199–1236.

38. Kayumov L, Brown G, Jindal R, Buttoo K, Shapiro CM. A randomized, double-blind, placebo-controlled crossover study of the effect of exogenous melatonin on delayed sleep phase syndrome. *Psychosom Med.* 2001;63:40–48.

39. Bonacci JM, Venci JV, Gandhi MA. Tasimelteon (Hetlioz): a new melatonin receptor agonist for the treatment of non-24-hour sleep-wake disorder. *J Pharm Pract.* 2015;28:473–478.
40. Mundey K, Benloucif S, Harsanyi K, Dubocovich ML, Zee PC. Phase-dependent treatment of delayed sleep phase syndrome with melatonin. *Sleep.* 2005;28:1271–1278.
41. Erland LA, Saxena PK. Melatonin natural health products and supplements: presence of serotonin and significant variability of melatonin content. *J Clin Sleep Med.* 2017;13:275–281.
42. Mason M, Welsh EJ, Smith I. Drug therapy for obstructive sleep apnoea in adults. *Cochrane Db Syst Rev.* 2013;5:CD003002.
43. Strollo PJ. Solriamfetol for the treatment of excessive sleepiness in OSA: a placebo controlled randomized withdrawal study. *Chest.* 2019;155:364–374.
44. Stoschitzky K, Sakotnik A, Lercher P, et al. Influence of beta-blockers on melatonin release. *Eur J Clin Pharmacol.* 1999;55:111–115.
45. Schweitzer PK, Randazzo A. Drugs that disturb sleep and wakefulness. In: Kryger MH, Roth T, Dement WC, eds. *Principles and Practices of Sleep Medicine*, 6th ed. St Louis, MO: Elsevier Saunders; 2016:480.

PART IV

Sleep Assessment and Those Who Assess

22

Polysomnography and
Other Technologies

IAN M. COLRAIN, STEPHANIE CLAUDATOS,
AND MASSIMILIANO DE ZAMBOTTI ∎

INTRODUCTION

Polysomnography is the use of multiple biological signals to describe or define sleep states and stages or other physiological processes that might demonstrate abnormal activity during sleep. The word *polysomnography* comes from the Greek "poly," meaning "many"; the Latin word for sleep "somnus"; and the Greek work "grapho," meaning "to write" (more literally "to scratch," which was, after all, how the ancient Greeks wrote). So, parsing the word from its multiple derivations, polysomnography (PSG) is writing (or scratching) lots of things about sleep. For those of us who started in sleep research before laboratories became computerized, this was a more meaningful and obvious word to use. Nights in the sleep lab were spent accompanied by the background noise of ink-filled pens writing data onto continuous rolls of paper.

The study of sleep and its potential relationship to health dates back nearly three millennia in the Western tradition. The ancient Greeks even had sleep temples in which people would spend the night, perhaps in a drug-induced sleep state, to have their dreams interpreted by priests of the cult of Asklepios (the god of medicine). Modern scientific study of sleep commenced in the late 19th century. The first edition of the world's oldest physiology journal *Pflügers Archiv* (now the *European Journal of Physiology*) in 1868 contained an article on sleep disordered breathing [1]. Other articles published around that time included studies of narcolepsy [2] and insomnia [3]. The first major text on sleep was probably *Le problème physiologique du sommeil* (The Physiologic Problem of Sleep) by Henri Piéron, published in Paris in 1913 (and sold for 10 francs). Sixteen years later, Nathaniel Kleitman published a major review in *Physiological Reviews* [4], in which he limited himself to papers published after Piéron's book. Kleitman's article cited 137 papers, many in German and French, a heroic effort in the days before PubMed, the Internet, PDFs, and email. This review also highlights the rapid growth of interest in sleep, although the studies of human sleep at that time were limited to direct observation of individuals' behavior by researchers or crude forms of activity measurement.

HISTORY OF POLYSOMNOGRAPHY

A major breakthrough in the development of PSG came the same year Kleitman's paper was published, when Hans Berger published the first paper describing scalp-recorded brain activity in humans [5]. As its discoverer, Berger had naming rights for the new technique and called it electroencephalography (abbreviated as EEG). The first waveform he described was a single frequency rhythmic waveform close to 10 cycles per second, seen when the subject (usually himself, or his son Klaus) had their eyes closed. He called this waveform "alpha" and described a second pattern of faster activity, logically called "beta," that replaced alpha when the eyes were opened. Within 6 years of Berger's paper, EEG was recorded during sleep, in a private laboratory in the upstate New York mansion of Alfred Lee Loomis. Working with a Princeton professor E. Newton Harvey, and a local HAM radio enthusiast, Garret A. Hobart III, Loomis built his own amplifiers and pen chart recording system (see Figure 22.1) and reported findings of EEG activity during sleep in two 1935 papers in *Science* [6, 7]. In 1937, Loomis, Harvey, and Hobart published a paper in which they and outlined a scoring system to distinguish different states or levels of sleep and, in a subsequent series of papers,

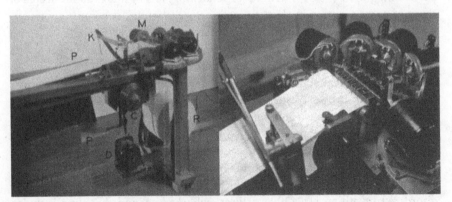

Figure 22.1 Left panel "paper cutting brain potential recorder" showing the motor (D) driven continuous feed pen chart recorder used in the Loomis laboratory. Right panel, an enlarged view of the electromagnets that drive the 13 pens used to record data. SOURCE: Loomis A, Harvey E, Hobart G. Distribution of disturbance-patterns in the human electroencephalogram, with special reference to sleep. *J Neurophysiol.* 1938;1:413–430.

described a number of other features of sleep such as K-complexes [8] (isolated large, >75 μV slow oscillation of about 0.8 Hz) and sleep spindles [7] (brief transient burst of about 12–15 Hz). Work in the Loomis laboratory stopped in 1939 when Loomis directed his attention to the development of radar for the British and US governments during World War II.

Before describing the Loomis scoring system, we should pause to describe the characteristics of scalp-recorded EEG. Figure 22.2A provides a simplified description of the different types of EEG waveforms studied with PSG and Figure 22.2B, a reproduction of the Loomis scoring system. Figure 22.3 shows example data from the Loomis laboratory recording system.

Electrooculography (EOG) is recorded by placing electrodes near the eyes. It does not measure eye muscle movement but rather takes advantage of a potential difference (voltage) between the retina at the back of the eyeball and the cornea at the front. If electrodes are placed above and below the eye, when the eye looks up, the electrode above the eye is closer to the positive end of the voltage (cornea) and the electrode below the eye is closer to the negative end of the voltage (retina). Likewise, looking left and right can be measured by placing electrodes to the sides of the eyes (in most people the eyes move together). This measure played an important role in the 1953 discovery of rapid eye movement (REM) sleep and its relationship to dreaming by Aserinsky and Kleitman [9].

Kleitman's laboratory at the University of Chicago was one of several in the United States, and around the world, studying sleep. Following the paper by Aserinsky and Kleitman, further work was conducted by another of Kleitman's students, William "Bill" Dement, who would go on to found the world's first sleep clinic at Stanford University. Dement and Kleitman [10] sought to extend the Loomis lab's description of sleep and came up with their own four-stage system, (cunningly labeled stage 1, stage 2, stage 3, and stage 4) in which they indicated that throughout the night, some episodes of stage 1 were associated with REMs. A summary of their scoring system is presented in Figure 22.2C, and hypnograms from 3 nights are reproduced from their paper in Figure 22.4.

STANDARDIZATION OF POLYSOMNOGRAPHY: RECHTSCHAFFEN AND KALES

In 1968, a remarkable series of meetings occurred under the auspices of the University of California, Los Angeles Brain Information Services. The meetings were of 12 men who had formed an ad hoc committee to formalize and standardize the recording methods and scoring of PSG data. The resulting document was the "bible" for sleep researchers and clinicians for 3 decades and became known simply as Rechtschaffen and Kales, or more typically "the R&K," for the committee co-chairs, Alan Rechtschaffen from the University of Chicago and Tony Kales from UCLA [11]. In addition to providing a benchmark for sleep researchers, the R&K guidelines normalized the terminology used with that of the broader neuroscience research community, adopting the EEG definitions [12]

A) Properties of EEg frequencies relevant to polysomnography			
Waveform	**Frequencies**	**State**	**Scalp Locations**
Alpha	8-12 Hz (single frequency)	Eyes closed, awake	Occipital
Beta	13-30 Hz	Eyes open, awake	Widespread
Theta	4-7 Hz	Sleep	Widespread
Delta	1-3 Hz	Deep sleep	Widespread but largest over Frontal
Sleep Spindle (Sigma)	13-16 Hz (single frequency)	Sleep	Central, top of the head
K-complex	Single Delta wave	Sleep	Widespread but largest over Frontal

B) Five stage system proposed by Loomis et al. (1938)	
Levels	**Description**
A	Alpha — alpha rhythm trains, eyes may be rolling under the lids
B	Low voltage — no alpha, only low voltage EEG Rolling of the eyes may occur
C	Spindles — 14Hz spindles of 20-40 V every few seconds
D	Spindles plus random — spindles with large random potentials. Random voltages may be as high as 300V
E	Random — spindles become inconspicuous but large random potentials persist and come from all parts of the cortex

C) Four-five stage system proposed by Dement and Kleitman (1955)	
Stages	**Description**
1	Absence of spindles — activity included in Loomis' A and B; any activity between Wake and spindles
2	Spindles and a low voltage background; includes biparietal humps or K-complexes
3	High voltage slow waves (delta) with some spindles
4	At least half or more of the record associated with slow waves 1-2 Hz, greater than 100 V
1 + rapid eye movements Stages	As per the state 1 description above, but with rapid eye movements

D) Five stage system (with division into REM and non-REM sleep) proposed by Rechtschaffen and kales (1968)	
Stages	**Description**
W (wakefulness)	EEG contains alpha and/ or low voltage, mixed frequency activity
MT (movement time)	Polygraph record is obscured by movements of the subject
1	A relatively low voltage, mixed frequency EEG, without rapid eye movements
2	Sleep spindles and K-complexes on a background of relatively low voltage, mixed frequency EEG
3	Moderate amounts of high amplitude, slow wave activity
4	Large amounts of high amplitude, slow wave activity
REM	Low voltage mixed frequency EEG in conjunction with episodic REMs and low amplitude EMG

Figure 22.2 Panel A: Types of EEG waves relevant to polysomnography, their frequency bands, the state(s) in which they are most prominent, and scalp location(s). Panel B: The sleep scoring system developed by the Loomis laboratory [8]. Panel C: Further refinement of the Loomis system by Dement and Kleitman [10], after their discovery that rapid eye movements occur episodically throughout sleep. Panel D: Further refinement (presented in summary form) of the Dement and Kleitman system, by the committee led by Rechtschaffen and Kales [11].

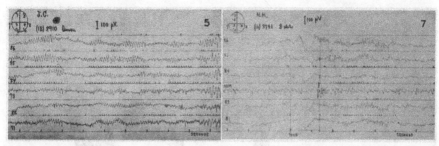

Figure 22.3 Left panel: Alpha activity during wake from 6 different EEG derivations. The numbers (86, 75, etc.) relate to the numbered electrode positions in the drawing in the top left of the image. Thus, sites 1 and 2 are left and right frontal electrode, 3 and 4 are left and right central electrodes, and 5 and 6 are left and right occipital electrodes. Traces 7 and 8 represent the neutral left and right mastoid processes behind the ears, from which it is assumed that not much EEG activity can be seen. Thus, derivation 86 is right occipital EEG referenced to the right mastoid, etc. Right panel: A different subject, this time in the "B" state of sleep. These data are from an experiment in which tones were presented. A K-complex is seen in the period following the tone, and before the subject awoke, was associated with an arm movement recorded on the fourth trace down.
SOURCE: Loomis A, Harvey E, Hobart G. Distribution of disturbance-patterns in the human electroencephalogram, with special reference to sleep. *J Neurophysiol.* 1938;1:413–430.

and the electrode placement standards [13] of the International Federation for Electroencephalography and Clinical Neurophysiology.

The techniques were specific to the most advanced pen chart recorder technology of the day and specified minimum paper speed, filter settings, and minimum pen deflection for known EEG amplitude and other features. Given that the best equipment available consisted of eight channels, which were often split between two recorded individuals, standards for four-channel PSG were defined. A four-channel "montage" included one EEG channel (either a left central electrode with active site referenced to the right ear or mastoid—considered a neutral or electrically stable site—or a right central electrode, referenced to the left ear or mastoid). It also included two EOG channels for eye movements and one channel to measure muscle activity from on, or under, the chin. This last channel of electromyography was needed to measure the phenomenon, first seen in animals, that postural muscles become hyperpolarized when rapid eye movements occur, and the mental (chin) or submental (under the chin) muscles were convenient places to measure this phenomenon. A summary version from their paper is presented in Figure 22.2D.

The reason the Rechtschaffen and Kales manual remained the gold standard well past our use of pen chart recorders was the exquisite detail in which the EEG, EOG, and electromyographic features of each state and stage were defined, with 39 full-page figures demonstrating the phenomena. However, with the advent of multiple channel amplifier systems and their eventual digitization, with computer screens replacing ink pens and reams of paper, other signals were added to the PSG and other scoring systems became needed.

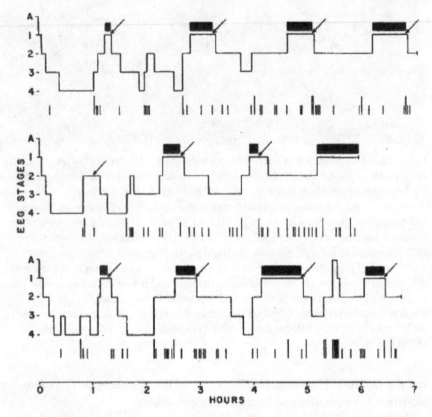

Fig. 3

Continuous plotting of the EEG patterns for three representative nights. The thick bars immediately above the EEG lines indicate periods during which rapid eye movements were seen. The vertical lines below stand for body movements. The longer vertical lines indicate major movements, changes in position of the whole body, and the shorter lines represent minor movements. The arrows indicate both the end of one EEG cycle and the beginning of the next.

Figure 22.4 This figure shows the hypnogram of progression through the different stages of sleep as defined by Dement and Kleitman (see Table 22.3) and including the Stage 1 periods when eye movements occurred.

SOURCE: Reproduced from Dement W, Kleitman N. Cyclic variations in EEG during sleep and their relation to eye movements, body motility, and dreaming. *Electroencephalogr Clin Neurophysiol.* 1957;9:673–690.

THE DEVELOPMENT OF CLINICAL POLYSOMNOGRAPHY

The annual sleep conference in the United States has been referred to as the APSS since its first iteration in 1960 (it has been more formally known as SLEEP since 1986). In 1960, a handful of participants attended and APSS stood for the Association for the Psychophysiological Study of Sleep. In 2018 the meeting included nearly 5000 participants and APSS became the Associated Professional

Sleep Societies. While the modern conference still features both basic and human science, a large number of clinicians also attend and the meetings includes an abundance of clinical presentations on treatable pathologies associated with sleep, primarily the obstructive sleep apnea (OSA) syndrome. OSA receives the greatest attention not because it is the most common sleep disorder (that dubious distinction belongs to insomnia), but rather because it is easy to diagnose in a laboratory (or in home study) and has treatment options, even if a cure remains elusive.

Apnea means "without breath," and thus sleep apnea refers to cessation of breathing during sleep. The most common form of sleep apnea is OSA, caused by an obstruction of the collapsible part of the human airway, somewhere between the back of the hard palate in the mouth and the start of the trachea in the chest. Obesity is a predisposing factor for OSA. Charles Dickens is often credited with the first description of obesity-related OSA, in his description of Fat Joe in his novel *The Pickwick Papers*. This led to a medical condition known as Pickwickian syndrome, recognized by Sir William Osler, one of the founders of Johns Hopkins University. However, it is likely that the link between obesity and apnea has been known since antiquity [14].

In 1976, Christian Guilleminault at Stanford University wrote an important paper, co-authored by Bill Dement, describing OSA syndromes [15]. In their review, these authors indicated that daytime sleepiness and potential changes in heart function were related to large numbers of apneas during sleep, that OSA could occur in people who were not morbidly obese and that the apneic events were associated with decreases in blood oxygen levels and increases in blood carbon dioxide levels. In short, they defined a complex medical syndrome associated with OSA. Unfortunately, the only treatment option at that time was to surgically bypass the collapsible segment of the upper airway with a tracheostomy. Five years later and over 7000 miles from Stanford, a groups of Australian physician scientists published a paper demonstrating a nonsurgical treatment. The paper by Colin Sullivan and colleagues [16] reported data from five subjects who had positive pressure applied to their noses during sleep, which completely eradicated their OSA. Within 5 years an important medical syndrome had been reported, and its effective treatment identified. This led to an explosion of clinical sleep medicine as a field and the urgent need to add a series of additional measures to PSG.

A NEW STANDARD: AASM GUIDELINES

Development of clinical PSG and the transition from pen chart recorders to computerized PSG required a new approach to PSG. In 2007, the American Academy of Sleep Medicine released new guidelines for the visual scoring of sleep in adults. While largely based on the original work by Rechtschaffen and Kales, the new guidelines formally added frontal and occipital EEG to the central site previously defined. This montage allows better measurement of specific sleep events and characteristics that are magnified at different frontal (e.g., slow oscillation), central (e.g., spindles), or occipital (e.g., drop in alpha across the wake-to-sleep transition) derivations. The new guidelines also removed the distinction between stage 3 and stage 4 of non-REM sleep (now renamed N3 sleep) and tweaked some rules about identification of features such as sleep spindles and K-complexes, as well as those defining the transitions between one state and another [17]. Another task force addressed issues relating to the scoring of respiratory events during sleep [18], a topic not covered by Rechtschaffen and Kales [11]. Others dealt with digital recording and analysis [19], measurement of movement disorders [20], visual scoring of sleep in infants and children [21], scoring of cardiac events during sleep [22], and scoring of brief arousals [23]. The end result was that standard clinical PSG now consists of many signals, as shown in Figure 22.5.

PSG clearly provides a wealth of data from multiple EEG signals and multiple measurement of the cardiorespiratory system (See Figure 22.6). It is the state-of-the-art method for diagnosing sleep-related breathing disorders (also see Chapter 17 of this chapter) and other issues such as narcolepsy and sleep-related movement disorders (also see Chapter 23 of this chapter). It provides detailed information about the amount and distribution of different sleep states and stages and can be useful in a multitude of contexts. It also requires a dedicated laboratory, trained staff, and expensive equipment; further, PSG can also only provide a snapshot (typically a single night of data) of an individual's sleep during their regular life. Because of these limitations, other technologies have been developed to assess sleep in the normal home environment, over multiple nights.

ACTIGRAPHY: USING MOVEMENT AS A MEASURE OF SLEEP

While there is a long history of studying movement during sleep [24], modern use of wrist-worn devices to estimate sleep dates to the 1970s, with work pioneered at the University of Pittsburgh [25–27]. This work, using handmade sensors that detected and recorded wrist movement, showed remarkable correlations with concurrent measures of wakefulness and sleep from PSG, on the simple assumption that motion indicated wakefulness and lack of motion indicated sleep. This basic principle is still used today, although updates include multidirectional accelerometers, light sensors, event markers, and batteries allowing up to 60 days of continuous use [28]. Algorithms are now used to convert activity into wake or sleep determinations. Some are proprietary to the device used (e.g., Philips Respironics, Inc. Bend, OR) and others publicly available (e.g., Cole–Kripk and Sadeh algorithms). Many have been validated against PSG in healthy and clinical populations, with ages ranging from infants to the elderly [29, 30].

When reading studies that have assessed the validity of actigraphy, it is important to first note whether the comparison was against PSG, which is still considered the gold standard. The key analysis to look for in quality assessments is that they compare the two signals on a minute-by-minute basis. The key outcome measures are "sensitivity"—the ability to accurately detect sleep (i.e., actigraphy

Polysomnography based on American of Sleep Medicine guidelines		
Signal	**Transducer**	**Purpose**
Frontal EEG	Electrodes	Sleep staging especially K-complex and delta activity, arousal measurement
Central EEG	Electrodes	Sleep staging, especially sleep spindles, arousal measurement
Occipital EEG	Electrodes	Sleep staging especially alpha activity, arousal measurement
Left eye EOG	Electrodes	Sleep staging especially REM sleep
Right eye EOG	Electrodes	Sleep staging especially REM sleep
Chin EMG	Electrodes	Sleep staging especially REM sleep
Air flow	Thermistor	Apnea detection
Air pressure	Nasal cannula	Hypopnea detection
Chest movement	Piezo-electric band	Obstructive apnea/hypopnea detection
Abdominal movement	Piezo-electric band	Obstructive apnea/hypopnea detection
Oxygen saturation	Finger photo-cell	Obstructive apnea/hypopnea detection
Limb movement	Electrode or piezo electric sensor	Periodic limb movement detection
Body position	Gravity switch or 3-way accelerometer	Body position during sleep
Sound	Microphone	Snoring detection
ECG	Electrodes	Heart rate and heart rhythm abnormalities

Figure 22.5 Typical signals now recorded with polysomnography, following adoption of the 2007 American Academy of Sleep Medicine guidelines.

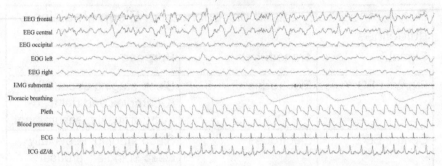

EEG frontal
EEG central
EEG occipital
EOG left
EEG right
EMG submental
Thoracic breathing
Pleth
Blood pressure
ECG
ICG dZ/dt

Figure 22.6 Signals recorded in a research polysomnography study evaluating autonomic nervous system functioning during sleep. This montage includes 3 channels of EEG, 2 of EOG, and an EMG signal. A piezo-electric band for measuring thoracic breathing, photoplethysmograph, and blood pressure outputs from a Portapres continuous blood pressure monitor (TNO TPD Biomedical Instrumentation, Amsterdam, The Netherlands) and an ECG and the output of an impedance cardiograph (Bio-Impedance Technology, Inc., Chapel Hill, NC). Data were recorded using a Compumedics Grael Amplifier system and Profusion 4 Software (Compumedics, Abbotsford, Victoria, Australia).

scores a minute as sleep, when sleep is shown on PSG), "specificity"—the ability to accurately detect wakefulness (i.e., actigraphy scores a minute as wake, when wake is shown on PSG), and overall accuracy—combined ability to detect wake and sleep.

Although the majority of studies report high sensitivity and accuracy, the specificity of actigraphy is inherently impaired; in other words, actigraphy is less capable of identifying wakefulness when the individual is not moving (e.g., when they are lying in bed, still and awake, actigraphy can misidentify this as sleep) [31–33].

Despite this known limitation, actigraphy is widely accepted and used in research, when long periods of data collection are needed, and has some utility for the clinical assessment of circadian rhythm disorders. However, an Academy of Sleep Medicine review in 2003 indicted that "the time has arrived for standards to be established, similar to those developed for PSG by Rechtshaffen and Kales (1968)" (p. 346) [34]. This group urged the development of defined standardized units of measurement that would permit comparison of different devices and algorithms. No such standards have been developed, despite updates in recommended practice parameters for actigraphy use [35].

RECENT DEVELOPMENTS IN CONSUMER WEARABLE TECHNOLOGY

The digital health revolution of the past decade has seen many sophisticated and relatively inexpensive devices marketed directly to public consumers. The first generation of devices originated as fitness trackers with a motion sensor to derive parameters such as number of steps and time spent active. The most recent generation includes multiple sensors, with which their manufacturers claim to also record physiological indices such as heart rate and variability and skin temperature and conductance (offering a window on autonomic functioning). Sleep quickly became an "accessible" feature that many of these companies claim their devices are able to measure. A recent position statement by the American Academy of Sleep Medicine acknowledges the usefulness of consumer sleep technology in enhancing the patient–clinician interaction around sleep issues and their ability to increase awareness of the importance of sleep [36]. However, the authors caution that without detailed knowledge of how these devices measure sleep, and without evaluation by the US Food and Drug Administration, they should not be used for clinical assessment. It is interesting to note, however, that this position paper failed to cite the growing body of work that has compared different consumer sleep technologies to PSG.

THE FUTURE OF SLEEP MEASUREMENT?

Our group recently published a state-of-the-art review of wearable technology in clinical and research settings [37], which provides detailed information on multiple devices and the extent to which they have been shown valid. The first generation of consumer sleep wearables were essentially consumer-grade actigraphy devices, using algorithms to measure movement and estimate whether someone was awake or asleep, and as such they suffered from many of the same limitations as scientific-quality actigraphy, with a poor ability to detect motionless wakefulness [38, 39]. The more recent generation of multisensory devices appeared at first to be more promising for measuring sleep/wake, and their manufacturers even claimed an ability to estimate sleep stages. The use of additional signals, especially heart rate variability, offered, at least in theory, the ability to discriminate between sleep stages using a combination of motion and autonomic nervous system activity features. This led to the development of algorithms to estimate different sleep stages, in particular REM versus non-REM sleep [40, 41]. While these do not show perfect concordance with PSG measures, they hold potential—although it is important to note that neither these devices nor the claims of the companies that manufacture them are regulated by any authoritative source.

The widespread use of consumer wearable nonetheless allows the future possibility of using such "big data" on the science of sleep, with millions of data points coming in a continuous flow, night after night, potentially allowing evaluation of longitudinal changes and variations in sleep associated with illness and other significant life events. For example, continuous data collection would allow integration with ecological momentary assessment and potentially advance our understanding of relationships between sleep and biopsychosocial factors, including health behaviors.

The current challenge is to navigate the complex capitalist incentives and business models of the companies producing the devices—and their desire to maintain ownership of their proprietary analysis techniques—while remaining focused on the needs of sleep clinical and research communities. The sleep community hopes to find a way to use this technology without compromising standards (see [37] for a detailed discussion about the issues and challenges in using consumer wearables in clinical and research settings). To facilitate this, we need new ways of conducting, reviewing, and rapidly publishing validation studies. Currently, by the time a paper is published, the device that was evaluated has often been replaced by new hardware and software, which now require new validation. Further, the ethical and privacy issues surrounding use of wearable technology cannot be ignored and deserve proper discussion. While the use of consumer devices for sleep assessment is currently very controversial [42–45], the promise of sleep assessment on a scale that could not have been imagined by Loomis or Kleitman is too important to be left to profit-focused companies alone.

CONCLUSIONS

The desire to observe sleep has been documented for over 2000 years, from the temples of Asklepios to modern corporate headquarters. Over the past 100 or so years, sleep researchers have been rapid adopters of the latest technology, which has itself informed our questions about what sleep is and why we need it. It is hard to imagine what will come next. Perhaps, in the coming decade, quantum sensors will allow us to accurately and inexpensively measure brain function on a nightly basis [46]. One thing is certain, whatever new technologies are developed, sleep researchers will be there to use them. Sleep is too important to forego any opportunity for advancement.

REFERENCES

1. Pfluger E. Ueber die ursache der athemewegunen, sowie der dyspnoe und apnoe [On the causes of breathable tumors, dyspnoea and apnea]. *Pflugers Archiv* 1868;1:61–106.
2. Heath C. Narcolepsy. *Brit Med J* 1889;16:358–359.
3. de Manaceine M. Obervations experimentales sur l'influence de l'insomnie ablsue. [Experimental observations on the influence of complete insomnia]. *Archive Italiennes de Biologie* 1894;11:322–325.
4. Kleitman N. Sleep. *Physiol Rev.* 1929;9:624–665.
5. Berger H. Über das elektrenkephalogramm des menschen. [About the human electroencephalogram]. *Archiv Forschung Psychiatrie* 1929;87:527–570.
6. Loomis AL, Harvey EN, Hobart G. Further observations on the potential rhythms of the cerebral cortex during sleep. *Science.* 1935;82:198–200.
7. Loomis AL, Harvey EN, Hobart G. Potential rhythms of the cerebral cortex during sleep. *Science.* 1935;81:597–598.
8. Loomis A, Harvey E, Hobart G. Distribution of disturbance-patterns in the human electroencephalogram, with special reference to sleep. *J Neurophysiol.* 1938;1:413–430.

9. Aserinksy E, Kleitman N. Regularly occurring periods of eye motility, and con-comitant phenomena, during sleep. *Science.* 1953;118:273–274.

10. Dement W, Kleitman N. Cyclic variations in EEG during sleep and their rela-tion to eye movements, body motility, and dreaming. *Electroencephalogr Clin Neurophysiol.* 1957;9:673–690.

11. Rechtschaffen A, Kales K. *A Manual of Standardised -Terminology, Techniques and Scoring Systems for Sleep Stages of Human Subjects.* Washington, DC: U.S. Government Printing Office; 1968.

12. Brazier MA. Preliminary proposal for an EEG terminology by the Terminology Committee of the International Federation for Electroencephalography and Clinical Neurophysiology. *Electroencephalogr Clin Neurophysiol.* 1961;13:646–650.

13. Jasper HH. The ten-twenty electrode system of the International Federation. *Electroencephalogr Clin Neurophysiol.* 1958;10:371–375.

14. Kryger M. From the needles of dionysius to continuous positive airway pressure. *Arch Intern Med.* 1983;143:2301–2303.

15. Guilleminault C, Tilkian A, Dement WC. The sleep apnea syndromes. *Annu Rev Med.* 1976;27:465–484.

16. Sullivan CE, Issa FG, Berthon-Jones M, Eves L. Reversal of obstructive sleep apnoea by continuous positive airway pressure applied through the nares. *Lancet.* 1981;1:862–865.

17. Silber MH, Ancoli-Israel A, Bonnet MH, et al. The visual scoring of sleep in adults. *J Clin Sleep Med.* 2007;3:121–131.

18. Redline S, Budhiraja R, Kapur V, et al. The scoring of respiratory events in sleep: re-liability and validity. *J Clin Sleep Med.* 2007;3:169–200.

19. Penzel T, Hirshkowitz M, Harsh J, et al. Digital analysis and technical specifications. *J Clin Sleep Med.* 2007;3:109–120.

20. Walters AS, Lavigne G, Hening W, et al. The scoring of movements in sleep. *J Clin Sleep Med.* 2007;3:155–167.

21. Grigg-Damberger M, Gozal D, Marcus CL, et al. The visual scoring of sleep and arousal in infants and children. *J Clin Sleep Med.* 2007;3:201–240.

22. Caples SM, Rosen CL, Shen WK, et al. The scoring of cardiac events during sleep. *J Clin Sleep Med.* 2007;3:147–154.

23. Bonnet MH, Doghramji K, Roehrs T, et al. The scoring of arousal in sleep: relia-bility, validity, and alternatives. *J Clin Sleep Med.* 2007;3:133–145.

24. Tyron WW. *Activity Measurement in Psychology and Medicine.* New York, NY: Plenum Press; 1991.

25. Kripke DF, Mullaney DJ, Messin S, Wyborney VG. Wrist actigraphic measures of sleep and rhythms. *Electroencephalogr Clin Neurophysiol.* 1978;44:674–676.

26. Kupfer DJ, Detre TP, Foster G, Tucker GJ, Delgado J. The application of Delgado's telemetric mobility recorder for human studies. *Behav Biol.* 1972;7:585–590.

27. Kupfer DJ, Foster FG. Sleep and activity in a psychotic depression. *J Nerv Ment Dis.* 1973;156:341–348.

28. Koninklijke Philips NV. Actiwatch Spectrum Plus. https://www.usa.philips.com/healthcare/product/HCNOCTN445/actiwatch-spectrum-plus-get-the-actiwatch-advantage/specifications. Accessed February 26, 2020.

29. Sadeh A. The role and validity of actigraphy in sleep medicine: an update. *Sleep Med Rev.* 2011;15:259–267.

30. Van de Water AT, Holmes A, Hurley D.A. Objective measurements of sleep for non-laboratory settings as alternatives to polysomnography: a systematic review. *J Sleep Res.* 2011;20:183–200.

31. Kushida CA, Chang A, Gadkary C, Guilleminault C, Carrillo O, Dement WC. Comparison of actigraphic, polysomnographic, and subjective assessment of sleep parameters in sleep-disordered patients. *Sleep Med.* 2001;2:389–396.

32. Marino M, Li Y, Rueschman MN, et al. Measuring sleep: accuracy, sensitivity, and specificity of wrist actigraphy compared to polysomnography. *Sleep.* 2013;36:1747–1755.

33. Quante M, Kaplan ER, Cailler M, et al. Actigraphy-based sleep estimation in adolescents and adults: a comparison with polysomnography using two scoring algorithms. *Nat Sci Sleep.* 2018;10:13–20.

34. Ancoli-Israel S, Cole R, Alessi C, Chambers M, Moorcroft W, Pollak CP. The role of actigraphy in the study of sleep and circadian rhythms. *Sleep.* 2003;26:342–392.

35. Morgenthaler T, Alessi C, Friedman L, et al.; Standards of Practice Committee; American Academy of Sleep Medicine. Practice parameters for the use of actigraphy in the assessment of sleep and sleep disorders: an update for 2007. *Sleep.* 2007;30:519–529.

36. Khosla S, Deak MC, Gault D, et al., for the American Academy of Sleep Medicine Board of Directors. Consumer sleep technology: an American Academy of Sleep Medicine Position Statement. *J Clin Sleep Med.* 2018;14:877–880.

37. de Zambotti M, Cellini N, Goldstone A, Colrain IM, Baker FC. Wearable sleep technology in clinical and research settings. *Med Sci Sports Exerc.* 2019;51:1538–1557.

38. de Zambotti M, Baker FC, Colrain IM. Validation of sleep-tracking technology compared with polysomnography in adolescents. *Sleep.* 2015;38:1461–1468.

39. de Zambotti M, Claudatos S, Inkelis S, Colrain IM, Baker FC. Evaluation of a consumer fitness-tracking device to assess sleep in adults. *Chronobiol Int.* 2015;32:1024–1028.

40. de Zambotti M, Rosas L, Colrain IM, Baker FC. The sleep of the ring: comparison of the OURA sleep tracker against polysomnography. *Behav Sleep Med.* 2017;17:1–15.

41. de Zambotti M, Goldstone A, Claudatos S, Colrain IM, Baker FC. A validation study of Fitbit Charge 2 compared with polysomnography in adults. *Chronobiol Int.* 2018;35:465–476.

42. Khosla S, Deak MC, Gault D, et al. Consumer sleep technologies: how to balance the promises of new technology with evidence-based medicine and clinical guidelines. *J Clin Sleep Med.* 2019;15:163–165.

43. Magnusdottir S. The importance of evidence-based medicine and clinical guidelines: meaningful and clinically actionable information cannot be compromised for the convenience of consumer sleep data. *J Clin Sleep Med.* 2019;15:795–796.

44. Watson NF, Lawlor C, Raymann R. Consumer sleep technologies, clinical guidelines, and evidence-based medicine: this is not a zero-sum game. *J Clin Sleep Med.* 2019;15:797–788.

45. Watson NF, Lawlor C, Raymann R. Will consumer sleep technologies change the way we practice sleep medicine? *J Clin Sleep Med.* 2019;15:159–161.

46. Boto E, Meyer SS, Shah V, et al. A new generation of magnetoencephalography: room temperature measurements using optically-pumped magnetometers. *Neuroimage* 2017;149:404–414.

23

Subjective Assessments — How Well Do You Sleep?

KAREN SPRUYT ■

INTRODUCTION: QUESTION THE QUESTION!

You will have seen several references throughout this book to sleep researchers' and clinicians' use of questionnaires—we use them to assess everything from symptoms of sleep disorders to general sleep amounts and quality. This chapter is partnered with Chapter 22 of this volume, which addresses objective methods we use to assess sleep and wake.

There is significant power of efficiency and cost-effectiveness to using questionnaires for measuring a wide range of problems. However, using them can also become a real hindrance—and may even lead to inadequate screening or misdiagnoses, which can result after the appropriate steps for developing, administering, and/or interpreting a questionnaire are either ignored or insufficiently scrutinized. Establishing the desired level of objectivity based on a subjective tool entails maintaining the standard size of the "unit amount." For example, a questionnaire intended to measure sleep-disordered breathing should consistently assess disturbed breathing during sleep, whether it is a 5-item Likert-scale tool or 21-item yes/no (binary) scale tool. Likewise, the construct of sleep-disordered breathing should be consistent whether we are assessing a 5-year-old or a 50-year-old and whether the person completing the questionnaire is the child's parent or the individual themselves. Thus, creating a high-quality questionnaire takes a great deal of time and effort upfront.

IMPORTANCE OF SUBJECTIVE INSTRUMENT DEVELOPMENT

Investigators often ponder whether subjective or objective measures are superior. To answer this, a distinction between variable type and measurement strategy is needed. For instance, to assess someone's health we may count their white blood cells, measure their physical activity, etc. However, assessing overall health also requires that we inquire about the individual's fatigue and daily functional activities. Thus, whether you focus on subjective and/or objective measurement essentially depends on your hypotheses. Keep in mind that symptoms are inherently subjective; that is, taking someone's temperature and inferring that they are ill relies on a theory or consensus, within which a range of error remains present. In addition, the determination of illness is based on professional recommendations that have been established to eliminate distortions in the unit amount (essentially, an attempt to eliminate as much subjectivity as possible) [1] (see Figure 23.1).

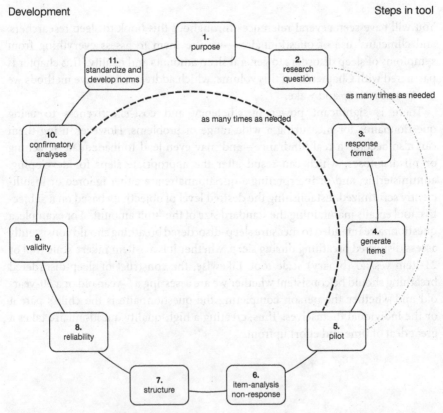

Figure 23.1 Steps in tool development.

PSYCHOMETRICS, THE MAGICAL KEY?

Despite this, a misconception still exists within the health sciences that "medical" data are "hard" data, whereas questionnaire data are "soft" data—with hard data presumably based on more rigorous standards. This need not be the case! As you know—or will learn—from the Chapter 22 of this volume, which describes the historic development of polysomnography, the functional state of sleep has been defined based on physiological measurement of brainwaves, eye movements, and cardiorespiratory features. These are scored based on clinical consensus. Although it is a monumental challenge, developing questionnaire instruments to collect sleep information should be no less rigorous. Any high-quality psychometric tool must satisfy certain criteria. Adhering to a standard process of roughly 11 development steps allows development of a tool that maintains its unit amount. In this chapter, we will review both the principles and practice of instrument development. Understanding these will make you a more well-informed consumer of the scientific literature in sleep—and, indeed, every other field in which questionnaire data are used.

INITIAL STEPS 1 AND 2

Step 1 is to reflect on the variable(s) of interest and targeted sample(s); in other words, the very beginning of the process of questionnaire development (and again later, in an iterative process) is to consider how the tool will be used and why. Following on that (and, ideally, in a parallel framework), Step 2 is to consider the research question that the instrument will be used to address. Thus, the goal of this step is to reflect on whether the tool will be suitable to collect the type of data required to address your hypothesis.

STEPS 3 AND 4—RESPONSE FORMAT AND RESPONSE ITEMS

These steps build on the two preceding. They allow us to reflect not only on which questions and which answers assess the variable(s) of interest, but also on how a question is formulated and how it can be answered. Tools may greatly vary in terms of the types of questions/answers options used, as well as in the number of questions/answers they include. Steps 3 and 4 are meant to work together and are best kept consistent across the tool, to facilitate the jobs of both the respondent and the individual later scoring and analyzing the completed questionnaire.

The common goal of steps 1 to 4 is that we want the underlying concepts and/or assumptions contained in the questions, such as language (e.g., jargon), meaning, and interpretation of the wording to be identically understood by all respondents. Getting as close as this ideal as possible will minimize errors of comprehension and completion. The field of sleep research and clinical medicine has struggled with using words such as "snoring," "gasping," and "apnea" on questionnaires—if we use these tools to help diagnose sleep-disordered breathing, then it is essential that everyone (i.e., those completing our questionnaires and all researchers and clinicians) have a common understanding of these terms. Ways of meeting these goals include careful reflection on the purpose of the tool, its target sample/population, how it will be administered, how long it will be, etc.

There are several tips for succeeding in this process that are used by experts. These are valuable for both constructing a questionnaire and for interpreting the data that were obtained from them (i.e., the next time you are reading a scientific publication) They include keep wording simple, avoid double-barreled questions, avoid loaded (i.e., emotionally charged words) questions, avoid negative wording, and avoid easy "yea/nay" questions (i.e., ask similar question but with reversed meaning so that participants are not answering every question the same way).

The answer format should also fit the question. You may opt for (partially) open/closed-ended questions, although several other rating scale options do exist. *The visual analogue scale* is the most commonly used graphic rating scale; for this method, a mark is made along a continuous (e.g., 10 cm) line and either anchored or unanchored by adjectives. Semantic differential scales measure responses to words or concepts on a scale labeled with two contrasting adjectives. Likert scales are relatively standard, ranging from three to seven, or even nine, response option alternatives (the rule of thumb favors unpaired options with five or seven alternatives). Labeling (i.e., the adjectives) is particularly important and should be selected carefully. Namely, in addition to the number of options, the labels restrict (and force) the respondents' range of responses. Note that many other scale formats exist; for example, see the Thurnstone scale and the Guttman scale.

The influence of the order of the questions should also be carefully considered. Namely, respondents rationalize their own behavior (or attitude, habit, symptom, etc.) through their answers. Sometimes funneling questions might be the best option to prevent an influence of the order in which questions are asked. Alternatively, filter questions can be used such that general questions are used to determine whether questions that are more specific need to be answered (e.g. "If yes . . ."). Lastly, how you plan to administer the tool (e.g., interview, mail, online, etc.) will certainly influence how you proceed through these first four steps.

There are some creative approaches to meeting these goals. One example is the "think aloud" approach, for which potential test respondents state (aloud) what they think as they read the questions and/or how they navigate through each part of the questionnaire. A qualitative approach such as focus groups, expert panels, or parent/patient groups may also help you, as does using previously validated tools as resources. However, keep in mind that tools lose validity (more on this in the following discussion) when used beyond the context in which they were developed.

When translating tools to other languages, a forward–backward translation is a necessity. This also requires a tedious process of evaluating and fulfilling conceptual equivalence and item/content equivalence, as well as semantic equivalence, operational equivalence (i.e., the way data was collected), and measurement (i.e., psychometric properties) and functional (i.e., equivalence throughout the development steps) equivalence. It is certainly not a mere translation. Hence, pretesting and piloting your tool can be superfluous until you have completed steps 1 to 4; yet, after these steps are completed, pilot testing becomes essential.

STEP 5—PILOT STUDY OR STUDIES

Pilot trials allows us to define and refine the tool and are essential for tuning a questionnaire to its purpose, including allowing us to further reflect on the order of the questions, their flow, the language used, layout, clarity, etc. Piloting also prevents disasters with the actual data collection. During piloting we can think critically about, and statistically analyze, the correspondence between the reported and actual variable of interest (e.g., sleep habit) we intend to measure. Several factors determine the size of pilot samples, including the size of the target population, the complexity of the topic, the estimated refusal rate and how sensitive the topic may be. As a rule of thumb, fewer than 100 respondents are generally used in a final pilot study (we also use 5%–10% of the targeted population, or a minimum of 5 to 10 respondents per question). Descriptive statistics such as measures of central tendency and measures of variability or dispersion (e.g., percentage, kurtosis, skewness, outliers, extreme scores, missing data) in combination with qualitative feedback (or even text mining) will guide this process.

Steps 2 to 5 should be an iterative process, meaning that we do them repeatedly, until a consensus has been reached among experts and/or respondents. Basic descriptive statistics can be calculated to reassure us that this process is on track and to test modifications as we progress through these steps. As soon as a good draft of the tool has been developed, it can be put to the test via a pilot study!

STEP 6—ITEM ANALYSIS AND NONRESPONSE ANALYSES

Assessing the performance of individual test items, separately and as a whole, is the next step. In addition to descriptive analyses (e.g., classical test theory approach) and missing data analyses, one may use item-response theory (IRT) analyses. IRT establishes how well the item differentiates (discrimination parameter), its suitability (difficulty parameter), and the pseudo-guessing parameter (i.e., those with and without the problem/symptom/etc.). General rules of thumb are that a questionnaire is doing its job based on the rates: ratings at ≥80% and ≤20% of items are weak discriminators; ratings at 85% are "easy"; >51 and <85% are "moderate"; and ≤50% are "difficult." To use an example with which you're probably very familiar, 25% is the pure chance rate on a multiple-choice item with four possible responses.

Assessing the performance of individual tool items, separately and as a whole, based on the assumption that the overall quality of a tool depends on the quality of its items (i.e., questions and response format) is done via item analysis. There are two main approaches to item analysis: *classical test theory* and the IRT, either of which should be combined with missing data analysis. The minute details about these are beyond the scope of this chapter—but suffice it to say here that these are intricate and essential aspects of determining the overall quality of the instrument [1–3]. They also highlight the importance of not extracting one or two items from an instrument and using them independently.

Missingness

Since it is impossible to ensure that every respondent will respond to every item on a questionnaire, anyone who uses questionnaires will need to deal with missing data. Item non-response can occur for many reasons, including sensitivity of the item, respondent fatigue (which is why it's important that the tool not be too long), lack of knowledge/interest, the appropriate answer not being available, questions or answers not being applicable, etc. The solution to handling missing values depends on randomness. If missing values are *completely at random* and if the number of the cases is less than 5% of the sample, one may consider excluding the missing cases. To assess its randomness, split your data set into one containing the missing values and the other containing the nonmissing values and compare them via basic statistical techniques. In addition, a pairwise or a listwise deletion of missing value cases in your analyses can be used to pursue the effect of randomness. However, when you have data missing *at random*—that is, missing data values being distributed within one or more subsamples—then more elaborate steps are needed. In this case, you have nonignorable missing values, which are the most problematic form of missing data. Time to consult a statistician. Although imputation, or replacing missing values based on the existing data through mathematical algorithms, may seem tempting, never forget you are, in fact, fabricating data in a biased data set.

In short, Step 6 is your quality control check before you go into production.

STEP 7—REVEAL THE STRUCTURE

The next step is about identifying the underlying concepts of the tool. Only rarely is a questionnaire unidimensional. Whether your data are suitable for structure (i.e., multiple components or factors) detection can be assessed using Kaiser–Meyer–Olkin measure of Sampling Adequacy or Bartlett's test of sphericity. These statistics indicate the proportion of variance in your variables that might be caused by one or more underlying factors/concepts. Based on a Kaiser–Meyer–Olkin value higher than 0.5, or a significant Bartlett's test, one can assess the structure with principal component analysis or factor analysis. Weak items with loading scores <0.40 should be excluded, a process also guided by screen plots (i.e., a line segment plot that shows the fraction of total variance in the data) and with Kaiser criterion of eigenvalue (i.e., a scalar associated with a linear system of equations) >1, the components or factors can be defined. Subsequent identification (and interpretation) of underlying concepts, or subscales, and verifying their stability should be done via exploratory factor analyses, which is one of the next steps in instrument development. The terms principal component analysis/ factor analysis, exploratory factor analysis, and confirmatory factor analyses are often used interchangeably; however, the confirmatory factor analysis technically assumes an underlying, pre-defined construct that you will be confirming. The exact method by which you perform this data reduction will affect its interpretation, scoring, and use. So, it is important to read up on some statistics before starting this adventure. The last three steps focus on the widespread use of the tool, hence its applicability.

STEPS 8 AND 9—RELIABILITY AND VALIDITY

Reliability (step 8) refers to the consistency of a measurement, and *validity* (step 9), to how accurately it represents the target concept (i.e., variable of interest). Reliability does not imply validity, although a tool cannot be considered valid if it is not reliable. Several statistical, or psychometric, tests allow us to assess a tool's reliability and validity (indeed, there are entire textbooks written on this topic). The most common approaches are summarized in the following discussion. Overall, their purposes are to help us determine where a tool fits into the "Robin Hood scenario" describing reliability and validity:

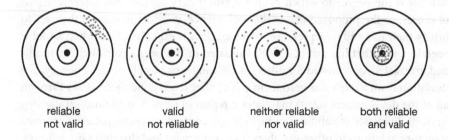

| reliable | valid | neither reliable | both reliable |
| not valid | not reliable | nor valid | and valid |

Reliability

For each total score, subscore, or combination of scores that are to be interpreted, relevant reliabilities and standard errors of measurement must be established. Ensuring many types of a tool's consistency are prerequisite to its large-scale use. These include its consistency over time (test–retest reliability), across items (internal consistency), across different raters/observers (inter-rater reliability), and across similar tools (parallel forms reliability). Hence, there are several indexes of reliability.

The most commonly used reliability test in the sleep research field is internal consistency, which is assessed using Cronbach's coefficient alpha (α), which should reach at least 0.80 (although during the preliminary stages of tool development 0.70 is generally accepted). Of note, this is a generalization of Kuder–Richardson 20 index, which ranges (in theory) from 0.0 to 1.0, with a 0.7 being sufficient. However, caution is needed as the Kuder–Richardson 20 (and thus the α) is, in part, a function of test length, particularly when merely relying on the α estimate for item deletion from the tool. Consequently, a critical eye should be kept on the coefficient α based on the raw scores, the corresponding 90% to 95% confidence intervals and the overall standardized α. The split-half correlation is also popular, which involves splitting the items into two sets with a correlation of 0.80 or greater generally considered good.

The repeatability coefficient, or test–retest reliability, is a measure of precision, for which differences between initial and later scores should be due solely to measurement error. Precision may be flawed for many reasons, including an interval that is too short between the initial test and the retest, with a potential carry-over effect (e.g., respondents may remember their original answers). Agreement among raters (e.g., caregiver and expert) can also be assessed in various ways, including Cohen's kappa, Scott's pi, Fleiss' kappa, inter-rater correlation, concordance correlation coefficient, intraclass correlation, and Krippendorff's alpha (please consult appropriate handbooks or a statistician about these less-used analyses).

Validity

Validity is the degree to which evidence and theory support our interpretations of scores, or the proposed use of the tool. Hence, it is incumbent on the user to justify their use and interpretation of a tool. This is especially true when a tool is used in a way that has not been well validated or has been (even slightly) modified, translated, or adjusted for different age ranges or samples, etc. Generally, any deviation from a tool's standard format (i.e., after it has gone successfully through all of the development steps) mandates a repeat of steps 6 to 10 (and ideally step 11, too). Evidence of validity can include test content, response patterns, internal structure, relations to other variables (i.e., convergent and discriminant validity), test criterion relationships (i.e., objective measures), validity generalization, and, finally but very important, evidence based on consequences of testing (e.g., [mis] diagnosis). In other words, a tool is valid when the resulting score is meaningful. Revision/iteration is thus a major part of the process in developing a reliable *and* valid tool.

An item analysis, previously described for reliability assessment, should not be mistaken for item validity. Similarly, internal consistency does not imply validity. Thus, in step 9, the key is to psychometrically proof that the tool/item is doing what it claims to do. When a tool does not appear to be measuring what it is supposed to be measuring, it has low face validity. When a tool is covering the theoretical construct or concept (e.g., sleep duration) it is supposed to assess, it is said to show content validity. Because, like face validity, content validity is not usually assessed quantitatively, it is consequently the most difficult to assess when developing a tool.

Critical reflection upon the "criterion" definition (e.g., sleep duration) is warranted to evaluate both. When the tool scores are compared to another criterion (i.e., another measurement tool that has been previously validated), criterion-related validity can be demonstrated. For example, a temporal relationship between the tool and the criterion, or concurrent validity, can be established, such as when we compare actigraphic data to polysomnography [2] (also see Chapter 22 of this volume). This is in contrast to predictive validity, for which an independent follow-up measurement with a criterion was performed to validate the tool. When several other measures of the same construct or criterion are used, we can establish convergent validity. Additionally, when scores are not correlated with conceptually distinct tools, we establish discriminant validity. Multitrait–multimethod approaches can also be used to establish this step. Finally, classification accuracy statistics can be applied and are especially important when the purpose of a tool is to use it to make diagnoses; receiver operator curves are the preferred statistical approach in this case (e.g., see [3]).

After that, it is time to put the tool to the test.

STEP 10—CONFIRMATORY ANALYSES

Confirmatory analyses are about verifying the stability, or robustness, of the aforementioned steps. This relatively straightforward step may involve an additional pilot study or performing random subsampling using a large, pre-existing data set. Such "tool tryouts" should be done using samples that have the same characteristics as the group, or population, for which the tool is intended. As you undoubtedly now understand, navigating the process of developing items and combining them to form a tool (or modification/adaptation) requires expert knowledge, skill, and interest in a specific field, as well as statistical acumen.

The confirmatory analysis is the penultimate step, when the tool's final psychometric quality is determined. This is also when the developer publishes the questionnaire's objective, how it was developed, the timeframe followed, the number of questions and their time to complete, instructions to respondents, scoring, and score interpretation. In other words, this is the information that you can examine on your own as you evaluate whether a tool is worthwhile.

Confirmatory analyses do not require fancy or complex modeling, as some expect (i.e., structural equation modeling is not required). To this point, we have been exploring the underlying structure, mistakes, and missing values; establishing the key variables; spotting abnormalities or extreme values; evaluating statistical assumptions; and so forth. You may even have tested some hypotheses in relation to predictive models (e.g., group differences) and margins of error. As its name suggests, by using confirmatory analyses, it is now time to put your chosen (i.e., developed) tool to the final test. That is, via new (pilot) data collection, random subsampling, or even bootstrapping/cross-validation techniques, you are now in a position to assess the robustness of your previous psychometric findings. It is the step in which you assess the significance, inference, and confidence (i.e., minimal measurement error) of your tool, using the sample(s) for which it was designed.

STEP 11 — STANDARDIZATION AND NORM DEVELOPMENT

It is now time for large-scale usage of your tool. Norms should be based on a theoretically sound, representative, scientific sample of sufficient size. That is, the validity of norm-referenced interpretations is, in part, determined by the appropriateness of the reference group to which tool scores are compared. Standardization and norming are a critical step; it involves establishing scores that enhance the users' ability to compare scores and different respondents' performances/responses, as well as to establish one or more cut-points dividing the score ranges. Such cut-points may have significant repercussions, such as when they are used for diagnostic labeling, financial reimbursements, eligibility to participate in an intervention program, etc. Consider the lessons from the story of intelligence tests as a warning of these perils.

If step 10 sticks, you can start collecting normative data, which is a separate set of data collection. In this step, you particularly need to take care with your sampling method (e.g., simple random sampling, clustered sampling, stratified sampling, etc.). Namely, norm-referenced tools yield information regarding a respondent in comparison to a norm or average of comparable respondents (e.g., age, gender, disease). In other words, these are the steps to use (or to look for in others' reports of their procedures):

1. Identify your population of interest and devise a cost- and labor-effective procedure for drawing a sample from the population of interest.
2. Report the most critical statistics and their amount of sampling error (upon estimating the minimum sample size).
3. Compute the norm (group) statistics of interest and their standard errors.
4. Identify the types of normative scores (i.e., percentiles, standard scores, developmental scales, ratios and quotients) and prepare normative conversion tables.
5. Document the norming procedure and write the guidelines for interpretation of the norms. Then, publish your results.

Finally, a couple notes of caution. Now that you've been through all 11 laborious steps, you must also be aware of the well-described Flynn effect, or the aging of your norms (tool), which may potentially invalidate its scores or use. Finally, culture-free and culture-fair tools are difficult to attain; therefore, be very intentional as you work with culture-related content.

CONCLUSION: GOOD SLEEP OR NOT—IS THAT THE ANSWER?

Armed with the previously discussed set of principles, you can start your questionnaire search, and if you feel brave enough, dive into questionnaire development. In 2011, the first comprehensive reference guide to all pediatric sleep questionnaires that were available that year was published [4]. We are now in the process of publishing a state-of-the-art update [5]; as a state-of-the-art perspective on our field, I offer highlights from that paper, which is based on 113 published reports that describe a combined 64 tools.

Regarding Steps 1 to 4, of the papers, 21.2% developed a new tool, whereas around 31% were translations, and the remainder were psychometric evaluations or adaptions/modifications of existing tools. In the years since publication of the original systematic review [1, 4], a tendency toward improved psychometric assessment of tools is evident. Especially, reports of structure analysis, internal consistency and test–retest reliability, and convergent validity are apparent. Almost half reported some degree of piloting.

Yet extra efforts in tool development is still needed for tools that assess children outside the 6- to 12-year-old age range, as well as for tools with respondents other than the parent (primarily mother). Most tools aim at questioning sleep disorders or problems (73.5%), followed by sleep–wake patterns (50.4%) and sleepiness (53.1%). Likert-answer format was most commonly chosen, ranging from 3 to 10 response options.

Regarding Step 5, more studies provide the details of piloting, yet sampling was often a convenience sample or potentially underpowered. Overall, sample sizes reported for general psychometric evaluation varied from 20 to 9198. Findings regarding steps 6 to 9 remain scattered across tools across newly developed tools, translations/modifications, or psychometric evaluation. That is, regarding the statistical reporting of each step, findings are dispersed. We found that NARQoL-21 [6] and SNAKE [7] underwent all 11 steps, the Sleep Disturbance Scale for Children [8] underwent nearly all steps except step 3, followed by Obstructive Sleep Apnea-18 [9], Continuous Spike and Wave During Sleep [10] and Children's Sleep Assessment Questionnaire [11] which only lacked step 11. Step 10 is generally unsuccessful during translation/modification. For step 11, the following 9 instruments underwent norming: Children's Sleep Health Questionnaire [12], Japanese Sleep Questionnaire for Elementary Schoolers [13, 14], NARQoL-21 [6], Omnibus Sleep Problems Questionnaire [15], Sleep Disturbance Scale for Children [8, 16], Sleep Comics [17], and SNAKE [7], but they may not have demonstrated all the other steps.

In closing, it should now be clear that answering the question "How well do you sleep?" involves a great deal of work and much reflection, based on each of the 11 important steps. I therefore pose the question I find most important: *How well do you ask about sleep?*

ACKNOWLEDGMENTS

This overview of tools in pediatric sleep research is based on the systematic review performed by Tabitha Sen under my mentorship during her stay in my lab.

REFERENCES

1. Spruyt K, Gozal D. Development of pediatric sleep questionnaires as diagnostic or epidemiological tools: a brief review of dos and don'ts. *Sleep Med Rev.* 2011;15:7–17.
2. Spruyt K, Gozal D, Dayyat E, Roman A, Molfese DL. Sleep assessments in healthy school-aged children using actigraphy: concordance with polysomnography. *J Sleep Res.* 2011;20:223–232.
3. Spruyt K, Gozal D. Screening of pediatric sleep-disordered breathing: a proposed unbiased discriminative set of questions using clinical severity scales. *Chest.* 2012;142:1508–1515.
4. Spruyt K, Gozal D. Pediatric sleep questionnaires as diagnostic or epidemiological tools: a review of currently available instruments. *Sleep Med Rev.* 2011;15:19–32.
5. Sen T, Spruyt K. Pediatric sleep tools: an updated literature review Currently re-submitted to Frontiers in Psychiatry, special section on Sleep Disorders for the Special Issue on Sleep Tools. Submitted for publication.
6. Chaplin JE, Szakacs A, Hallbook T, Darin N. The development of a health-related quality-of-life instrument for young people with narcolepsy: NARQoL-21. *Health Qual Life Outc.* 2017;15:135.
7. Blankenburg M, Tietze A, Hechler T, Hirschfeld G, Koh M, Zernikow B. Snake: the development and validation of a questionnaire on sleep disturbances in children with severe psychomotor impairment. *Sleep Med.* 2013;14:339–351.
8. Putois B, Leslie W, Gustin MP, et al. The French Sleep Disturbance Scale for Children. *Sleep Med.* 2017;32:56–65.
9. Soh HJ, Rowe K, Davey MJ, Horne RSC, Nixon GM. The OSA-5: development and validation of a brief questionnaire screening tool for obstructive sleep apnoea in children. *Int J Ped Otorhinolaryngol.* 2018;113:62–66.
10. LeBourgeois MK, Harsh JR. Development and psychometric evaluation of the Children's Sleep–Wake Scale. *Sleep Health.* 2016;2:198–204.
11. Chuang HL, Kuo CP, Liu CC, Li CY, Liao WC. The development and psychometric properties of the Children's Sleep Assessment Questionnaire in Taiwan. *J Ped Nurs.* 2016;31:e343–e352.
12. Irwanto, Rehatta NM, Hartini S, Takada S. Sleep problem of children with autistic spectrum disorder assessed by Children Sleep Habits Questionnaire-Abbreviated in Indonesia and Japan. *Kobe J Med Sci.* 2016;62:E22–E26.
13. Kuwada A, Mohri I, Asano R, et al. Japanese Sleep Questionnaire for elementary schoolers (JSQ-ES): validation and population-based score distribution. *Sleep Med.* 2018;41:69–77.
14. Shimizu S, Kato-Nishimura K, Mohri I, et al. Psychometric properties and population-based score distributions of the Japanese Sleep Questionnaire for Preschoolers. *Sleep Med.* 2014;15:451–458.

15. Biggs SN, Kennedy JD, Martin AJ, van den Heuvel CJ, Lushington K. Psychometric properties of an omnibus sleep problems questionnaire for school-aged children. *Sleep Med.* 2012;13:390–395.

16. Huang MM, Qian Z, Wang J, Vaughn MG, Lee YL, Dong GH. Validation of the sleep disturbance scale for children and prevalence of parent-reported sleep disorder symptoms in Chinese children. *Sleep Med.* 2014;15:923–928.

17. Schwerdtle B, Kanis J, Kübler A, Schlarb A, Kübler A, Schlarb AA. The Children's Sleep Comic: psychometrics of a self-rating instrument for childhood insomnia. *Child Psychiatr Hum Dev.* 2016;47:53–63.

Sleep as a Profession — Clinical Psychologist

SARAH M. HONAKER ■

INTRODUCTION

When I tell people I am a sleep psychologist, they often seem to imagine something quite mystical, such as dream interpretation. The reality of life as a sleep psychologist is actually much different. Sleep psychologists usually have some combination of three roles: (i) seeing patients with sleep difficulties; (ii) conducting research about sleep; and/or (iii) teaching or training students about sleep. One of my favorite things about my job is the variety of activities I do—every day is different! (Table 24A2) As you know from previous chapters, people need enough high-quality sleep to be their best selves. Helping those who are having trouble sleeping, either through research or by working directly with patients, can really improve people's lives.

WHAT DO SLEEP PSYCHOLOGISTS ACTUALLY DO?

Clinical Work

Many sleep psychologists work with patients to treat their sleep problems. The most common disorder sleep psychologists treat is insomnia, but others include circadian rhythm sleep disorders, nightmares, hypersomnia, night-time fears or anxiety, narcolepsy, and difficulty wearing a sleep apnea mask. There are many evidence-based sleep treatments that have been shown through research studies to improve people's sleep [1, 2]. Psychologists will often work with patients to choose and carry out a treatment plan to help their specific sleep problem. The following are some simplified examples of the types of patients who a sleep psychologist might see.

- Henry is a healthy 18-month-old boy. His parents brought him to a sleep psychologist because he wakes up four times each night and cries for a parent. A sleep psychologist might work with Henry's parents to try some strategies at home to help him learn to put himself back to sleep when he wakes during the night.
- Destiny is a 10-year-old girl who has an anxiety disorder. Her fears and worries at night make it difficult for her to fall asleep at bedtime; as a result, she keeps getting out of bed and going to her parents' room. A sleep psychologist might teach Destiny some skills to manage her worries and fears at bedtime and guide her parents on how to respond if she comes to them at night.
- Bella is a 17-year-old female who has trouble falling asleep on school nights because she does not feel tired. She struggles to awaken for school and is very sleepy in her morning classes. A sleep psychologist works with Bella to gradually shift her circadian timing system earlier, using sleep scheduling and light therapy.
- Jim is a 50-year-old company executive. He experienced a stressor at work several months ago that kept him awake worrying at night. Now that stressful event is over, but he continues to struggle to fall asleep even when tired. A sleep psychologist might treat his insomnia with a validated treatment approach called cognitive-behavioral therapy for insomnia [3], which involves strategies such as sleep scheduling changes and relaxation.
- Beverly is a 79-year-old female who was recently the victim of a crime. She has vivid nightmares and, as a result, dreads falling asleep at night. A sleep psychologist might use a nightmare treatment called imagery rehearsal therapy [4] to help reduce her nightmares.

Research

Sleep psychologists may conduct research on sleep and sleep disorders. The following are some examples of research studies done by sleep psychologists, assisted by their teams—often including many trainees at different levels—around the world.

- Azizi Seixas, PhD, Assistant Professor at New York University, and colleagues developed and evaluated a sleep education website for black adults at risk for obstructive sleep apnea [5].
- Lisa Meltzer, PhD, Associate Professor at Jewish National Health, and trainee Chris Donoghue published an article on the link between bullying and poor sleep in adolescents [6].
- Penny Corkum, PhD, Professor at Dalhousie University in Canada, and colleagues studied the effectiveness of an online treatment for children with sleep difficulties [7].

- Michael Gradisar, PhD, Professor at Flinders University in Australia, and colleagues measured the stress hormone cortisol in infants to see if interventions involving crying increased stress hormones (they didn't) [8].

Sleep psychologists may play any variety of teaching roles involving learners at all stages, ranging from undergraduate students to licensed professionals who are continuing their training. While a sleep psychologist working in a psychology department at a university is most likely to teach psychology students, those working in medical centers often teach both psychology and medical trainees, such as medical students. The following are some examples of the types of teaching that a sleep psychologist might do.

- Teach a course on sleep.
- Mentor students who are conducting a sleep research study.
- Lecture medical students on sleep issues.
- Train students and other psychologists on how to treat nightmares.
- Allow a psychology or medical trainee to observe while they see patients.
- Observe a psychology or medical trainee seeing a patient with a sleep disorder, and provide feedback to help improve their skills.

WHERE DO SLEEP PSYCHOLOGISTS WORK?

Sleep psychologists typically work in the same settings in which you would generally find psychologists: academic medical centers, healthcare organizations, colleges and universities, private practices, community mental health centers, and private research corporations. The following are examples of some of the most common settings in which sleep psychologists work.

- I work at an academic medical center as a pediatric sleep psychologist. I am a faculty member at Indiana University School of Medicine, where I conduct research, and I treat sleep disorders in children at Riley Children's Hospital.
- Michael Fukasawa Schmitz, PsyD, works for a regional health system, Fairview Health Services, where he leads the Insomnia and Behavioral Sleep Health Program focusing on population-based strategies to manage insomnia and expanding the availability of behavioral treatment within primary and specialty care settings.
- Hawley Montgomery-Downs, PhD (the editor of this textbook), was trained as a developmental psychobiologist and works in a university psychology department where she teaches undergraduate and graduate sleep courses, mentors students, and conducts sleep research.
- Sleep and Health psychologist, Ryan Wetzler, PsyD, DBSM, ABPP, owns a private practice, Sleep Health Center. He and his employees treat insomnia and other sleep-related disorders in adults and children.

HOW DO YOU GET THAT JOB?

Sleep psychologists start by becoming psychologists. While there are many professionals who provide psychology services like counseling or therapy, such as licensed counselors or licensed clinical social Workers, to become a *psychologist* there is a specific training path. Psychologists must earn a doctoral degree, such as a PhD or a PsyD. See Table 24A.1 for a list of specific steps. What makes one a *sleep* psychologist is the special sleep training or experience they pursue, either in graduate school or once they are working as a psychologist.

Table 24A.1 HOW TO BECOME A SLEEP PSYCHOLOGIST

Step 1: Finish this course and complete your undergraduate degree! If you think you want to complete a PhD program, which focuses more on research training, it will be very helpful to gain some research experience as an undergraduate. This will help you get into graduate school and will also give you the opportunity to make sure that you enjoy research.

Step 2: Earn your doctoral degree in Psychology. There are four main graduate school options for those who are interested in becoming a psychologist:

1. *PhD programs in Clinical Psychology* train students to become both researchers and clinical psychology providers (i.e., to see patients). These programs are highly competitive and often require research experience. If you think you want to be a sleep psychologist, it makes sense to go to a graduate program where you will have a research mentor who does sleep research.

2. *Schools of Professional Psychology* offer a PsyD degree (Doctor of Psychology). While there are some research requirements, those programs focus mostly on teaching you how to care for patients.

3. Some students begin by completing a program that offers a *Master's Degree in Psychology*, and then apply to a doctoral (PsyD or PhD) program. A master's degree program may be a helpful step for students who are unsure they want to earn a doctoral degree, or who may not have enough experience for admission to a doctoral program.

4. For those interested in mainly sleep research and do not want to treat patients, there are *PhD programs in other areas of psychology* such as Developmental, Physiological, and Social Psychology.

Step 3: Earn a license to practice psychology. If you want to see patients as a sleep psychologist, you will need to earn a license to practice psychology from your state or government. In the United States, the requirements vary from state to state, but almost always involve passing one or more exams.

Step 4: Get a job! There are *so* many different settings where you can work as a sleep psychologist. You can do research at a college or university, at an academic medical center, or for a private company. You can see patients in a private practice, a company, or a hospital/medical center.

Table 24A.2 A WEEK IN THE LIFE OF A SLEEP PSYCHOLOGIST WORKING IN AN
ACADEMIC MEDICAL SETTING

Day	Activities	Explanation
Monday	Pediatric Sleep Psychology Clinic —*Appointments with eight patients* —*Provide an intern clinical training*	You see children and teens with sleep problems who come for an appointment at the Children's Hospital. An intern is there to learn sleep psychology by observing and helping you.
Tuesday	Adult Sleep Psychology Clinic —*Appointments with 8 patients*	You treat adults with sleep problems who come for appointments at the hospital.
Wednesday	Research Day —*Research team meeting* —*Work on a grant application*	You meet with your research team, trainees and employees working on the study you are leading. You then work on writing a grant to earn money for your next research project.
Thursday	Research Day —*Prepare a lecture for a conference* —*Work on a manuscript*	You are attending a conference in Orlando next week to present your research, so you work on slides for that presentation. In the afternoon you work on an article for a journal describing a research study.
Friday	Specialty (Sleep Apnea) Clinic —*Treatment team meeting* —*Appointments with 8 sleep apnea patients*	You work with a physician and a respiratory therapist to see patients who need to wear a continuous positive airway pressure mask to treat sleep apnea. Your role is to motivate patients to wear the mask, and teach children who are afraid of the mask.

An academic medical setting is a hospital system affiliated with a medical school. Psychologists in these settings usually see patients at the hospital and are faculty members at the medical school. The activities are a schedule for a psychologist who does both research and clinical work. Some sleep psychologists will only do research and others may only do clinical work. This psychologist sees both adults and children; some psychologists will only see adults or children.

REFERENCES

1. Morgenthaler TI, Owens J, Alessi C, et al. Practice parameters for behavioral treatment of bedtime problems and night wakings in infants and young children. *Sleep*. 2006;29:1277–1281.
2. Morgenthaler T, Kramer M, Alessi C, et al. Practice parameters for the psychological and behavioral treatment of insomnia: an update. An American Academy of Sleep Medicine report. *Sleep*. 2006;29:1415–1419.

3. Edinger JD, Means MK. Cognitive–behavioral therapy for primary insomnia. *Clin Psychol Rev.* 2005;25:539–558.

4. Krakow B, Zadra A. Clinical management of chronic nightmares: imagery rehearsal therapy. *Behav Sleep Med.* 2006;4:45–70.

5. Seixas AA, Trinh-Shevrin C, Ravenell J, Ogedegbe G, Zizi F, Jean-Louis G. Culturally tailored, peer-based sleep health education and social support to increase obstructive sleep apnea assessment and treatment adherence among a community sample of blacks: study protocol for a randomized controlled trial. *Trials.* 2018;19(1):519.

6. Donoghue C, Meltzer LJ. Sleep it off: bullying and sleep disturbances in adolescents. *J Adolesc.* 2018;68:87–93.

7. Corkum PV, Reid GJ, Hall WA, et al. Evaluation of an internet-based behavioral intervention to improve psychosocial health outcomes in children with insomnia (Better Nights, Better Days): protocol for a randomized controlled trial. *JMIR Res Protocol.* 2018;7(3):e76.

8. Gradisar M, Jackson K, Spurrier NJ, et al. Behavioral interventions for infant sleep problems: a randomized controlled trial. *Pediatrics.* 2016;137(6):e20151486.

Sleep as a Profession—
Sleep Physician

JENNIFER L. MARSELLA AND KATHERINE M. SHARKEY ■

INTRODUCTION

In this chapter, we will discuss the path to becoming a sleep medicine physician and what we do as sleep medicine physicians, as well as opportunities to become more involved within the field. Sleep medicine is a relatively new specialty; although disturbed sleep and abnormal sleep behaviors have been described for hundreds of years, sleep monitoring and sleep as a medical discipline were only established after the 1950s [1, 2]. This chapter is focused on the American system of sleep medicine, but there are pathways to specialize in sleep medicine and become a member of sleep societies in other countries. The authors of this chapter are colleagues who have collaborated on scholarly projects since 2018. Dr. Katherine Sharkey trained in a combined Internal Medicine and Psychiatry residency and is director of a sleep lab and a sleep researcher focusing on women's health. Dr. Jennifer Marsella is a neurologist and sleep medicine specialist who recently completed her sleep medicine fellowship and is early in her academic career. We hope that this chapter gives readers a flavor of what it is like to practice this intellectually stimulating specialty.

THE PATH TO BECOMING A SLEEP MEDICINE PHYSICIAN

Sleep medicine is a multidisciplinary field, and physicians can become specialized in sleep medicine through a variety of avenues. Figure 24B.1 shows the process of becoming a sleep medicine doctor. After earning an undergraduate degree, aspiring sleep medicine physicians must complete medical school. This is

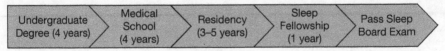

Figure 24B.1 Training path to becoming a board-certified sleep medicine physician.

a wonderful time to learn about different medical specialties and try an elective in sleep medicine. Medical students who are interested in sleep will need an elective to supplement the 2 to 4 hours of formal sleep medicine education provided in most medical school curriculums—an insufficient amount of instruction given the high prevalence of sleep disorders in the population [3]. Many institutions have Sleep Medicine Interest Group (SMIG) chapters [4]. SMIG membership allows medical students the opportunity to learn more about sleep and sleep medicine, participate in community outreach, and become connected with the field's national professional organization, the American Academy of Sleep Medicine (AASM) [5]. For those institutions that do not have a SMIG chapter, medical students can start one at their school and can reach out to the AASM for assistance in finding advisors and mentors for their SMIG.

Toward the end of medical school, medical students match into a residency program based on their interests. Unlike many medical or surgical subspecialty fellowships, those interested in a sleep medicine fellowship have a choice of many residency programs, as shown in Table 24B.1. Some internal medicine or pediatric residents who have completed a fellowship in pulmonology and/or critical care will also choose to further specialize in sleep medicine.

Sleep medicine fellowships are 1 year in length. These interdisciplinary training programs focus on normal sleep physiology, pathophysiology of sleep disorders, diagnosis and treatment of sleep disorders, and interpretation of sleep procedures, such as various types of sleep studies (also see Chapter 22 in this volume). The training is multidisciplinary, including exposure to medicine, pediatrics, neurology, psychiatry, surgery, dentistry, and psychology. See Table 24B.2

Table 24B.1 Sleep Medicine Fellowship Residency Requirements

To apply for a sleep medicine fellowship, applicants must complete one of the following residency programs:
  Anesthesiology
  Family Medicine
  Internal Medicine*
  Medicine/Pediatrics*
  Otolaryngology
  Pediatrics*
  Psychiatry
  Neurology*

*In these specialties it is not uncommon for doctors to complete a fellowship in another specialty, either before or after starting a sleep medicine fellowship.

Table 24B.2 SLEEP MEDICINE FELLOWSHIP SCHEDULE

Jul	Aug	Sep	Oct	Nov	Dec	Jan	Feb	Mar	Apr	May	Jun
Throughout: adult sleep medicine continuity clinic and interpretation of sleep studies											
Score	E/D	Peds	CBT-I	Peds	E/D	Peds	CBT-I	Peds	E/D	Peds	CBT-I
Didactics in normal sleep physiology and sleep disorders, research in sleep medicine											
• Adult sleep medicine continuity clinic: evaluate and treat adult patients with sleep disorders. • Interpretation of sleep studies: read and interpret in-lab and home sleep studies. • Score: learn how to score sleep studies according to the AASM scoring guidelines [6]. • E/D: spend time in otolaryngology (ENT) and dentistry clinics; see evaluations for surgery for OSA and go to the OR to see drug-induced sleep endoscopies and surgeries for OSA, spend time with dentists who specialize in dental appliances to treat OSA. • Peds sleep clinic and Peds sleep study interpretation. • CBT-I: learn from psychologists and counselors who treat insomnia with CBT-I.											

E/D, ENT and Dentistry; Peds, pediatrics. CBT-I, cognitive-behavioral therapy for insomnia; AASM, OSA, obstructive sleep apnea; OR, operating room.

for an example of a year-long schedule for a fellowship in sleep medicine and Table 24B.3 for an example of a more detailed schedule for one week of training.

A sleep medicine fellowship provides clinical training, as well as research experience, if desired. This training program is for those who plan to practice adult and/ or pediatric sleep medicine. Although it is extremely beneficial to be exposed to the process of performing overnight sleep studies, the majority of a sleep fellow's clinical experience is in the outpatient setting during the daytime. After completion of the fellowship program, physicians are eligible to become board certified in sleep medicine. To become certified to practice sleep medicine, physicians must pass a standardized test sponsored by the AASM that tests knowledge and competency in diagnosis of sleep disorders and interpretation of test results.

The AASM has many opportunities for education and mentorship for those interested in sleep medicine and those training in sleep medicine. On the AASM website [5], there is a section called "Choose Sleep," with resources for people

Table 24B.3 SCHEDULE FOR 1 WEEK DURING ENT/DENTISTRY BLOCK

Monday	Tuesday	Wednesday	Thursday	Friday
AM: Adult sleep medicine clinic	AM: Adult sleep medicine clinic	AM: Adult sleep medicine clinic	AM: ENT clinic	AM: Didactics and conferences
PM: Interpret sleep studies	PM: Research	PM: Interpret sleep studies	PM: ENT OR	PM: Dental clinic

at different stages of training, from undergraduate students to faculty early in their sleep medicine career. The AASM mentor program is an opportunity for individuals at any level of training with an interest in sleep medicine to be paired with a mentor in the field. Through this program, mentees create meaningful relationships with their mentors as they are guided in career growth through professional development, knowledge transfer, and networking. Being paired with a mentor can give the junior colleague a leg up as they advance in their careers, but it is not a one-way street. Mentors also learn a lot from their mentees and find these relationships to be stimulating and rewarding. The authors of this chapter can speak to the success of this program as they were connected through it.

For those interested in research activities, the AASM holds an annual Young Investigators Research Forum, a career development program for young investigators with promising careers in clinical and translational sleep medicine research to gain specific knowledge and skills related to performing sleep research and competing successfully for grant funding. Another national professional sleep society that focuses more on research and scientific investigation than clinical practice, the Sleep Research Society (SRS) [7], organizes an annual Trainee Symposia Series to promote scientific investigation in sleep and circadian research.

Also, on the national level, the AASM and SRS hold an annual meeting of the Associated Professional Sleep Societies. At this conference, trainees and those interested in sleep medicine can learn about trends in the field and begin to form connections with others in sleep medicine.

WHAT IS LIFE LIKE FOR A SLEEP MEDICINE PHYSICIAN?

The practice of sleep medicine is exciting and engaging because it has ample variety. One of the most common patient encounters is performing an initial evaluation of an individual referred by another physician or clinical provider, or who scheduled an appointment on their own because they are experiencing a sleep problem.

Typical issues among new patients include not sleeping well at night, feeling excessively sleepy during the day, snoring and experiencing apneas (breathing pauses) at night, and unusual/unwanted movements or behaviors at night. Sometimes a sleep doctor can make a diagnosis and recommend treatment based on the history and physical exam alone. Other times, depending on the symptoms reported by the patient, a sleep physician may order a sleep study. For example, in a patient whose bed partner or roommate reports loud snoring or witnessed breathing pauses, a home sleep test for sleep apnea would be an appropriate next step. A patient who experiences dream enactment, on the other hand, requires an in-laboratory sleep study. In patients with severe daytime sleepiness, narcolepsy might be on the differential diagnosis (i.e., process of differentiating between conditions with similar signs and/or symptoms), and a multiple sleep latency test would be ordered to assess daytime sleepiness. Finally, in cases of a suspected circadian rhythm sleep–wake disorder or insomnia, wrist actigraphy to monitor several days of sleep patterns is a very helpful test. Laboratory blood tests and neuroimaging are also sometimes needed at the time of initial workup of a sleep disorder.

Following diagnosis, patient education is a key responsibility of a sleep medicine physician. Since many sleep disorders are chronic (e.g., narcolepsy, restless legs syndrome, sleep apnea) or can be recurrent (e.g., psychophysiologic insomnia), patients need to understand the implications of their diagnosis, the first-line treatment and any available alternatives, and the risks/side effects of the various treatments and of not treating.

The focus of return visits also depends on the patient's diagnosis. In a patient who has obstructive sleep apnea (OSA), for example, positive airway pressure (PAP) may be prescribed, and the patient needs information about the practical aspects of using the device (i.e., supplies, cleaning) as well as feedback on their patterns of PAP use and its efficacy. In a patient with insomnia, the first-line treatment, cognitive-behavioral therapy for insomnia (CBT-I), requires the patient to make behavioral changes. Thus, follow-up visits in patients treated with CBT-I tend to focus on the patient's success in implementing strategies like sleep restriction and stimulus control (also see Chapter 18 of this volume).

In patients who are treated with medications, the sleep medicine physician will check in about whether the patient is taking the medicine, efficacy, and side effects. Many pharmacologic treatments are expensive, and it is useful for physicians to inquire about whether patients can afford the prescribed medications, as sometimes more cost-effective options (e.g., generic medications or another brand) may be available. Additionally, some medications are not recommended for long-term use, and the physician and patient must decide together whether the benefits of the medication outweigh the risks and whether continuing is appropriate.

During follow-up visits, a sleep doctor may recommend additional testing and/or further referral. For instance, OSA can be treated with a mandibular advancement device in some patients, and this requires referral to a dentist who specializes in fitting these appliances, or with surgery, which requires referral to an otolaryngologist.

Interpreting sleep studies is another important role fulfilled by the sleep medicine physician. Tests including diagnostic laboratory polysomnography, overnight titration of continuous PAP pressures, multiple sleep latency testing, maintenance of wakefulness testing, wrist actigraphy, home sleep tests for obstructive sleep apnea, and laboratory blood testing. Test reports interpreting the results, relating the diagnosis, and making treatment recommendations are sent to the referring clinician and are often required by insurance companies to approve treatment payments.

Sleep doctors may also have administrative and leadership tasks. A sleep laboratory medical director oversees the 24-hour operations of the sleep center, including hiring and leading sleep center staff, maintaining lab standards, completing accreditation requirements, and ensuring timely communication of results to other practitioners. Because of the multidisciplinary nature of sleep medicine, sometimes practitioners see patients with medical issues not related to sleep. For instance, a pulmonologist may care for patients with asthma or chronic obstructive pulmonary disease in addition to patients with sleep disorders. Sleep medicine is an outpatient specialty and sleep doctors generally do not see inpatients in the hospital. Most sleep doctors take overnight call and must be available by phone or pager to answer questions or provide medical orders for the registered polysomnographic technologists (see discussion later in this chapter) who work with patients at night.

Sleep medicine doctors often have the opportunity to be of service to the sleep field at large. In addition to caring for patients, they can advance sleep science and clinical practice by performing research studies and publishing their findings in scientific journals or by peer-reviewing grant applications and journal articles about other scientists' research results. Sleep medicine physicians help train future sleep medicine doctors by teaching medical students, residents and fellows. They may also serve on committees related to sleep education or sleep health. This can range from local boards, focused on community education about driving safety or student mental health, to national committees making decisions about grant funding or public policy. National committees may be sponsored by the AASM, SRS, or other entities.

Sleep medicine physicians who are AASM members for at least 5 years and who contribute significantly to the scientific literature or make other advances in the sleep medicine field may be given the status of "Fellow of the American Academy of Sleep Medicine." This distinction recognizes contributions to sleep medicine in the domains of scholarship, service, education, and public awareness and is considered a professional honor.

The job of a sleep medicine physician is very rewarding. Sleep doctors care for a wide variety of patients and manage a range of diseases and disorders. Sleep doctors often care for the same patients for years, given the chronic nature of many sleep disorders. Helping patients improve their sleep quality and daytime functioning can impact their health significantly, and many sleep doctors find this to be a gratifying part of the job. Although the path to becoming a sleep medicine physician takes many years, it is worth it to be able to help people with such an important part of their daily lives.

CONCLUSION

For us, our profession as sleep medicine physicians is extremely rewarding. We are specialists but also work within a multidisciplinary field, allowing us to work with a wide variety of colleagues and affording us the opportunity to tailor our paths based on our interests. Sleep medicine doctors improve the quality of their patients' sleep and lives. As such a new specialty, more sleep physicians are needed to evaluate and treat patients, as well as research the many unknowns of normal sleep and circadian rhythms and their disorders. This is an exciting time to be a sleep medicine physician.

REFERENCES

1. Shephard JW, Buysse DJ, Chesson AL Jr, et al. History of the development of sleep medicine in the United States. *J Clin Sleep Med*. 2005;1(1):61–82.
2. Schulz H, Salzarulo P. The development of sleep medicine: a historical sketch. *J Clin Sleep Med*. 2016; l12(7):1041–1052.
3. Rosen R, Zozula R. Education and training in the field of sleep medicine. *Curr Opin Pulm Med*. 2000;6(6):512–518.
4. American Academy of Sleep Medicine. Sleep Medicine Interest Groups. https://aasm.org/professional-development/choose-sleep/sleep-medicine-interest-groups/. Accessed May 20, 2019.
5. American Academy of Sleep Medicine. [Home page]. https://aasm.org/ Accessed May 20, 2019.
6. Iber C. *The AASM Manual for the Scoring of Sleep and Associated Events: Rules, Terminology and Technical Specifications*. Westchester, IL: American Academy of Sleep Medicine; 2007.
7. Sleep Research Society. [Home page]. https://www.sleepresearchsociety.org/. Accessed May 20, 2019.

Sleep as a Profession— Polysomnographic Technologist

KATHRYN M. JOHNSON ■

INTRODUCTION

As a member of the sleep medicine team, the polysomnographic (PSG) technologist, also known as the "sleep technologist" or "sleep tech," plays a vital role in both the diagnosis of sleep disorders and their treatments. While the technical skills required to perform these complex medical procedures can be taught, the "people skills" of the successful tech are just as important. Most, if not all, patients evaluated in a clinical sleep lab are chronically sleep deprived and suffer from all of its detrimental effects. From calming the fears of a frightened child, to introducing a reluctant patient to continuous positive airway pressure (PAP) therapy for the first time, the sleep tech must respond to everything in a professional manner while also demonstrating empathy and carrying out the needed procedures and tests for the patients in their charge.

JOB DUTIES

Sleep techs must be comfortable working with patients of all ages, from newborns and young children to teens, adults, and older adults. Sleep techs work in a variety of settings, including hospital-based or free-standing sleep centers, medical supply or equipment companies, and academic research institutions; however, most start their career watching people sleep in a traditional sleep laboratory. This is a demanding, but rewarding, job as it offers the opportunity to literally watch a patient's sleep improve.

Sleep labs or centers might be located within a hospital, a physician office, or in a free-standing location (e.g., a hotel). In the traditional sleep lab, technologists initially orient the patient to the sleep lab environment and educate them on the procedure they are about to undergo. Often, this orientation includes helping patients overcome their fears of sleeping in a strange place, covered in sensors and wires, with their every move monitored and recorded.

Technologists must frequently clarify the reasons the physician has ordered the sleep test, how the testing procedures provide valuable information about their health, and, often, the results of previous testing. Building a rapport with the patient is imperative to overcoming their nervousness, and in this context, patients often disclose pertinent information to their technologist that was not revealed to their physician. Technologists must be able to identify and overcome a variety of barriers, including language differences, visual or hearing deficits, and developmental or learning disabilities, to find ways to provide information to patients who might otherwise be unable to understand what is happening to them. The ability to think on one's feet and alter a procedure while meeting testing goals is a valuable skill. For example, when a tech begins preparing a patient for their sleep recording and must decide where to attach sensors for monitoring limb movement when they realize their patient is a double amputee!

An informative sleep study starts with a good "hook-up" (a regretful, yet professional term in this field). This process must be done with a very high level of accuracy, using multiple types of electrodes and sensors to measure (at a minimum) brain wave activity, eye movements, muscle activity, respiration, respiratory effort, and blood oxygen levels. Sensor application must be secure enough to withstand movements during sleep as well as restroom breaks (sometimes numerous) throughout the night. This challenge is multiplied when the patient is a child or an individual with other conditions that reduce their ability to understand and cooperate with the hook-up procedures. Failure to optimally apply the electrodes and sensors will result a poor recording of little diagnostic value and/or multiple intrusions to reapply sensors, disrupting and fragmenting the patient's sleep.

Another vital aspect of the sleep tech's job is maintaining the recording equipment. Use of digital equipment has simplified equipment upkeep compared to pre-digital paper and ink, but modern technology has introduced new requirements for computer skills and an understanding of networking and electronic data storage.

While most patients in the sleep lab are able to perform their own activities of daily living, they often have other medical conditions which require additional care by, or assistance from, the technologist. For example, patients may need help with testing their blood sugar, using their nebulizer, or to ambulate if they have limited mobility. While in years past the typical patient in the sleep lab would have been relatively healthy, our patient population has shifted to include those with significant respiratory, cardiac, and/or neurologic diseases. While rare, sleep technologists must be prepared to respond to patient emergencies. An understanding of vital signs (e.g., blood pressure, pulse, respiratory rate) as well as knowledge of normal and abnormal cardiac rhythms is essential to determine when a patient needs a higher level of care, and the tech must make a decision to send them to the emergency room. Cardiopulmonary resuscitation and/or basic life support are universal requirements and an understanding of how to respond to unusual sleep behaviors, such as seizures or parasomnias, is an essential skill set. All of this requires a tech who is not only multitalented, competent, and caring, they must also be someone who can stay alert all night while most of the world is sleeping. Indeed, these are very special professionals.

In recent years, there has been a move toward ambulatory (also known as "home-based" or "out of center") sleep testing. This type of recording provides limited information compared to full, attended PSG and may often result in a lower quality study due to the absence of a technologist to intervene when sensors are dislodged or other problems arise during the study night [1]. However, out-of-center testing may be a viable alternative when in-lab testing is not feasible (e.g., for patients unable to travel to the sleep center) and is idea for follow-up testing to determine the efficacy of some therapeutic interventions, such as surgical correction or use of a dental device for obstructive sleep apnea. It should be noted, unattended testing is best utilized in younger patients without significant comorbidities. These home studies are less expensive and may be the preferred by some insurance companies. In these cases, the technologist must provide the patient with clear, easy-to-understand instructions on how to apply the equipment at home. This education must be provided to patients of varied ages as well as maturity and education levels, and a technologist must be available by phone to answer questions that may come up during the study night, because questions will come up.

Following Dr. Colin Sullivan's 1981 publication [2] showing that nasal PAP could effectively eliminate obstructive apnea during sleep, sleep technologists moved from a purely diagnostic role to also having a role in the treatment of sleep-disordered breathing. Today, titration of PAP therapy is a major responsibility for sleep technologists, one that includes both establishing a patient's optimal therapy mode and pressure settings, as well as finding the best interface for comfortable and effective delivery of PAP therapy. Equally important, techs provide their patients with reassurance and encouragement during their first experience using PAP therapy. Often, this first experience is the key to ongoing compliance with treatment; thus, the sleep technologist is largely responsible for success or failure with this therapy.

Not all sleep techs work at night. Another important sleep technologist job is responsibility for sleep study "scoring." This is sometimes performed during the study night, but it may be a "day tech" job. Determining the quantity and quality of a patient's sleep is accomplished by viewing the entire night's recording in 30-second segments, or epochs, and assigning each the proper sleep stage. This "staging" follows a set of detailed and highly standardized rules, originally compiled by Drs. Rechtschaffen and Kales during the late 1960s [3]. These rules have since been updated and expanded by the American Academy of Sleep Medicine (AASM) [4]. The expansion of the original "R&K" rules added methods we now use to recognize and classify other sleep-related events, such as changes in breathing and movements during sleep. The majority of sleep labs use these standardized conventions for staging of sleep and sleep-related events, which allow for easy comparison between sleep laboratories, whether across the city or on the other side of the world [5]. The technologist must also be able to accurately identify events that occur during sleep, including respiratory events, limb movements, cardiac arrhythmias, unusual sleep behaviors, abnormal electroencephalographic discharges or electrocardiographic patterns. Identification of sleep-related events is considered one of the most important skills for the sleep technologist and is highly dependent on achieving a stable and precise sensor placement. Once staging and scoring of the study is complete, the technologist compiles a report for the interpreting physician that quantifies sleep efficiency and quality, as well as respiratory events and/or limb movements, and includes the tech's observations on events during the study night. The technologist commentary is extremely important to the interpreter, since not all events are reflected in the numerous tables of a sleep study report. These technical remarks might include additional information and observations, which may or may not be pertinent to the recording or to the patient's complaints. While the focus may be on the patient's sleep, there are many additional factors that impact their quality of sleep; a sensitive sleep technologist will often discover factors. For example, they may learn that the patient normally sleeps sitting upright, that they are a night shift worker, and that they always sleep with their 100-pound German Shepherd.

Sleep techs also conduct daytime PSG studies, including the multiple sleep latency test, the maintenance of wakefulness test, and standard PSG for night shift workers who routinely sleep during the day. These so-called day tech can also provide valuable assistance to clinicians and may even see patients for follow-up to discuss compliance issues and fit PAP interfaces. Using technologists in these ways can markedly improve the efficiency of a sleep clinic, allowing the clinicians to use their time more effectively while also giving patients access to additional help so they can meet day-to-day challenges with their treatment. Dentists who provide oral appliances for treatment of obstructive sleep apnea may also hire sleep techs to assist with patient evaluation, treatment, and follow-up.

Sleep centers and durable medical equipment companies (which supply treatment devices such as PAP machines) often hire sleep technologists to provide equipment set up, pressure adjustments, interface fitting, desensitization procedures, and compliance reporting. Importantly, having an experienced sleep technologist available to communicate with insurance representatives may be the difference between obtaining authorization for procedures or not. Technologist interaction with staff and providers in the region who might refer patients can also greatly enhance a sleep center's practice. Techs are wonderful at educating the public about sleep services at community wellness events and often move into management roles as they expand their expertise.

Research is another professional area in which sleep techs may be found, either as an exclusive research laboratory role or by adding a research element to an otherwise clinical laboratory. The field of sleep medicine is still relatively new, and there are many opportunities to participate in a variety of research studies, including investigating new drugs or treatments, and continuing research to expand our knowledge of sleep and its effect on our lives: How would you like to work on a research project studying sleep in space [6]? Sleep technologists are often recruited to work in a variety of capacities for equipment or supply manufacturers, most commonly in equipment sales or customer support but they may also be involved in new product research and development: Who better to ask about what is needed in the field than a sleep tech?

TRAINING AND EDUCATION

Where should you start if you're interested in entering the field of sleep technology? There are many pathways to becoming a sleep technologist. When this book was published, the Commission on Accreditation of Allied Health Education Programs (CAAHEP) listed 43 accredited programs for PSG technology, with an additional 7 neurodiagnostic programs that have an add-on PSG component [7]. These programs are typically 12 to 24 months in length and award either a diploma/certificate or associate degree upon completion. The Commission on Accreditation for Respiratory Care has four programs with a PSG component [8].

In addition to traditional training programs for students with little or no medical background, there are condensed courses for medical professionals who are seeking training in sleep medicine. These courses, which can last a few days to 2 or more weeks, are well suited for those who are actively working in a healthcare occupation, such as respiratory therapy, electroneurodiagnostics, or nursing, and provide an easy pathway to add PSG to an existing skill set.

On-the-job training (OJT) continues to be a frequently utilized method for those interested in a sleep technologist career. While formal training programs may be the method employers prefer, the demand for techs currently outpaces the number these schools can supply. OJT is frequently supplemented by an online education program by the AASM, the Accredited Sleep Technologist Education Program (A-Step), or another online or in-person training program. Completion of the A-Step program, which consists of 80 hours of instruction and a 3-hour online examination, will help OJT techs fulfill the eligibility requirements for a credentialing examination. One should keep in mind that talented and dedicated technologist trainees may be found in a variety of places, not just in the previously mentioned medical professions but also in seemingly unrelated occupations such as computer science, clerical, or even housekeeping. Often OJT techs are the most passionate about their work and feel they have been given a wonderful gift: a profession they love and at which they excel.

CREDENTIALS AND LICENSURE

Many organizations offer credentialing for sleep technologists. The most widely recognized is the Board of Registered Polysomnographic Technologists, which offers a temporary, entry-level credential, the Certified Polysomnographic Technologist, as well as the Registered Polysomnographic Technologist credential.

In recent years, the Board of Registered Polysomnographic Technologists has responded to the expanded role for sleep techs with the Certification in Clinical Sleep Health credential, which qualifies the holder, similar to a nurse navigator, to provide education and support for sleep patients and the community. Respiratory therapists have the option of adding a Sleep Disorders Specialty to their credential thru the National Board for Respiratory Care, designating their additional training and expertise in sleep technology. The American Board of Sleep Medicine has also established a testing process that provides the successful candidate with the Registered Sleep Technologist credential. Eligibility for these exams differs from group to group but all are designed to demonstrate competency in providing sleep medicine services to patients.

Several states in the United States have established licensure for sleep technologists, and these licensure laws have varying educational, credentialing, and experience requirements. A list of the states that currently require licensure can be found on the AASM website [9]. Some third-party payers also require that credentialed technologists provide sleep medicine services as a condition of payment.

So, you are interested in becoming a sleep technologist? There are many pathways to this career, and the eligibility requirements are frequently updated, so take some time and do your research on the current requirements for your location. The gold standard training in the United States is one of the CAAHEP-accredited programs, which provide both the didactic and clinical components necessary to learn the practice of sleep technology. Graduation from a CAAHEP program assures that you will be prepared and qualified to take the registry exams. If you are unable to enroll in one of these formal training programs, look for a local sleep center that is willing to provide OJT or consider volunteering in a sleep lab to gain a better understanding of the duties of a sleep tech.

Sleep technology is a fascinating field and is one that continues to evolve as we learn more about the impacts that sleep disorders have on our lives. This career can give you some of the most rewarding moments. For example, I once received a call from the daughter of a patient with dementia to say her mother dressed herself for the first time in years after using continuous PAP for just one night. Or you may be the first to recognize that a patient is having morning headaches because he taped over his exhalation port so the air wouldn't blow on his wife. You might treat a pediatric patient for severe central sleep apnea and later see him graduate from college or see your patient with narcolepsy celebrate getting her driver's license because her sleepiness has been adequately treated. As a sleep technologist, sleep center manager (and a sleeper), I have to say I have never regretted the effort I put into learning about sleep medicine or that I put my knowledge into practice every day.

REFERENCES

1. Portier F, Portmann A, Czernichow P, et al. Evaluation of home versus laboratory polysomnography in the diagnosis of sleep apnea syndrome. *Am J Resp Crit Care Med.* 2000;162:814–818.

2. Sullivan CE, Berthon-Jones M, Issa FG, Eves L. Reversal of obstructive sleep apnoea by continuous positive airway pressure applied through the nares. *Lancet.* 1981;1:862–865.

3. Rechtschaffen A, Kales A, eds. *A Manual of Standardized Terminology, Techniques and Scoring System for Sleep Stages of Human Subjects.* Los Angeles, CA: Brain Information Service/Brain Research Institute, University of California; 1968.

4. Iber C, Ancoli-Israel S, Chesson A, Quan SF, eds. *The AASM Manual for the Scoring of Sleep and Associated Events: Rules, Terminology and Technical Specifications.* 1st ed. Westchester, IL: American Academy of Sleep Medicine; 2007.

5. Magalang UJ, Chen N-H, Cistulli PA, et al. Agreement in the scoring of respiratory events and sleep among international sleep centers. *Sleep.* 2013;36:591–596.

6. Wu B, Wang Y, Wu X, Liu D, Xu D, Wang F. On-orbit sleep problems of astronauts and countermeasures. *Mil Med Res.* 2018;5:17.

7. Commission on Accreditation of Allied Health Education Programs. Find a program. https://www.caahep.org/Students/Find-a-Program.aspx. Accessed April 29, 2019.

8. Commission on Accreditation for Respiratory Care. Accredited program listing https://www.coarc.com/Students/Find-an-Accredited-Program.aspx. Accessed April 29, 2019.

9. American Academy of Sleep Medicine. State policy directory. https://aasm.org/advocacy/state-policy-directory/.Accessed April 29, 2019.

ADDITIONAL RESOURCES

BOOKS

Morin CM, Espie CA, eds. *The Oxford Handbook of Sleep and Sleep Disorders*. New York, NY: Oxford University Press; 2012.

Wolfson A, Montgomery-Downs H, eds. *The Oxford Handbook of Infant, Child, and Adolescent Sleep and Behavior*. New York, NY: Oxford University Press; 2013.

Walker M. Why We Sleep: *Unlocking the Power of Sleep and Dreams*. New York, NY: Scribner; 2018.

WEBSITES

Official site of the World Sleep Society. https://worldsleepsociety.org/

Official site of the International Pediatric Sleep Association http://www.pedsleep.org/

Official site of the Sleep Research Society. https://www.sleepresearchsociety.org/

Official site of the Society of Behavioral Sleep Medicine. https://www.behavioralsleep.org/

Official site of the American Academy of Sleep Medicine. https://aasm.org/

ABOUT THE EDITOR AND AUTHORS

EDITOR

Professor Hawley E. Montgomery-Downs embarked on her sleep research journey as an undergraduate student at Humboldt State University, when Professor John Morgan allowed her to test the effects of sleeping in a sauna-like environment. This led her to graduate school at the University of Connecticut, where she studied infant sleep using nonintrusive observation techniques under the mentorship of Professor Evelyn Thoman. After earning her doctorate in Developmental Psychobiology in 2001, she joined the polysomnography and neurobehavior laboratory of Professor David Gozal at the University of Louisville, where she completed a 4-year postdoctoral fellowship in Pediatric Sleep Medicine. From 2005 through 2019, she was a member of the psychology, pediatric, and neuroscience departments at West Virginia University. While there, she had the privilege of teaching the course Psychobiology of Sleep to hundreds of exceptionally motivated undergraduate students. She and her team of talented doctoral students also addressed issues surrounding postpartum families, pediatric sleep-disordered breathing, and more. Their cumulative work was supported by federal, nonprofit, industrial, and institutional grants. Hawley has been an active member of the Sleep Research Society, the International Pediatric Sleep Association, and the World Sleep Association and is a past president of the West Virginia Sleep Society. She is also mom to three amazing people. She is now independently employed as a consultant and freelance scientific editor.

AUTHORS

Sabra M. Abbott, MD, PhD, is a sleep medicine physician and assistant professor of Neurology at the Northwestern University Feinberg School of Medicine. Dr. Abbott's research and clinical practice focus on the diagnosis and management of circadian rhythm sleep–wake disorders.

Shilpa M. Agraharkar, MD, is a psychiatrist practicing in New York, New York. Dr. Agraharkar graduated from New York University School of Medicine.

Marco Angriman, MD, works as a consultant in the Child Neuropsychiatry Unit of the Department of Pediatrics at the regional Hospital in Bolzano, Italy. Dr. Angriman's main clinical and research interests focus on pediatric sleep disorders (insomnia, restless legs syndrome), attention-deficit/hyperactivity disorder (ADHD; neurobiological aspects of ADHD, especially the comorbidity between ADHD and sleep disorders in children), neurological disorders of the newborns, and neurodevelopmental disabilities.

Hrayr Attarian, MD, is a professor of neurology and director of the Center for Sleep Medicine at Northwestern University. He completed undergraduate degree and medical school at the American University of Beirut and residency at SUNY Upstate Medical University in Syracuse, New York. He finished two fellowships, one in neurophysiology at University of Rochester and one in Sleep Medicine at University of Minnesota. He has published 78 peer-reviewed papers and numerous chapters and edited three textbooks. His interests are sleep health in underprivileged groups globally as well as sleep health and sleep disorders in women.

Fiona C. Baker, PhD, is Senior Program Director of the Human Sleep Research Laboratory at SRI International, a nonprofit research organization in Menlo Park, California. She also holds an appointment as Honorary Professorial Research Fellow in the Brain Function Research Group, School of Physiology, at the University of the Witwatersrand, Johannesburg, South Africa. Her research focuses largely on sleep and related physiology in women across the lifespan. She also studies maturational changes in sleep and brain structure/function in adolescents, considering sex differences and whether deficits in neuromaturation and sleep health precede or follow variations in adolescent behaviors, including alcohol and other substance use.

Siobhan Banks, PhD, is co-director of the Behaviour–Brain–Body Research Centre at the University of South Australia. Professor Banks's research sits at the nexus of biology (fatigue and circadian rhythms), behavior (individual and team performance), and technology (human center design). She has expertise in the objective measurement of fatigue, designing tools and protocols to investigate the biological and behavioral responses to sleep deprivation, irregular work hours and stress.

Argelinda Baroni, MD, is an assistant professor at the NYU Langone, where she studies the relationship between sleep and psychiatric conditions. Clinically, she sees children and adolescents in Bellevue psychiatric emergency department for psychiatric emergencies. She completed a fellowship in child and adolescent psychiatry and in sleep medicine at NYU. Dr. Baroni teaches an large undergraduate course on sleep and a smaller class on Internet addiction at NYU. She sleeps better when she charges her phone in the kitchen overnight and encourages everyone to do the same.

Chiara Bartolacci, PhD, is a psychologist and psychotherapist in formation. Dr. Bartolacci holds her degree in psychology and cognitive science. In her early career, she focused on sleep in elderly, sleepiness while driving, sleep and cognition, electrophysiological correlates of dream experience, cognitive-behavioral therapy for insomnia. She currently works the Sapienza University of Rome on human factors and behavior analysis.

Bei Bei, PhD, PsyD, is a Senior Research Fellow at Turner Institute for Brain and Mental Health, Clinical Psychologist and Research Lead at Monash University Healthy Sleep Clinic, and Honorary Senior Research Fellow at the Centre for Women's Mental Health, Royal Women's Hospital. She holds a doctor of psychology (clinical) and a PhD from University of Melbourne. Her research and clinical work focuses on the individual differences in sleep–wake behaviors, the relationship between sleep and mental health, and psychological interventions for better sleep, especially in women and adolescents.

Oliviero Bruni, MD, is a full professor in child neurology and psychiatry at the Sapienza University of Rome. He is founder and past president of the International Pediatric Sleep Association, field editor (pediatrics) of *Sleep Medicine*, past member of the Board of Directors of the Italian Association of Sleep Medicine and was elected as chair of the Childhood Sleep Disorders and Development Section of the American Academy of Sleep Medicine (AASM). He is currently involved in the scientific committees of the AASM, European Sleep Research Society, and World Sleep Society. He organized, acted as faculty member, and participated as invited lecturer in several international congresses. He has been involved in sleep research and clinical care in children for over 30 years and has published around 200 peer-reviewed papers, in addition to books, book chapters, and abstracts.

Stephanie Claudatos is a PhD student in clinical psychology at Palo Alto University and a researcher in the Human Sleep Research Program at SRI International. Her research interests include the intersection of sleep and developmental psychopathology, with a clinical focus on health psychology and behavioral medicine.

Ian M. Colrain, PhD, founded the Stanford Research International Biosciences Division, Human Sleep Research Laboratory in 2001; this group partners with organizations worldwide to bring new medicines and devices to market through basic research, pharmaceutical and technology discovery, preclinical development, and clinical translation. He is an associate editor for *Sleep* and a member of the Medical Advisory Board for Compumedics Pty. Ltd., a leading manufacturer of sleep diagnostic equipment. Previously, he was the clinical senior research fellow in the Stanford University Sleep Disorders Center and held tenured faculty appointments at Auckland University in New Zealand and the University of Melbourne in Australia, where he is currently a professorial fellow.

Keren Armoni Domany, MD, graduated medical school at the Technion–Ruth and Bruce Rappaport Faculty of Medicine in Haifa, Israel. She did her pediatrics residency at the Dana Children's Hospital, Tel Aviv Sourasky Medical Center. Following her residency, she did a fellowship in pediatric pulmonology at the Dana Children's Hospital, and then she spent 2 years in research fellowship in sleep medicine at Cincinnati Children's Hospital Medical Center, Cincinnati, Ohio. Her main research focus is obstructive sleep apnea in children.

Jeanne F. Duffy, MBA, PhD, is a clinical researcher and neuroscientist in the Division of Sleep and Circadian Disorders at Brigham and Women's Hospital in Boston and is an associate professor of medicine in the Division of Sleep Medicine at Harvard Medical School. Dr. Duffy's research interests focus on basic and applied aspects of circadian physiology in humans, including how the circadian timing system impacts sleep, waking performance, and hormone release. Her studies investigate individual differences in sleep timing, duration, need, and response to sleep loss and the role of the biological clock in those individual differences.

Jason G. Ellis, PhD, is a professor of sleep science and director of Northumbria Sleep Research in the United Kingdom. He is a qualified somnologist and expert in behavioral sleep medicine, certified by the European Sleep Research Society, and a practicing psychologist under the Health and Care Professions Council. He splits his time between his basic research interests in the pathophysiology of sleep disorders (insomnia, restless legs syndrome, and circadian rhythm disorders) and his applied work on cognitive behavioral therapy for insomnia (CBT-I). Within the latter framework he examines the impact of novel adjunct therapies, the influence of social factors on adherence, and the effective delivery of CBT-I in complex cases and environments. He has worked within the National Health Service in the United Kingdom, delivering CBT-I to individuals with a range of physical and psychological conditions and serves on the editorial boards of *Behavioral Sleep Medicine* and *Sleep Health*.

Raffaele Ferri, MD, is the current president of the Associazione Scientifica Italiana per la Ricerca e l'Educazione nella Medicina del Sonno, past president of the Italian Association of Sleep Medicine, and member-at-large of the International Restless Legs Syndrome Study Group; he has been secretary and vice-president of the European Restless Legs Syndrome Study Group. Dr. Ferri has been, for years, an active member of the Italian Society of Psychophysiology being a member of its Board of Directors for more than 10 years and its representative for the Federation of the European Psychophysiology Societies for which Dr. Ferri has also been secretary. He has published more than 450 papers in international peer-reviewed scientific journals, in addition to book chapters and abstracts. He is an associate editor for *Sleep, PLOS One,* and the *International Journal of Psychophysiology*.

Luigi De Gennaro, PhD, Sapienza University of Rome, is a full professor of physiological psychology at the Department of Psychology, Sapienza University of Rome and director of the sleep laboratory of Sapienza University of Rome. He is author of more than 170 articles on international peer-reviewed journals. He is associate editor of the *Journal of Sleep Research* and a member of the editorial board *PLOS One, Frontiers of Psychology,* and *Frontiers in Neurogenomics,* among many others.

Kevin Gipson, MD, is a pediatric pulmonologist and sleep medicine physician who specializes in the care of infants, children, and adolescents with complex respiratory and sleep disorders. He earned his medical degree from Louisiana State University School of Medicine in New Orleans in 2012 and completed his residency in general pediatrics at Children's Hospital New Orleans in 2015. He completed fellowship training in pediatric pulmonology at Massachusetts General Hospital in 2018, followed by a fellowship in sleep medicine at Stanford University in 2019.

Marc P. Halperin, MD, is a child, adolescent, and adult psychiatrist in private practice in New York City. He serves as a clinical instructor within the Departments of Psychiatry and Child & Adolescent Psychiatry at NYU Langone Health. Dr. Halperin has both clinical and academic interests in sleep disorders, LGBTQ populations, perinatal mental health, family systems, medical student/resident education, and psychodynamic psychotherapy.

Sarah M. Honaker, PhD, DBSM, is an assistant professor of pediatrics at the Indiana University School of Medicine, where she provides behavioral sleep services for children and conducts health services research. Dr. Honaker's research examines the development and implementation of strategies to promote evidence-based care for children's sleep disorders. She has over 15 peer-reviewed publications in this area and has received research funding from the National Institute of Health and the American Academy of Sleep Medicine Foundation.

Rosemary S. C. Horne, PhD, DSc, is a Senior Principal Research Fellow and heads the Infant and Child Health research theme within the Ritchie Centre, Hudson Institute of Medical Research and Department of Paediatrics, Monash University, Melbourne Australia. Her research interests focus on numerous aspects of sleep in infants and children. Rosemary has published more than 200 scientific research and review articles. She is chair of the physiology working group of the International Society for the Study and Prevention of Infant Deaths, a director of the International Pediatric Sleep Association, and is on the editorial boards of the *Journal of Sleep Research, Sleep,* and *Sleep Medicine.*

Defne Inhan, BSc, is a graduate of the inaugural class of New York University Shanghai, where she completed a neural science and psychology degree with a focus on child and adolescent mental health studies. Studying within NYU's Global Network in Shanghai, New York, and Accra, she grew an appreciation for cultural and societal dimensions of mental health and development. During and following her education, she has engaged in research on language processing, memory and how early childhood development influences the brain at the Developmental Affective Neuroscience Laboratory at Columbia University. Currently, she is a policy officer at the representation of the Bahá'í International Community to the European Union and plans to advance her academic career in child and adolescent mental health from a global perspective.

Kathryn M. Johnson, AS, R.EEG/EP T., RPSGT, FASET, is the manager of the Regional Sleep Center at St. Mary's Medical Center in Huntington, West Virginia. She is responsible for the day-to-day operations of the Neurophysiology Department, which includes EEG, EMG/NCV, and the Sleep Center, which has been in operation since 1993. Ms. Johnson has 46 years of experience in the field of neurodiagnostics, including 30 years in sleep medicine. She is a founding member of the West Virginia Sleep Society, currently serving as an advisor to their board of trustees, and is active with ASET, the Neurodiagnostic Society. She is a frequent speaker at conferences on the state, regional, and national level.

John D. Kennedy is a pediatric respiratory physician specializing in child sleep disorders. His research interests include the impact of sleep disordered breathing on daytime performance, neuromuscular functioning and cardiovascular health. He advises on public health policies addressing sleep disorders in childhood and is a pediatric medical school educator.

Kurt Lushington, MPsych, PhD, is a researcher and clinical psychologist. His interests include the psychopathology and treatment of sleep disorders, the role that sleep plays in brain development, and the impact of fatigue on workplace performance. Professor Lushington is past chair and currently serves on the Behavioural Medicine Sleep Disorders Committee of the Australasian Sleep Association and is the current Head of School of the School of Psychology, Social Work, and Social Policy at the University of South Australia.

Anastasia Mangiaruga, PhD, holds her degree in psychology and cognitive sciences. Her main research interest is the link between sleep and cognition. In her early career, she focused on dream experience and parasomnias, in the hypothesis that abnormal sleep-related behaviors could be considered as a covert manifestation of the ongoing cognitive processing. At the University of Bologna, she works on the psychosocial impact of the central disorders of hypersomnolence.

Carolina Z. Marcus, MD, is a practicing sleep medicine physician and is associated with the University of Rochester Medical Center. Dr. Marcus diagnoses and manages sleep disorders, including obstructive sleep apnea, central sleep apnea, insomnia, sleep–wake cycle disorders, restless legs syndrome, parasomnia disorders, and narcolepsy.

Jennifer L. Marsella, MD, is an academic neurologist specializing in sleep medicine. Dr. Marsella is a senior instructor at University of Rochester. She has a special interest in sleep disorders in women, across the lifespan, and the menstrual cycle. Additionally, she enjoys educating students about sleep medicine and helping them improve their own sleep health.

Alfred J. Martin is a pediatric respiratory physician specializing in childhood sleep disorders. His research interests include sleep disordered breathing, cystic fibrosis, and noninvasive ventilation in children. He is the director of the Department of Respiratory and Sleep Medicine at the Women's and Children's Hospital, Adelaide, Australia.

James J. McKenna, PhD, a Fellow in the American Association for the Advancement of Science, a biological anthropologist first to study and continues to study the physiology and behavior of mother–infant co-sleeping and breastfeeding in relationship to SIDS risk factors (what he calls, breastsleeping) for over 30 years.

He remains one of the leading experts in, and spokesman for, safe infant sleep with over 155 refereed scientific articles published in prestigious medical journals worldwide. His most recent book is entitled *Safe Infant Sleep: Answers to Your Cosleeping Questions* (Platypus, 2020).

Jacob E. Medina, BS, has almost a decade's worth of research experience. He earned his degree in psychology from Colorado State University where he researched social psychology and cognitive neuroscience. He later worked at Brigham & Women's Hospital in Boston studying sleep and circadian biology. Currently, Jacob works at the Ridley-Tree Cancer Center in Santa Barbara, CA conducting oncology research.

Maria Grazia Melegari, MD, is child and adolescent neuropsychiatrist and worked as Chief of the Childhood Mental Health Service in Ospedale La Scarpetta in Rome. She was director of clinical, diagnostic, therapeutic, and rehabilitation activities related to early childhood for several years and was awarded the title High Professionalism in Psychiatric Disorders of Early Childhood and Preschool Age. She is the coordinator of the Regional Reference Center of ADHD and Autism. She is also a senior lecturer at the Sapienza University and Lumsa University of Rome. Her main research interests focus on psychiatric disorders of early childhood like ADHD (mainly comorbidity between ADHD and sleep disorders in children) and autism or other neurodevelopmental disabilities.

Yvonne Pamula, PhD is a Sleep Scientist who has been managing the scientific and technical operations of the Children's Sleep Disorders Unit at the Adelaide Women's and Children's Hospital for over 20 years. She is interested in the normal development of sleep across childhood, the role of sleep in brain development and how sleep disorders impact sleep physiology and behavior.

Rafael Pelayo, MD, is a clinical professor at Stanford University School of Medicine and has been a part of the Stanford Sleep Disorders Clinic since 1993. William Dement appointed him as his successor to teach Sleep and Dreams, which was first university-level course created to teach undergraduates the science of sleep and its impact on their health.

Kevin R. Peters, PhD, is an associate professor of psychology at Trent University, Peterborough, Ontario, Canada. He has taught a third-year undergraduate course on sleep and arousal for the past 12 years. He has published in the area of sleep, memory, and aging.

Alexandria M. Reynolds, PhD, received her doctoral degree in experimental psychology from the University of South Carolina. She is an assistant professor of psychology and director of the NeuroCognitive Sciences Laboratory at the University of Virginia's College at Wise. Her main areas of research include sleep and cognition, sleep extension, and aging.

Jason Rihel, PhD, received his doctoral degree in 2004 from Harvard University. From 2004 to 2012, Jason developed methods to study sleep in zebrafish at the

NYU School of Medicine and Harvard University. He is currently a reader in behavioral genetics at University College London, where he has led a research lab on sleep research since 2012. Jason has received numerous grants and awards for his research, including the prestigious Investigator Award from the Wellcome Trust, a Starting Grant from the European Research Council, and the Excellence Fellowship from University College London.

Serena Scarpelli, PhD, IRCCS, is a psychologist and psychotherapist and has been a member of the Laboratory of Sleep Psychophysiology, Sapienza University of Rome, for 10 years. Dr. Scarpelli's main research interests include the electrophysiological correlates of dream experience; sleep, memory and neural plasticity; sleep and Alzheimer's disease; sleep and neurodevelopmental disorder; and cognitive-behavioral therapy for insomnia. She is the author of 27 articles in international peer-reviewed journals and serves as referee and editor for scientific journals. She is a member of the editorial board of the Italian Association of Sleep Medicine.

Michael K. Scullin, PhD, completed his doctoral degree in psychological science at Washington University in St. Louis and a postdoctoral fellowship in sleep at Emory University School of Medicine. He is a recipient of the National Science Foundation CAREER award and an associate professor of psychology and neuroscience at Baylor University. His research focuses on sleep, education, and cognitive aging.

Katherine M. Sharkey, MD, PhD, FAASM, FACP, is a sleep medicine physician and associate professor of medicine and psychiatry and human behavior and assistant dean for Women in Medicine and Science at the Alpert Medical School of Brown University. Dr. Sharkey's research focuses on sleep and circadian rhythms as they relate to mood regulation and women's health. Her research is supported by grants from the National Institute of Mental Health and the Hassenfeld Institute. Dr. Sharkey is an associate editor of behavioral sleep medicine and serves on the editorial board of *Sleep Health*.

Jess P. Shatkin, MD, MPH, leads the educational efforts of the Child Study Center at Hassenfeld Children's Hospital at NYU Langone Health, where he is vice chair for education and professor of child and adolescent psychiatry and pediatrics at the NYU Grossman School of Medicine. Dr. Shatkin teaches undergraduates, medical students, residents, and practicing physicians about sleep medicine, in addition to providing treatment for all manner of psychiatric and sleep-related illnesses. Dr. Shatkin has written three books and more than 100 articles addressing medical education, adolescent risk and resilience, and sleep.

Karen Spruyt, PhD, has been researching and lecturing in the field of sleep medicine, developmental (neuro)psychology, and statistics for more than 15 years. She has published her research in high-impact, peer-reviewed journals and has authored two widely used books on pediatric sleep problems. Dr. Spruyt collaborates with multidisciplinary research teams around the world and performs translational research in her domains of interest: child development and somnopathology.

Riva Tauman, MD, graduated medical school at the Sackler Faculty of Medicine at the Tel Aviv University. She did her pediatrics residency at the Dana Children's Hospital, Tel Aviv Souraski Medical Center. Following her residency, she did clinical and research fellowship at the Kosair Children's Hospital, Louisville, Kentucky, and passed the American Boards of Sleep Medicine. She practices sleep medicine in adults and children since her return from fellowship. She is the president of the Israeli Sleep Research Society and the head of the Sleep Medicine Center at the Tel Aviv Medical Center. She has published 60 peer-reviewed papers, three review papers, and six chapters in textbooks. Her research focus is the effect of sleep-disordered breathing on the fetus during pregnancy.

Kristin P. Tully, PhD, is engaged in a program of research that centers around safety in patient transitions through maternity care, patient–provider communication, breastfeeding experiences, parent–infant nighttime interactions, and health care innovation. Broadly, she is interested in engaging new families, clinicians, and other key stakeholders to identify unmet patient needs and co-develop effective, sustainable, and scalable solutions.

Erin J. Wamsley, PhD, began her academic career as a liberal arts student at Guilford College in North Carolina, before completing her doctoral studies at the City University of New York in 2007. Subsequently, Dr. Wamsley began a postdoctoral fellowship in the Division of Sleep Medicine at Harvard Medical School and was later promoted to instructor of psychiatry at Harvard Medical School, where she served until 2014. In her current role as associate professor and director of the sleep laboratory at Furman University, Wamsley and her research group study how the brain processes memories during sleep and resting wakefulness, as well as the relationship of sleep-dependent memory processing to dream experiences. Dr. Wamsley has published over 50 scientific articles on these topics and delivered numerous lectures both nationally and internationally.

Amy R. Wolfson, PhD, is a professor of psychology at Loyola University Maryland. She has been engaged in child and adolescent sleep research for over 30 years with a focus on adolescents' and emerging adults' sleep and cognitive, behavioral, and emotional well-being. Her work examines interventions aimed at improving adolescents' sleep at a systemic level such as delaying school start times and at an individual/group level, such as the Sleep Smart Program. Most recently, her scholarship has turned to understanding sleep health for vulnerable children and adolescents including youth residing in juvenile justice and foster care settings. When she is not teaching, mentoring, and doing research, she loves spending time with her family whether hiking, running, or enjoying great food.

Crystal L. Yates, PhD, focuses her research on the impact of sleep loss and circadian misalignment (interruption to the body's daily rhythms) on fatigue, performance, and metabolism. Dr. Yates's specifically investigates how sleeping and eating at nonstandard times affects shift workers' metabolism, food preference, and perceived taste and cognitive performance. She is also researching what countermeasures could reduce the negative impact of night shifts on health and well-being.

Margaret Yu, MD, is from Chicago and completed undergraduate, medical school, and residency at Northwestern University. After completing a stroke fellowship, she plans to work as a neurohospitalist with a focus on inpatient quality improvement.

Massimiliano de Zambotti , PhD, is the lead of the Translational Sleep Technology Unit of the Human Sleep Research Program at SRI International. He is an expert in normal and pathologic sleep, with a focus on the interaction between sleep cortical, autonomic, and cardiovascular regulation during sleep. Dr. de Zambotti has advanced expertise in the sleep technology field, in the development and testing of sleep-tracking and sleep-augmenting technologies.

Terra Ziporyn, PhD, is the executive director and co-founder of Start School Later, a nonprofit dedicated to school hours compatible with healthy sleep, as well as an historian of medicine and science writer whose books include *The New Harvard Guide to Women's Health, The Women's Concise Guide to Emotional Well-Being*, and *Nameless Diseases*. Formerly an associate editor at the *Journal of the American Medical Association*, she has received science writing fellowships from the American Association for the Advancement of Science, the American Chemical Society, and the Woods Hole Marine Biological Laboratory and has written extensively on a wide range of health and medical issues for both popular and professional audiences.

Tables, figures and boxes are indicated by *t*, *f* and *b* following the page number

For the benefit of digital users, indexed terms that span two pages (e.g., 52–53) may, on occasion, appear on only one of those pages.